6140159838

Abdelhamid H. Elgazzar · Orthopedic Nuclear Medicine

Springer-Verlag Berlin Heidelberg GmbH

Abdelhamid H. Elgazzar

Orthopedic Nuclear Medicine

With a Foreword by Edward B. Silberstein

With 212 Figures in 398 Parts and 78 Tables

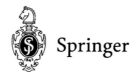 Springer

Abdelhamid H. Elgazzar, MD, FCAP
Diplomate, American Board of Pathology
Diplomate, American Board of Nuclear Medicine
Professor and Chairman
Department of Nuclear Medicine, Faculty of Medicine
Kuwait University Health Sciences Center
P.O. Box 24923, 13110 Safat/Kuwait

Contributor to chapter 6
Ezzuldin M. Ibrahim, MD, FRCP
Chairman, Department of Oncology/Hematology, King Faisal Specialist Hospital,
Jeddah, Saudi Arabia

Library of Congress Cataloguing-in-Publication Data
Elgazzar, Abdelhamid H., 1949-
Orthopedic nuclear medicine / Abdelhamid H. Elgazzar
p. ; cm.
Includes bibliographical references and index.
ISBN 978-3-642-62293-9   ISBN 978-3-642-18790-2 (eBook)
DOI 10.1007/978-3-642-18790-2
1. Bones--Radionuclide imaging. 2. Joints--Radionuclide imaging. 3. Radiography in orthopedics.
I. Ibrahim, Ezzuldin M. II. Title.
[DNLM: 1. Bone Diseases--radionuclide imaging. 2. Joint Diseases--radionuclide imaging.
3. Bone Diseases--radiotherapy. 4. Calcinosis--radionuclide imaging. 5. Joint Diseases--
radiotherapy. 6. Radiopharmaceuticals. WE 225 E41o 2004]
RC930.5.E447 2004
616.7'107575--dc21   2003054279

http.//www.springer.de

© Springer-Verlag Berlin Heidelberg 2004
Originally published by Springer-Verlag Berlin Heidelberg New York in 2004

Cover design: E. Kirchner, D-69121 Heidelberg
Typesetting: FotoSatz Pfeifer GmbH, D-82166 Gräfelfing
Printed on acid-free paper – SPIN: 10857297   21/3130 – 5 4 3 2 1 0

To my children, who gave me love and understanding

To my patients, who provided me with the opportunity to practice medicine humanely

To my sister Susan Elgazzar, whose courageous struggle to survive cancer has continued to inspire me

Foreword

It has been several years since the nuclear medicine community was presented with an outstanding text on bone scintigraphy. Over a span of three decades the value of this enormously important clinical modality has remained undiminished, despite the introduction of new techniques for examining bone, especially magnetic resonance imaging and positron emission tomography (PET). In fact the positron emitting sodium fluoride-F-18 was employed as a bone imaging agent over 30 years ago and now finds new value as a potent tool in PET diagnosis.

Dr. Elgazzar, a renowned nuclear medicine physician, researcher, author and teacher, has produced an important text on bone scintigraphy at a time when new concepts for use of this modality are on the horizon. His presentation is well grounded in the basic sciences and in pathophysiology, an approach which brings a remarkable coherence to the text. Correlative imaging concepts are also carefully threaded through these chapters.

The production of a quality bone scan, which will not miss relevant clinical findings because of errors in scanning technique, is not a simple matter, and Dr. Elgazzar emphasizes the caution and care with which the production of every bone scan must be approached, as well as the pitfalls in clinical interpretation.

Well illustrated, and containing many tables to succinctly summarize the concepts being covered, this text is remarkably accessible despite its depth and breadth.

The book is also distinguished by its extraordinarily thorough coverage of musculoskeletal disorders: both the common but difficult clinical problems faced in nuclear medicine departments daily, and also rare findings pertaining to a variety of metabolic and congenital disorders which have not received proper coverage and explanation elsewhere. In addition, an important and incisive chapter on the radiopharmaceutical therapy of a wide variety of bone and joint disorders appears in this text.

The author should receive the accolades of the international diagnostic imaging community for providing, in a single volume, a wise and comprehensive perspective on the current status of our ability to diagnose and treat disorders of the musculoskeletal system employing the multiple, complex techniques of nuclear medicine and related diagnostic modalities.

Edward B. Silberstein, M.D.
Eugene L. and Sue R. Saenger, Professor of Radiologic Health
Professor of Medicine, Emeritus
University of Cincinnati Medical Center
Cincinnati, Ohio, USA

Preface

Nuclear medicine is a specialty with great opportunities for innovation. There have been impressive advances in recent years with continuous and rapid scientific progress and expanding contributions to patient care and wellbeing. The role of nuclear medicine in orthopedics has grown to include many applications in diagnosis and treatment of various bone and joint diseases.

This text is designed to provide students and medical professionals with a comprehensive and clearly presented update on nuclear medicine applications in orthopedic medicine. The book begins with a chapter presenting fundamental anatomic, physiologic, pathologic, and technical concepts relevant to understanding orthopedic nuclear medicine and its use in clinical practice. Subsequent chapters cover diagnosis of skeletal infections, trauma, vascular disorders, metabolic bone diseases, neoplastic bone diseases, soft tissue calcifications, and joint disorders. The final chapter is devoted to the use of radionuclides in treatment of bone and joint diseases. This text is unique in its brief, yet comprehensive and in-depth approach to clarity through the creative use of numerous illustrations. Because an understanding of both normal and morbid pathophysiology is a prerequisite for successful use of orthopedic nuclear medicine, necessary pathophysiologic aspects are presented at the beginning of each chapter, followed by description of the use of scintigraphy for the various disease processes and correlative imaging issues.

This text is intended for all those interested in orthopedics, including radiologists, orthopedic surgeons, internists, pediatricians, other clinicians, and nuclear medicine professionals at all levels. My aim is to advance knowledge in orthopedic nuclear medicine and improve its use for patients with various bone and joint disorders.

Abdelhamid H. Elgazzar, MD, FCAP

Acknowledgements
It is with my deepest appreciation that I thank all who sincerely and willingly helped me to make this book a reality: Saif Abdelaziz, Veronica Cody, Fatma F Shitta, Ahmed Mahmoud, Sleiman Naddaf, Abdalla I Behbehani, Gloria Machado, Jeff Becker and all the technologists at NEMC, Abdulllatif A. Al-Bader, Mercy Mathew, Sati Gopinath, Jehan Al Shammari, Shihab Al-Mohanadi, Heba Esam, Fawzia Sanad, Azu Owanwanne, Fahd Maarafi, Essa Loutfi, James D'Almeida, Henry Fielding, David Collier, and Mostafa E. Ibrahim. To all of you I am grateful for your time and expertise.

Contents

Basic Sciences of Bone and Joint Diseases

Bone develops by intra-membranous and endochondral ossification. Intramembranous ossification occurs through the transformation of mesenchymal cells into osteoblasts, while in endochondral ossification a pre-existing cartilage forms first and then undergoes ossification. Two types of bone tissues form the skeleton; compact or cortical bone and cancellous, trabecular, or spongy bone. The spongy bone has a turnover rate approximately eight times greater than that of cortical bones. Bone is formed of three types of cells: osteoblasts, which produce the organic bone matrix; osteocytes, which produce the inorganic matrix; and osteoclasts, which are responsible for bone resorption. Bone marrow converts into yellow, or inactive, marrow, gradually reaching an adult pattern by the age of 25 years. Yellow marrow may reconvert due to the stress associated with several pathologic and physiologic processes. Joints develop in the mesenchyme between the ends of bones and are classified into several types according to their functional features as well as the nature of the adjoining tissue. The principal response of bone to injury, and disease, is reactive bone formation; this is the basis of increased uptake of bone-specific radiopharmaceuticals. Other specific bone and joint pathologic changes define the patterns of uptake of other radiopharmaceuticals used for imaging such diseases [e.g. gallium-67, labeled leukocytes, thallium-201, Tc99m methoxyisobutylisonitrile (MIBI) and F-18 fluorodeoxyglucose (FDG)]. The factors that ensure the best possible quality and interpretation of radiopharmaceutical investigation include obtaining the relevant clinical information; proper preparation of the patients (including sedation of pediatric patients); meticulous positioning of patients and adequate acquisition; familiarity of the normal appearance in different age groups (and normal variants); awareness of the technical pitfalls; and the strengths and limitations of each modality.

1.1
Introduction

Nuclear medicine plays a crucial role in the diagnosis and management of various skeletal diseases because of the ability of scintigraphy to reflect changes in bone physiology. This permits the early identification of diseases and injuries. The increasing use of this imaging modality for the investigation of benign bone disorders is noteworthy. Utilization and effective use of these modalities should be based on a basic understanding of bone anatomy and physiology, technical aspects of nuclear medicine techniques and sources of errors in conducting and interpreting these modalities.

1.2
Anatomy and Physiology of Bone

1.2.1
Bone Development

Bone develops by intramembranous and endochondral ossification. In some locations, such as the vault of the skull, intramembranous ossification alone occurs, while in other tissues, such as long bones, pelvis and skull base, both intramembranous and endochondral ossification occur. However, the process of bone formation is essentially the same and goes through the following steps [1]:

1. Osteoblasts differentiate from primitive mesenchymal cells.
2. Osteoblasts deposit a matrix that is subsequently mineralized.
3. Woven bone (primary spongiosa); this initial bone is characterized by an irregular network of collagen
4. This temporary woven bone is replaced by bone marrow in the marrow cavity, or by lamellar bone

Intramembranous ossification occurs through the transformation of mesenchymal cells into osteoblasts. This is seen in the flat bones of the skull, parts of the mandible and clavicle from which these bones form [2, 3]. Thickening of the cortex of other bones is due to intramembranous ossification beneath the periosteum leading to an increase in the diameter of bones. In *endochondral ossification*, a pre-existing cartilage forms first and then undergoes ossification. Most of the skeleton forms by this type of ossification [2].

The initial sites of ossification are called the centers of ossification. These can be further classified into primary, such as those located in the central portions of long bones (i.e. the diaphysis which forms most of the shaft), and secondary, such as those located in the epiphyses and apophyses of long bones (Fig. 1.1). Virtually all primary centers are present at birth. Secondary ossification centers develop later at the end of the growing long bone. The epiphysis is separated from the shaft of the bone by the epiphyseal growth cartilage or physis. An apophysis is an accessory, secondary ossification center that develops later and forms a protrusion from the growing bone. This is where tendons and ligaments insert or originate. Examples of apophyses include the ischial tuberosity. The metaphysis is the part of the bone between the diaphysis and the physis. The diaphysis and metaphysis are covered by periosteum, and the articular surface of the epiphysis is covered by articular cartilage (Fig. 1.2).

Growth Plate Development: Ossification progresses from the center towards the ends of the long bones where the frontier of intramembranous ossification advances and appears as an area of cellular activity that forms the growth plate (Fig. 1.3). This is the predominant site of longitudinal growth of bone. Later, the ossification centers of the epiphysis and metaphysis fuse at the growth line. This halts growth and can only be rec-

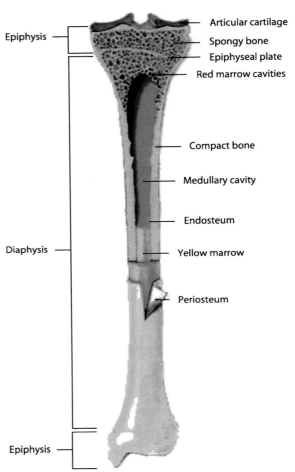

Epiphysis — Articular cartilage
— Spongy bone
— Epiphyseal plate
— Red marrow cavities

— Compact bone

— Medullary cavity

— Endosteum

Diaphysis — — Yellow marrow

— Periosteum

Epiphysis —

Fig. 1.2. The main elements of a long bone. The central region is the diaphysis which forms most of the shaft. The epiphysis is located at both ends of the bone separated from the shaft by the growth plate, or physis. The part of the shaft between the diaphysis and physis is the metaphysis. The shaft (diaphysis and metaphysis) is covered by the periosteum. The articular surface of the epiphysis is covered by articular cartilage (From Thibodeau. Patton KI (1999): Anatomy and physiology Mosby p190 with permission)

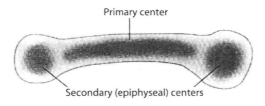

Primary center

Secondary (epiphyseal) centers

Fig. 1.1. Primary and secondary ossification centers (From Shipman et al. [50], with permission)

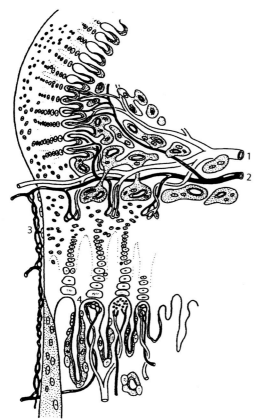

Fig. 1.3. The growth plate in a long bone. The diagram shows cartilage growth plate and adjacent metaphysis and epiphysis. Note the epiphyseal vein (*1*) and artery (*2*), the perichondral vascular ring (*3*), the terminal loops of the nutrient artery (*4*) in the metaphysis and ongoing endochondral ossifications in the physis and epiphysis. (From Gray's anatomy [3] with permission)

ognized as a faint line. The long bone lengthens at the metaphysis while it thickens at the periosteum. In children knowledge of the location of the ossification centers is essential to correctly interpret the activity seen on scintigraphic studies.

Apophyseal growth plates do not contribute to longitudinal growth of bone and are present in the iliac crest, anterior superior and inferior iliac spines, ischium and the lesser and greater trochanters (during the second decade). The apophyses fuse at variable ages (Table 1.1) and are particularly prone to avulsion [4].

1.2.2
Bone Anatomy
1.2.2.1
General Structural Features

Bone structure of normal adult bone can be summarized in four categories:

Gross Level

The skeleton consists of two major parts, the axial skeleton and the appendicular skeleton (Fig. 1.4). The axial skeleton includes the skull, spine and rib cage (ribs and sternum), while the appendicular skeleton includes the bones of the extremities, pelvic girdle and pectoral girdle (clavicles and scapulae).

Table 1.1. Sites and ages at fusion of the major apophyses

Site of apophysis	Age at fusion (years)	Attached muscle
Iliac crest	17–18	Abdominal wall muscles
Anterior superior iliac spine	16–20	Sartorius muscle
Anterior inferior iliac spine	25	Rectus femoris muscle
Symphysis pubis	20–25	Adductor group of muscles
Ischial tuberosity	20–25	Hamstring muscle
Lesser trochanter	18–19	Iliopsoas muscle
Greater trochanter	18–19	External rotators
Olecranon	18	Triceps
Distal radius	18	Brachioradialis

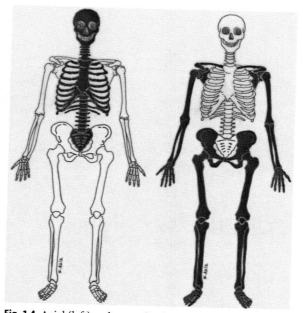

Fig. 1.4. Axial (left) and appendicular (right) skeletons

Tissue Level

Bone is divided into two types of tissues forming the skeleton: compact or cortical bone and cancellous, trabecular or spongy bone. The spongy bone has a turnover rate approximately eight times greater than the cortical bones and hosts hematopoietic cells and many blood cells. In mature bone, the compact bone forms an outer layer (cortex) which surrounds an inner one of loose trabecular, spongy bone in the medulla. The architecture is arranged in the haversian system (Fig. 1.5)

The spongy portion contains hematopoietic cells, which produce blood cells, fat and blood vessels. The compact bone constitutes 80% of the skeletal mass and contains 99% of the body's total calcium and 90% of its phosphorus.

The appendicular skeleton is composed predominantly of cortical bone. The cortical bone is thicker in the diaphysis than in the metaphysis and epiphysis of long bones (Fig. 1.6). The blood supply to the metaphysis is rich and consists of large sinusoids which slow the flow of blood. This is a feature that predisposes these

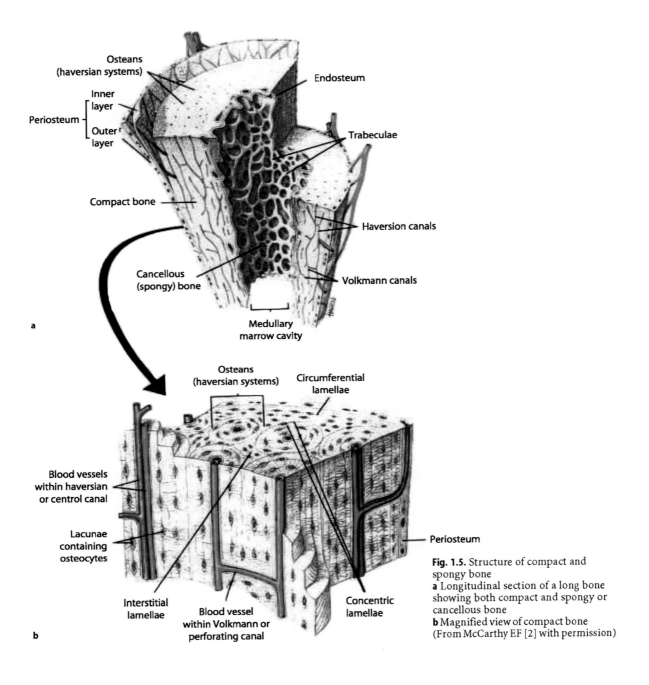

Fig. 1.5. Structure of compact and spongy bone
a Longitudinal section of a long bone showing both compact and spongy or cancellous bone
b Magnified view of compact bone (From McCarthy EF [2] with permission)

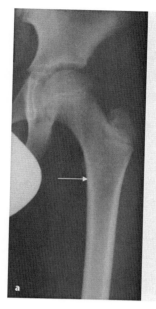
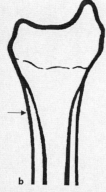

Fig. 1.6 a A radiograph of the proximal part of the femur illustrating the diaphyseal cortical bone that gradually thins in the regions of the metaphysis and epiphysis. **b** A schematic representation of this feature

Table 1.2. Bone structures and their functions

Major structural elements	Function
Bone cells	
Osteoblast	Production of Collagen and polysaccharide in bone.
Osteocytes	Produce bone matrix
Osteoclasts	Resorb bone, assist with mineral homeostasis
Bone matrix	
Organic matrix:	
Collagen fibers	Provide support and tensile strength
Proteoglycans	Control transport of ionized materials through matrix
Sialoprotein	Promotes calcification
Osteocalcin	Inhibits calcium/phosphate precipitation, promotes bone resorption
Laminin	Stabilizes basement membranes in bone
Osteonectin	Binds calcium to bones
Albumin	Transports essential elements to matrix
Inorganic matrix:	
Calcium	Provides rigidity and compressive strength
Phosphate	Regulates vitamin D and hence promotes mineralization

sites to bacterial proliferation. The spine, on the other hand, is composed predominantly of cancellous bone in the body of the vertebra and compact bone in the endplates and posterior elements.

Cellular Level

Three types of cells are seen in bone: (1) osteoblasts, which produce the organic bone matrix; (2) osteocytes, which produce the inorganic matrix; and (3) osteoclasts, which are active in bone resorption [5]. Osteoclasts are derived from the hemopoietic system, in contrast to the mesenchymal origin of osteoblasts. Osteocytes are derived from osteoblasts that have secreted bone around themselves [6].

Molecular Level

At the molecular level, bone matrix is composed primarily of organic matrix (approximately 35%), including collagen and glycoproteins, and inorganic matrix (approximately 65%), which includes hydroxyapatite,

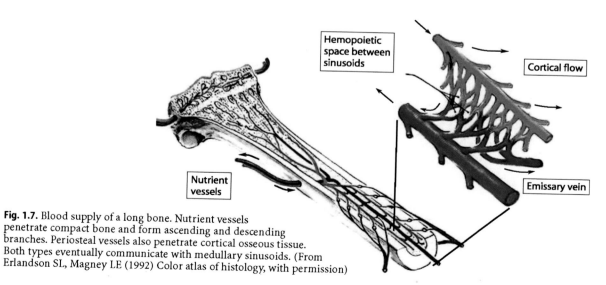

Hemopoietic space between sinusoids

Cortical flow

Nutrient vessels

Emissary vein

Fig. 1.7. Blood supply of a long bone. Nutrient vessels penetrate compact bone and form ascending and descending branches. Periosteal vessels also penetrate cortical osseous tissue. Both types eventually communicate with medullary sinusoids. (From Erlandson SL, Magney LE (1992) Color atlas of histology, with permission)

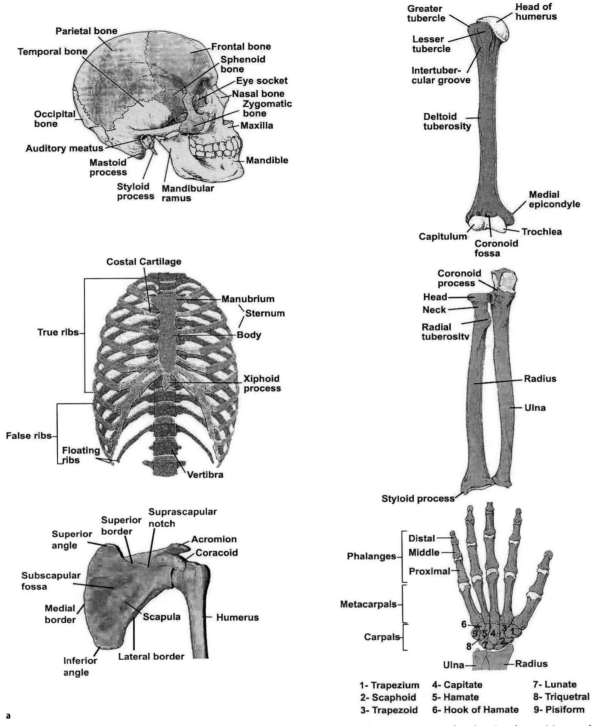

Fig. 1.8 a, b. Major bone of the human skeleton illustrating the main anatomic features necessary for planning the positions and the interpretation of the scintigraphic bone studies

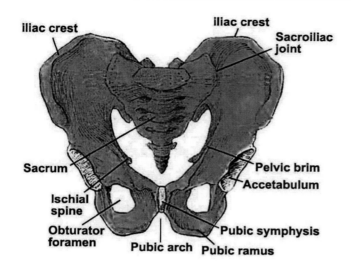

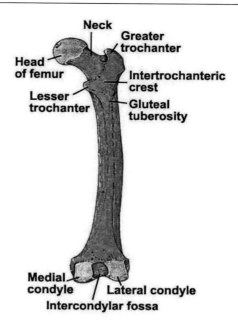

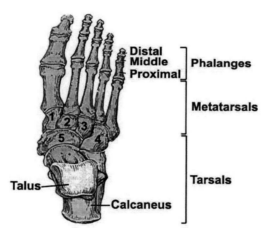

1, 2, 3- Medial, Intermediate, lateral cuneiform
4- Cuboid
5- Navicular

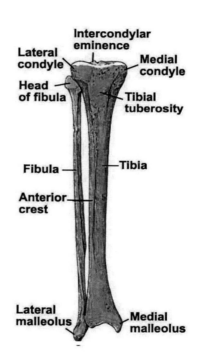

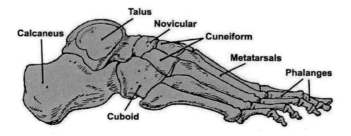

b

Fig. 1.8 (Cont.)

cations (calcium, magnesium, sodium, potassium and strontium) and anions (fluoride, phosphorus and chloride) [7, 8]. Table 1.2 summarizes the major constituents of bone and their function.

1.2.2.2
Blood Supply of Bone

Skeletal blood supply varies according to age. In children epiphyseal, metaphyseal and diaphyseal vessels are present. In adults all vessels inter-communicate. Nutrient and periosteal arteries feed a rich network of vessels to supply the cortex and medulla (Fig. 1.7) This vasculature takes the form of interconnecting capillaries, sinusoids and veins with hematopoietic spaces between sinusoids. It is estimated that blood flow to spongy bone containing marrow is 5–13 times higher than in cortical bone [9].

1.2.2.3
Features of Individual Bones

Familiarity with the anatomical features of individual bones is a prerequisite for the proper interpretation of scintigraphic studies and the correlation with other imaging modalities. Bones can be generally grouped in four categories, long, short, flat and irregular bones. Long bones include the femur, tibia, fibula, humerus, radius and ulna. Short bones include the metatarsals, metacarpals and phalanges. Flat bones include the ribs and sternum. Irregular bones include the vertebrae, pelvis and skull. The long bones consist of an epiphysis, metaphysis and diaphysis. The periosteum is a fibrous and membranous layer that covers the bone shaft and is rich in osteoblasts. A similar layer separates the marrow cavity of long bone from its cortical bone and is called the endosteum. Describing the detailed anatomical features of individual bone is beyond the scope of this text. However, a simple diagram illustrating the main features and parts of the major bones in addition to the bones of the hand and foot (Fig. 1.8) can serve as a quick reminder and reference for the interpretation and help with the swift identification of abnormalities. The availability of a skeletal model at the time of interpretation can also help localize the abnormalities shown by bone scintigraphy. Specific terms are used to describe locations of lesions on imaging modalities (including scintigraphy). Familiarity with these terms is important, and Fig. 1.9 summarizes the major descriptive terms used routinely.

1.2.3
Bone Physiology
1.2.3.1
Bone Function

Bone is a rigid connective tissue, which provides support and protection for the vital organs and tissue of the body. Within certain bones such as the skull, vertebrae and ribs, marrow cavities serve as sites of blood formation since these bones host the bone marrow. Bone has also an important function in mineral homeostasis.

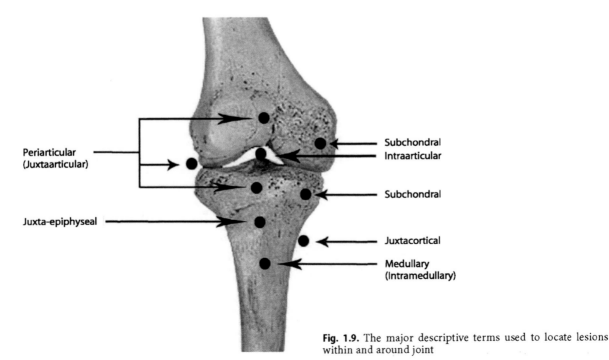

Fig. 1.9. The major descriptive terms used to locate lesions within and around joint

1.2.3.2
Bone Metabolism

Bone was previously thought to be inactive at the cellular level, but it is in fact a dynamic tissue. Its cells are involved in complex intercellular interactions in the process of continuous remodeling [10], whereby bone is removed slowly and then replaced by new bone.

Remodeling occurs throughout life with removal, and replacement, of bone at different rates in different parts of the skeleton. It is estimated that 18% of the skeleton is replaced every year in adults, indicating that almost the entire skeleton is replaced every 5 years. The process is more active in cancellous bone, with an approximate yearly replacement rate of 25% compared with 2% in compact bone [5]. Bone remodeling functions by removing injured bone (including aging bone, which becomes weaker); reinforcing bone in areas subject to abnormally increased stress; and, to a lesser extent, participating in calcium homeostasis by temporarily releasing calcium during the initial phase of remodeling [2]. Bone remodeling is carried out by teams of cells known as bone-modeling units (BMU) in a four-stage cycle that begins with an activation stage. This could be due to the effect of the protein, osteocalcin, and results in recruiting osteoclasts. This stage is followed by stage of resorption during which groups of osteoclasts remove bone, a stage that lasts for about 1 month. A reversal phase then follows which attracts osteoblasts to the resorption site by a coupling signal. This is again not clearly understood but could be due to the effect of the growth factors IGF (insulin growth factor) and TGF-B (transforming growth factor-B). This phase lasts for 1–2 weeks and is followed by the last phase of remodeling, the formation phase, which lasts for 5 months, during which time the osteoblasts line the resorption cavity and fill it with new bone (Fig. 1.10).

The bone remodeling cycles are highly regulated (by parathormone, vitamin D, and numerous other factors such as growth hormone) [11], with the result that in normal healthy individuals the amount of bone resorbed equals the amount of bone formed. The bone mass is thus unaltered. Under certain conditions, such as altered mechanical forces, metabolic bone disease, or metabolic and nutritional stress, this balance is disturbed [12]. Certain diseases are characterized by an increase in the rate of remodeling and are therefore known as high-turnover disorders; these may affect the entire skeleton or a single bone. Examples of such disorders include renal osteodystrophy and Paget's disease. In this group, both osteoblastic and osteoclastic activity is increased but the amount of bone formed is usually less than the bone removed resulting in osteopenia. An exception is Paget's disease, in the latter stages of which the osteoblastic activity exceeds the osteoclastic activity [13].

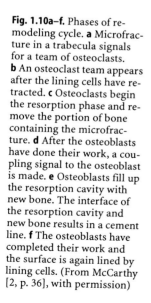

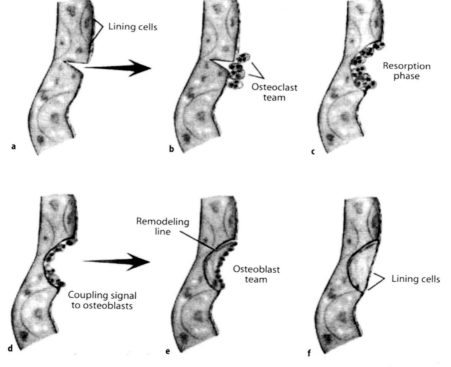

Fig. 1.10a–f. Phases of remodeling cycle. **a** Microfracture in a trabecula signals for a team of osteoclasts. **b** An osteoclast team appears after the lining cells have retracted. **c** Osteoclasts begin the resorption phase and remove the portion of bone containing the microfracture. **d** After the osteoblasts have done their work, a coupling signal to the osteoblast is made. **e** Osteoblasts fill up the resorption cavity with new bone. The interface of the resorption cavity and new bone results in a cement line. **f** The osteoblasts have completed their work and the surface is again lined by lining cells. (From McCarthy [2, p. 36], with permission)

1.3
Anatomy and Physiology of Bone Marrow

1.3.1
Development and Structure

Bone marrow is the soft tissue that lies in the spaces between the trabeculae of bones. Bone marrow generally consists of several elements, including blood vessels, nerves, mononuclear phagocytes, stem cells, blood cells at different stages of maturation, and fat [5]. There are two types of marrow, red and yellow. The red marrow has active hematopoietic cells, while the yellow marrow consists mainly of fat (Table 1.3) and is not hematopoietically active. The function of bone marrow is to provide blood cells, including red cells, white cells and platelets, based on the body's needs. Active bone marrow is present in adults in the pelvic bones (34%), vertebrae (28%), cranium and mandible (13%), sternum and ribs (10%), and proximal ends of humerus and femur (4–8%) [14].

Table 1.3. Bone marrow composition

Component	Red marrow	Yellow marrow
Water	40%	15%
Protein	20%	5%
Fat	40%	80%

1.3.2
Conversion and Reconversion

Bone marrow starts hematopoiesis in the 4th intrauterine month. It overrides the liver in this function by the 6th month (Fig. 1.11) and becomes fully responsible for hematopoiesis by birth [15]. Normally at birth almost the entire fetal marrow space is occupied by red (hematopoietic) marrow except the cartilaginous epiphyses (Fig 1.12) which later contain red marrow (on ossification) during the first few months of life. The conversion

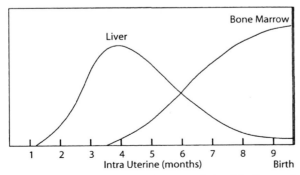

Fig. 1.11. Relationship between hematopoiesis of the liver and bone marrow before birth

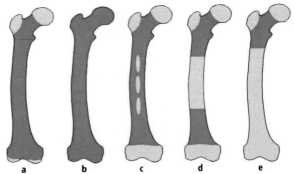

Fig. 1.12. Bone marrow distribution in a long bone illustrating changes during development over the years till the adult pattern is reached by about 25 years of age **a** birth; **b** 7 year-; **c** 14 year-; **d** 18 year-; **e** 25 year-old

from active red to yellow, non-hematopoietically active marrow starts in the immediate post-natal period, although it may begin just before birth in the terminal phalanges of the feet and hands. The conversion is a steady and progressive process that occurs at different rates in different bones as well as within an individual bone. The rate of conversion is fastest in the femora, followed by the ribs, sternum and vertebrae. Within the long bones, it is fastest in the midshaft. This process begins in the extremities and progresses, in general, from peripheral to central skeleton and from diaphyseal to metaphyseal regions in individual long bones. One year after birth the conversion is complete in the phalanges of the feet and hands. By the age of 7 years, conversion is significant in the distal epiphyses of long bones, and by age 12–14 years, conversion is clear in the mid-shaft of long bones with steady progress subsequently until the age of 25 (Fig. 1.12), by which point the conversion is complete in all bones, leaving red marrow in the vertebrae, sternum, ribs, pelvis, skull and the proximal portions of femora and humeri. A small amount may be detected in the calcaneus (Fig. 1.13). This normal adult pattern of hematopoietic bone marrow is not consistent and variations are frequently encountered. Some adults, for example, show red marrow in the distal third of the femora and humeri, or even sometimes in the entire shafts. Small islands of red marrow may also persist within the fatty marrow and are probably the basis of reconversion. Furthermore, with increasing demand for red cells, and due to certain pathological conditions (Table 1.4), reconversion of yellow to red marrow may take place. This process follows the reverse order of the initial red to yellow marrow conversion. It starts in the axial skeleton, followed by the extremities in a proximal to distal manner [15–17]. This process of reconversion is important since it also contributes to the variable distribution of bone marrow.

1.4
Anatomy and Physiology of Joints

Joints develop in the mesenchyme that is present between the ends of bones. They are classified according to their functional features as well as the nature of the adjoining tissue into several types (Table 1.5). The mesenchyme develops into fibrous tissue in fibrous joints; hyaline cartilage in synchondrosis; fibrocartilaginous tissue in the symphysis and into synovial membrane along with additional intra-articular structures in the synovial joints (Fig. 1.14). Familiarity with the major structural features of joints and their supporting structures (tendons, fasciae and ligaments), is a pre-requisite for the correct interpretation of nuclear medicine (and other types of) imaging. Synovial joints are considered to be specialized joints found mainly in the ap-

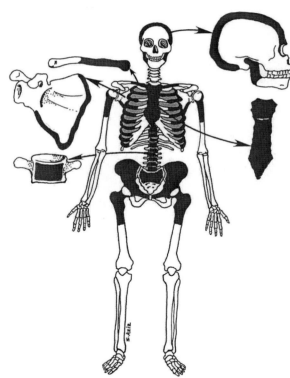

Fig. 1.13. Adult bone marrow distribution. This pattern is not consistent and there is natural variation which may be altered by many pathologic conditions

Table 1.4. Causes of reconversion of yellow to red marrow leading to alterations of marrow distribution

1. Chronic anemia, particularly hemolytic
2. Chronic heart failure
3. Myelofibrosis
4. Metastatic bone disease
5. Paget's disease
6. Multiple myeloma
7. Infarcts
8. Leukemia
9. Orthopedic surgery
10. Fractures
11. Infections
12. Possibly elevation of surrounding temperature

1.3.3
Alterations to Bone Marrow

In addition to the variability of marrow distribution at different ages and among adults, acquired alterations in the distribution of hematopoietic bone marrow may occur due to surgery, trauma, infection, and other destructive processes (Table 1.4). This is particularly important since it can explain the different findings from several nuclear medicine studies that might otherwise be thought to be abnormal (due to infection or replacement of bone marrow by an infiltrative processes) [15–19].

Table 1.5. Classification of joints

Basis, Major type	Types	Examples
Nature of adjoining tissue		
Fibrous		
	Suture	Skull sutures
	Syndesmosis	Radiolunar
	Gomphosis	Dental cement
Cartilaginous		
	Symphysis	Intervertebral disc, manubrio-sternal junction
	Synchondrosis	Growth plate
Synovial		Apophyseal joints, many extremity joints
Extent of motion		
Synarthroses (solid, nonsynovial), fixed or minimally movable	Fibrous and cartilaginous	Symphysis pubis
Diarthroses (cavitated), freely movable	Synovial	Knee, elbow

pendicular skeleton allowing free motion. The articulating surfaces of the opposing bones are separated by a cavity covered by a capsule with an articular cartilage covering the ends of both bones (Fig. 1.15). The inner surface of the joint capsule is formed by a synovial membrane which releases the synovial fluid (from a rich capillary network) into the articular cavity [20, 21]. The synovial fluid is a viscous fluid that serves to lubricate, nourish and cushion the avascular joint cartilage. When the synovial space is infected, bacterial hyaluronidase decreases the viscosity of the synovial fluid. Pain is then felt with stress on the joint capsule.

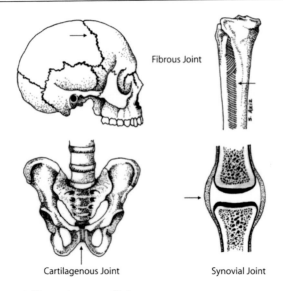

Fig. 1.14. The main types of joints

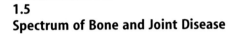

▷
Fig. 1.15. Synovial joint structure. (From Mourad [5], with permission)

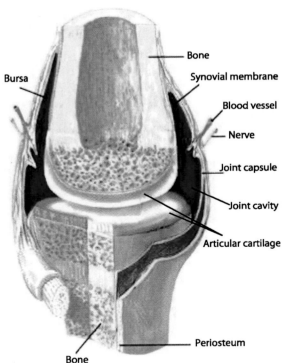

1.5
Spectrum of Bone and Joint Disease

A variety of bone and joint diseases exist which may be primary, or associated with other organ or systemic disease processes [2, 20, 21]. Consequently there are several ways to classify bone and joint diseases. Tables 1.6 and 1.7 show a simple classification for bone and joint diseases (with examples for further simplification).

1.6
Modalities for Imaging Bone and Joint Diseases

All the imaging modalities used for the diagnosis of bone and joint diseases fall into two complementary types, either morphological or functional (scintigraphic) modalities. Morphological modalities such as radiographs, ultrasonography, computed tomography (CT) and magnetic resonance imaging (MRI) depend mainly on structural changes, variations in density and differences in proton content in tissues. Functional modalities such as nuclear medicine techniques depend on the physiological changes. These modalities are numerous and no single modality is ideal in all situations. The choice of modality depends on the suspected condition, understanding of the strengths and limitations of each modality and an understanding of

Table 1.6. Classification of bone diseases

Type	Example
Nonneoplastic disorders	
Congenital disorders	Osteopetrosis
Circulatory disorders	Osteonecrosis
Traumatic disorders	Stress fractures
Infectious disorders	Osteomyelitis
Metabolic disorders	Osteoporosis
Bone changes in systemic disease	Neuropathic joint disease of diabetics
Neoplastic disorders	
Primary tumors	Osteogenic sarcoma
Metastatic tumors	Metastases of breast cancer

Table 1.7. Broad classification of joint disease

Type	Examples
Inflammatory joint disease	
a. Infectious	Infectious arthritis
b. Non-infectious	Rheumatoid arthritis, spondyloarthropathies
Non-inflammatory joint disease	
1. Primary osteoarthritis	Age related osteoarthritis
2. Secondary osteoarthrosis	Posttraumatic arthritis

the pathophysiology of the changes that occur in various pathological conditions and the associated co-morbidities (Table 1.8).

Table 1.8. Guideline to correlative imaging in bone disease

Disease condition	Standard radiograph	Scintigraphy	MRI	CT
Acute fractures	Modality of choice Both sensitive and specific	Limited role used in battered child, small bones of hands and feet and other locations where X-ray is not conclusive	Very useful in certain situations when other modalities are equivocal	
Stress fractures	Initial modality Low sensitivity (as low as 15%)	Modality of choice	Sensitive, may prove more specific than scintigraphy	
Skeletal infections	Initial examination	Modalities of choice	Suspected vertebral and probably diabetic foot infections	
Primary tumors	Initial examination	Limited role, determines multiplicity and metastases, specific diagnosis in some tumors (double density in osteoid osteoma, doughnut pattern in giant cell tumor and aneurysmal bone cyst)	Modality of choice	Osteoid osteoma, multiple myeloma
Metastases	Useful in multiple myeloma	Modality of choice	Determines local extent More sensitive than scintigraphy in purely lytic and vertebral lesions	
Assess tumor therapy	Limited role	Modalities of choice particularly PET. Tl-201 or Tc99m MIBI if PET is unavailable		

1.7
Diagnosis of Bone and Joint Diseases by Nuclear Medicine Techniques

The principle response of bone to injury and disease is reactive bone formation. The bone formed in this way develops in stages. Initially, it is disorganized, active, and is non-lamellar (woven), but later it may remodel to normal lamellar bone (Figs. 1.16 and 1.17). In comparison to normal lamellar bone, the woven bone has a much larger surface area and is lined by metabolically active osteoblasts. Additionally, in woven bone, the crystalline structures are smaller and have a larger surface area available for the absorption of bone radiopharmaceuticals [22, 23]. Accordingly, increased uptake of bone-specific radiopharmaceuticals is seen in such areas.

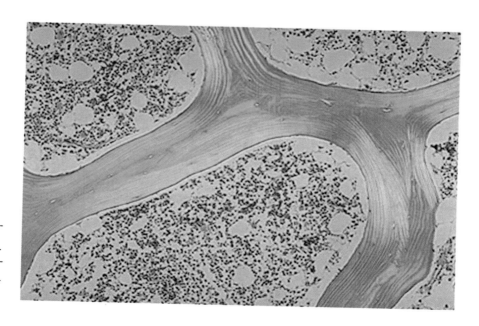

Fig. 1.16. Normal cancellous bone seen under polarized light which highlights the lamellar structure. The bony spicules are even, with occasional lacunae containing osteocytes. Cellular marrow is seen between the spicules of bone

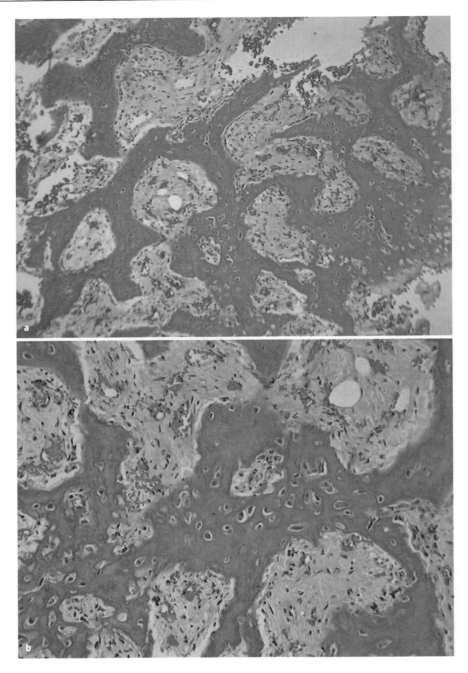

Fig. 1.17a–c. The irregular and disorganized nature of woven bone compared to lamellar bone depicted in Fig. 1.16. This is emphasized at different microscopic magnification levels: **a** ×10, **b** ×20, **c** ×40

Imaging should be correlative and tailored according to the individual characteristics of each case. Apart from bone scintigraphy using Tc99m diphosphonates, nuclear medicine modalities include a range of techniques used to image bone diseases. These include gallium-67, labeled white blood cells using indium-11 oxine or Tc99m HMPAO; Tl-201 imaging; Tc99m MIBI imaging; bone marrow imaging using Tc99m colloid; iodine-123 and I-131 MIBG; and PET imaging. Monoclonal and polyclonal antibody imaging are also used infrequently in bone disease, particularly in infections. The choice of a modality or combination of modalities is based on the individual case, the underlying disease and the pathophysiology of the suspected condition(s), as well as the knowledge of radiation exposure (Tables 1.9–1.15). Knowledge of radiation exposure is particularly important in the pediatric age group and in pregnant women. The commonly used bone scintigraphy

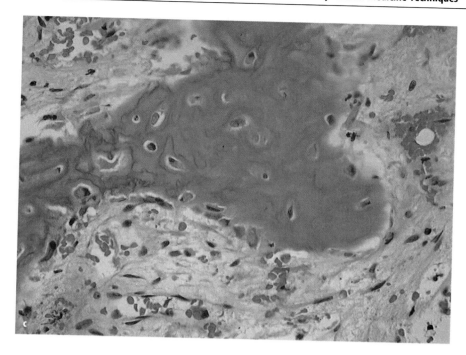

Fig. 1.17 (Cont.)

Table 1.9. Estimated radiation absorbed dose of Tc99m diphosphonates. Modified from Owunwanne et al. [47, p. 83], with permission

Organ	99mTc-MDP mGy/MBq	rad/mCi	99mTc-HEDP mGy/MBq	rad/mCi	99mTc-HMDP mGy/MBq	rad/mCi
Bone surface	0.061	0.23	0.036	0.13	0.091	0.34
Bladder wall	0.034	0.13	0.041	0.15	0.022	0.081
Bone marrow	0.0093	0.034	0.0094	0.035	0.013	0.048
Kidneys	0.0084	0.031	0.0066	0.024	0.0059	0.0022
Ovaries	0.0032	0.012	0.0037	0.014	0.0032	0.012
Testes	0.0022	0.0082	0.0025	0.0092	0.0023	0.0085
Whole body	0.0028	0.010	0.0026	0.0094	0.0036	0.013

Table 1.10. Estimated radiation absorbed dose of gallium-67 citrate

Organ	mGy/MBq	rad/mCi
Gastrointestinal tract		
Lower large intestine	0.24	0.90
Upper large intestine	0.15	0.56
Small intestine	0.097	0.36
Stomach	0.059	0.22
Bone marrow	0.156	0.58
Spleen	0.143	0.53
Liver	0.124	0.46
Skeleton and marrow	0.119	0.44
Kidneys	0.111	0.41
Ovaries	0.075	0.28
Testes	0.065	0.24
Total body	0.070	0.26

From [47, p. 122], with permission

Table 1.11. Estimated radiation absorbed dose of In-111-oxine leukocytes

Organ	mGy/MBq	rad/mCi
Spleen	5.5	20.35
Liver	0.21	2.63
Red marrow	0.69	2.55
Pancreas	0.52	1.92
Kidneys	0.33	1.22
Adrenals	0.31	1.15
Gastrointestinal tract		
Stomach wall	0.28	1.04
Small intestine	0.16	0.59
Upper large intestinal wall	0.16	0.59
Lower large intestinal wall	0.13	0.48
Heart	0.17	0.63
Ovaries	0.12	0.44
Uterus	0.12	0.44
Testes	0.045	0.17

From [47, p. 128], with permission

Table 1.12. Estimated radiation absorbed dose of thallium-201

Organ	mGy/MBq	rad/mCi
Heart wall	0.226	0.835
Gastrointestinal tract		
Upper large intestine	0.188	0.675
Lower large intestine	0.362	1.34
Small intestine	0.162	0.60
Gallbladder wall	0.022	0.081
Kidneys	0.537	1.99
Urinary bladder wall	0.036	0.135
Ovaries	0.120	0.445
Thyroid	0.250	0.925
Liver	0.176	0.65
Testes	0.562	2.835
Red marrow	0.176	0.65
Bone surface	0.338	1.25

Modified from [47, p. 75], with permission

Table 1.13. Estimated radiation absorbed dose of Tc99m sestamibi

Organ	mGy/MBq	rad/mCi
Heart wall	0.0048	0.018
Gastrointestinal tract		
Upper large intestine	0.043	0.139
Lower large intestine	0.030	0.111
Small intestine	0.026	0.096
Gallbladder wall	0.022	0.081
Kidneys	0.018	0.067
Urinary bladder wall	0.017	0.063
Ovaries	0.012	0.044
Thyroid	0.0057	0.021
Liver	0.0053	0.019
Testes	0.0028	0.011
Total body	0.0044	0.016

Modified from [47, p. 75], with permission

Table 1.14. Estimated radiation absorbed dose of Tc99m sulfur colloid

Organ	mGy/MBq	rad/mCi
Liver	0.0918	0.34
Spleen	0.0567	0.21
Bone marrow	0.0073	0.027
Ovaries	0.0015	0.0056
Testes	0.0003	0.011
Whole body	0.0051	0.019

Modified from [47, p. 86], with permission

Table 1.15. Estimated radiation absorbed dose of F-18 FDG

Organ	mGy/MBq	rad/mCi
Brain	0.029	0.107
Heart	0.045	0.166
Bladder wall	0.066	0.244
Kidneys	0.030	0.111
Liver	0.023	0.085
Spleen	0.022	0.081
Gastrointestinal tract		
Stomach wall	0.015	0.056
Small intestine	0.017	0.063
Upper large intestinal wall	0.017	0.063
Lower large intestinal wall	0.018	0.067
Bone surface	0.015	0.056
Testes	0.015	0.056
Thyroid	0.013	0.048
Red marrow	0.012	0.044

Modified from [47, p. 163], with permission

Table 1.16. Scintigraphic-pathologic correlation

Pathologic etiology	Scintigraphic pattern on bone scan
Increased vascularity	Increased flow and blood pool activity.
Angiogenesis	Increased blood pool activity
Osteoblastic response	Increased uptake
Bone destruction (infarction, rapidly growing tumor)	Cold areas
Large destructive lesion with rim of new bone formation.	Doughnut pattern
Paget's disease, some primary or metastatic tumors	Bone expansion
Arthritis, reflex sympathetic dystrophy (CR PS-1)	Periarticular increased uptake
Equilibrium of bone destruction and bone formation	Near normal appearance

1.8
Technical Considerations

1.8.1
Pre-imaging Considerations

1.8.1.1
Bone Imaging Radiopharmaceuticals

shows many patterns in a variety of benign and malignant bone diseases (some may be specific). Many of these patterns are better understood once the underlying pathophysiological changes are appreciated (Table 1.16) and the clinical condition of the patient is known. Paying attention to the clinical and technical details can make the imaging results more specific than just localizing an abnormality.

Strontium-85, strontium-87m and fluorine-18 were used as bone imaging radiopharmaceuticals before the introduction of technetium-99m to medicine in 1964. The first Tc99m-labeled bone imaging agent to be described was stannous-reduced Tc99m tripolyphosphate, followed by several other compounds with a higher bone uptake. The first was Tc99m pyrophosphate, which was introduced before the diphosphonates that are still being used as the agents of choice for routine bone scintigraphy [24]. In addition, gallium-67 citrate, indium-11 oxine or Tc99m HMPAO leukocytes, Tc99m colloids, Tl-201 imaging, Tc99m MIBI, F-18 FDG PET and Tc99m and In-111 labeled polyclonal and monoclonal antibodies have been introduced. With the increasing availability of PET scanners, F-18 will be used more for whole body bone scanning.

Common Diphosphonate Radiopharmaceuticals

Currently, Tc99m diphosphonates are the radiopharmaceuticals most commonly used for skeletal scintigraphy (Table 1.17). These agents concentrate predominantly in the mineral phase of bone (Table 1.18), which consists of crystalline hydroxyapatite and amorphous calcium phosphate. Using an in-vitro assay, Francis et al. [25] showed that the competitive adsorption of Tc99m diphosphonates in pure inorganic hydroxyapatite was 40 times that in pure organic bone matrix. These radiopharmaceuticals do not localize to a significant degree in osteoblasts or in the osteoid tissue. These various agents were found to have no significant difference in bone uptake (Fig. 1.18).

Several factors affect the uptake of diphosphonate in the skeleton, particularly the blood flow (an increased flow is matched by an increased uptake) and extraction efficiency. Pathological foci containing woven bone show an increased uptake due to a higher extraction efficiency. Other factors (Table 1.19) such as the action of vitamin D also influence diphosphonate uptake. Accordingly, in children uptake of the radiopharmaceutical is particularly seen at the costochondral junctions, the metaphyseal ends of the normal long bones and in the facial bones. When the skeleton has matured, this uptake disappears. Overall the skeletal accumulation of diphosphonate decreases with age particularly in the extremities [26]. In a study of 49 females aged 14–79

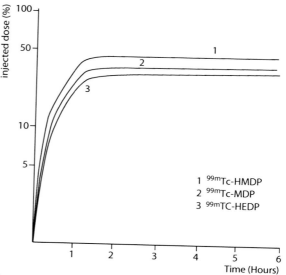

Fig. 1.18. Bone uptake over time by three types of Tc99m diphosphonates. Note that there is no significant uptake difference. Modified from [47], with permission

Table 1.19. Factors influencing skeletal accumulation of Tc-99m diphosphonates

Blood flow
Extraction efficiency
Vitamin D
Parathyroid hormone
Corticosteroids
Intraosseous tissue pressure
Capillary permeability
Acid-base balance
Sympathetic tone

years old and 47 males aged 6–89 years old with normal bone scans, the highest bone uptake in both sexes was obtained in individuals less than 20 years old with active epiphyseal growth plates. In men, bone uptake slowly decreased with age up to 60 years with a tendency towards increasing uptake values thereafter. In women, the mean uptake reached a minimum in the decade 20–29 years of age and then slowly increased with a positive linear correlation of uptake and age in those older than 55 years [27].

Proper Utilization of Tc99m Diphosphonates

The commonly used Tc99m diphosphonate compounds should be used optimally within 2 h and no later than 6 h after preparation since they decompose with time due to the oxidation-reduction process. This process results in excess free pertechnetate, which may

Table 1.17. Tc99m diphosphonate compounds

Tc99m methylene diphosphonate	Tc99m MDP
Tc99m hydroxyethylidene diphosphonate	Tc99m HEDP
Tc99m hydroxymethylene diphosphonate	Tc99m HDP
Tc99m dicarboxypropane Diphosphonate	Tc99m DPD
Tc99m dimethylamino diphosphonate	Tc99m DMAD

Table 1.18. Mechanism of uptake of diphosphonate bone-seeking radiopharmaceuticals [47]

1. Uptake in hydroxyapatite
2. Uptake in immature collagen
3. Uptake by enzyme receptor binding

Table 1.20. Administered activity of the current Tc99m diphosphonates and timing of imaging according to the patient age

Age	Activity of Tc99m diphosphonate	Time of imaging after injection
Pediatric age	According to weight	1.5 – 2 h
Adults		
Under 30 years	15 mCi	2 h*
30 – 50 years	20 mCi	3 h
Above 50 years	25 mCi	4 h

3 h, if extremities are the regions of interest

lead to uptake in the thyroid gland, salivary gland and gastric mucosa [24].

Amount of Administered Activity

Table 1.20 summarizes the recommended dose and timing of imaging at different ages. The amount of activity to be used for an adequate bone scan is dependent on several factors, the most important of which is the age of the patient; the bone activity and the renal function are closely related to the patient's age. Patients under 30 can be injected with approximately 15 mCi (600 MBq), patients between the ages of 30 and 50 are injected with 20 mCi (750 MBq), while patients over the age of 50 years can be injected with 25 mCi (900 MBq). In children the activity administered is modified according to the weight of the patient. The younger the patient, the lower the activity and the shorter the time between injection and acquisition of the images.

1.8.1.2
Patient Preparation

Patients must be properly prepared to achieve a diagnostically reliable study. The referring physician and nursing team should also be familiar with such preparations. For a routine bone scan the patient must be well hydrated depending on their clinical condition. The recommended ideal amount of fluid intake in adults between injection and imaging is 2000 ml, with a minimum of 500 ml [29]. The radiopharmaceutical activity and the time of imaging depend on the patient's age and underlying diseases.

Patients should be prepared differently for studies using other radiopharmaceuticals, such as F-18 FDG, and there may no need for any specific preparation, such as with use of labeled white blood cells and Tc99m colloids. For the best results, however, the procedure, its duration, risks and benefits of every study must be clearly explained to the patient.

Sedation for pediatric patients should be consid-

ered in order to obtain studies with good quality. This is particularly important in aiding interpretation in this age group. Sedation is frequently needed in patients below the age of 4 years and in older mentally retarded children. The most commonly used method is oral sedation using chloral hydrate, with a recommended dose of 75 – 100 mg/kg body weight to a maximum dose of 2.5 g. A lower dose of 50 mg/kg may not be sufficient in many cases, and adding a supplemental dose may not work in some patients, particularly if they have become agitated after the initial dose. Intravenous sedation using phenobarbital is another popular method. The recommended dose is 2.5 – 7.5 mg/kg body weight with a maximum of 200 mg. Other sedatives can also be used, as well as general anesthesia (in certain situations).

1.8.1.3
Patient History and Examination

Although a radiologist may read films with little history and no patient examination, bone scans cannot be adequately interpreted without detailed clinical information and a physical examination of the patient. A study illustrating this concept was conducted by Sundberg et al. [28], who found that the correct diagnosis of septic arthritis in children was achieved in 70 % of cases when clinical information was included in the interpretation. This fell to only 13 % when films were interpreted with no clinical information. Review of radiographs prior to the start of a study should be a routine practice, since it clarifies which special views might make the lesions more clearly visible. This also helps decide which areas may have a priority for radionuclide angiography and blood pool imaging. Table 1.21 summarizes the important specific information which is needed before obtaining and interpreting bone scans.

1.8.1.4
Time of Imaging After Injection

For patients under 30 years of age, the time of imaging generally is 2 h after injection. If the extremities are the areas of interest this increases to 3 h. For patients aged 30 – 50 years, imaging should take place at 3 h (again, if the extremities are the area of interest the imaging should be delayed an hour). For patients above 50 years of age, imaging is obtained at 4 h routinely. Further delay is needed if, in certain cases, there is delayed soft tissue clearance (e.g. kidney disease). Although adequate uptake by bone reaches adequate levels for imaging after 1 h, the additional delay is mainly related to the soft tissue clearance. This allows a better bone-to-background ratio for quality imaging.

Table 1.21. Essential relevant information in patient's history for quality bone scan plan and interpretation

Information	Reasoning
Prior trauma (including accidents), surgery (including biopsy) of bone and other tissue, presence of hardware with dates	Explain abnormal uptake and avoid confusion with current pathology
Whether the patient is left or right handed	Explain possible asymmetry of shoulder uptake as a normal variant and avoid false diagnosis
Occupation and physical activities	Explain certain findings such as joint uptake and help in the diagnosis of certain conditions such as fatigue, fractures in runners or ballet dancers
Therapy with steroids, etidronate or similar agents	Generalized decreased uptake
Tumors	Help in interpretation and explain certain findings such as dystrophic calcification
Patient body habitus fatty	Explain certain patterns as attenuation by tissue as in case of steatopygia
Chemotherapy with dates	Explain certain findings such as flare and expansion of bone marrow
Radiation therapy with dates	Explain early flare and late cold lesions to avoid misinterpretation
Prior imaging studies	Comparison and correlation with bone images
Pregnancy and delivery	Decision making regarding obtaining the study, explain certain postpartal findings in the pelvis such as diastasis

1.8.2
Imaging Considerations

1.8.2.1
Instrumentation

The clinical question being studied determines the use of single- or dual-head, wide field-of-view cameras which can be equipped with a variety of collimators. Dual-head cameras have the advantage of reducing the acquisition time and are particularly useful for routine whole body scans. For the best results, the highest resolution collimators should be used since resolution is important to recognize and localize abnormalities (Fig. 1.19). In addition to parallel-hole devices, pinhole and diverging collimators are used for the visualization of small skeletal structures or to image large patients respectively (Figs. 1.20, 1.21). A pinhole collimator is particularly useful in pediatric patients and in imaging the small bones of the hands and feet and abnormalities of the knee and ankle in adults, since it provides adequate magnification as well as resolution, which depends on the distance between the object and the collimator pinhole. This allows identification of details that may not be seen using a parallel-hole collimator or SPECT (Figs. 1.22 – 1.24).

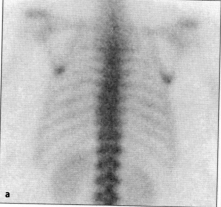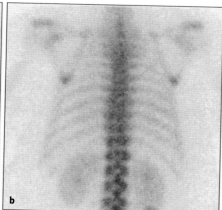

Fig. 1.19 a, b. Posterior Tc99m MDP images acquired for the same count using (**a**) general purpose and (**b**) high-resolution collimators for the same patient. Note the difference in resolution with more details seen on high-resolution collimator images

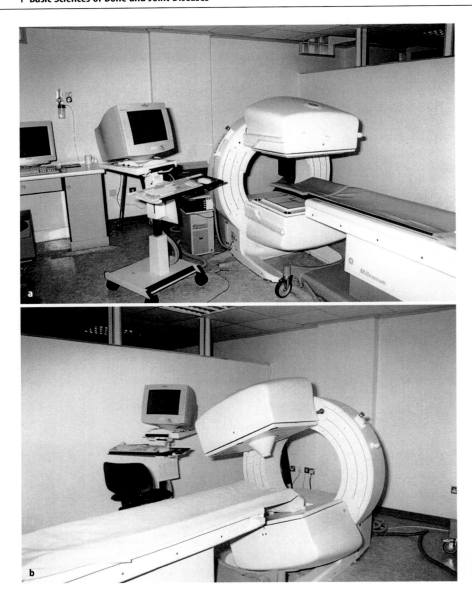

Fig. 1.20 a, b. Dual-head gamma cameras equipped with parallel (**a**) and pinhole collimator (**b**)

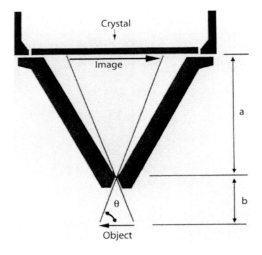

Fig. 1.21. The object magnification of a pinhole collimator. Crystal to pinhole distance (*a*), pinhole to object distance (*b*), angle at which photons pass through pinhole (θ) and pinhole diameter are all relevant parameters for determining magnification, sensitivity and resolution. (From Connolly et al. [49], with permission)

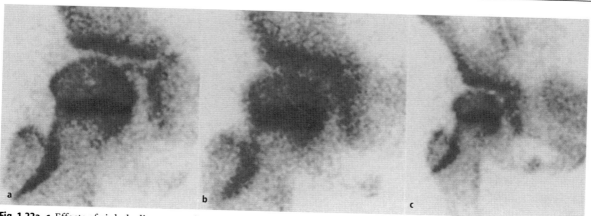

Fig. 1.22a–c. Effects of pinhole diameter and pinhole-to-patient distance on resolution and magnification. **a** Image of right hip was obtained using 3 mm insert with collimator approximately 2.5 cm from skin surface. Resolution is superior to that provided using 4 mm insert at the same distance from skin surface (**b**) and that provided using 3 mm insert approximately 10 cm from skin surface (**c**). Magnification is lower at greater distances. Count density is 150,000 for each image. (From Connolly et al. [49], with permission)

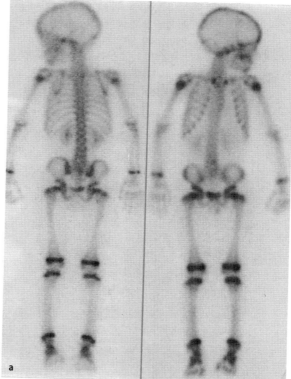

Fig. 1.23 a, b. Images of a hip using parallel-hole (**a**) and pinhole (**b**) collimators. Note the difference between the magnified pinhole view, showing clearly the photon-deficient abnormality (*arrow*), and the parallel-hole image in this patient with bilateral osteonecrosis of the femoral heads

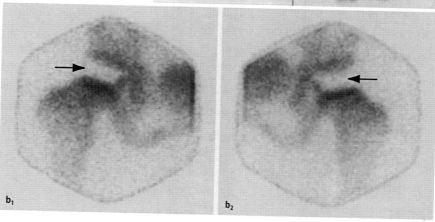

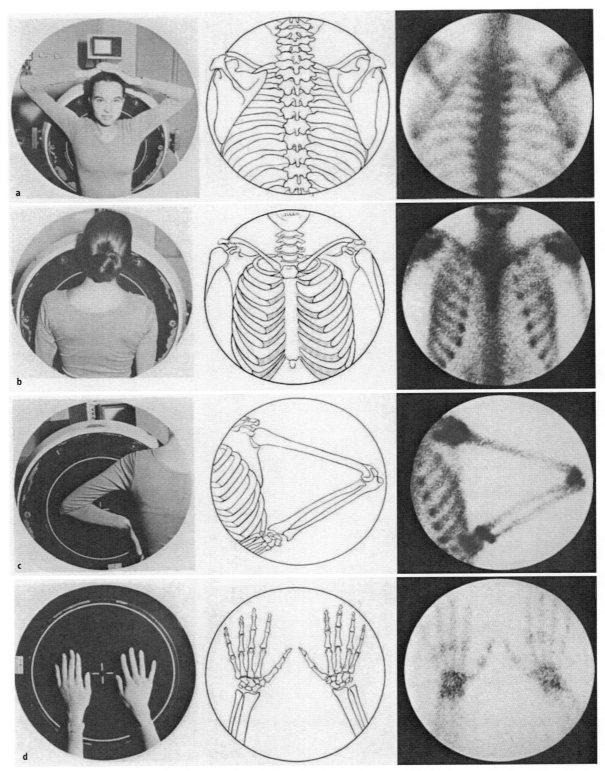

Fig. 1.24a–h. Proper positioning of major parts of the skeleton for adequate imaging. Illustrated are positioning of (**a**) posterior chest, (**b**) anterior chest, (**c**) arms, (**d**) hands, (**e**) anterior hip (pinhole), (**f**) anterior hip (pinhole) in a frog-leg position, (**g**) anterior knee and legs (note the internal rotation separating tibiae from fibulae), (**h**) dorsal feet (note internal rotation allowing symmetry, visualization of bones and minimizing overlap) (From Hughes; In Silberstein EB (ed): Bone scintigraphy [29], with permission)

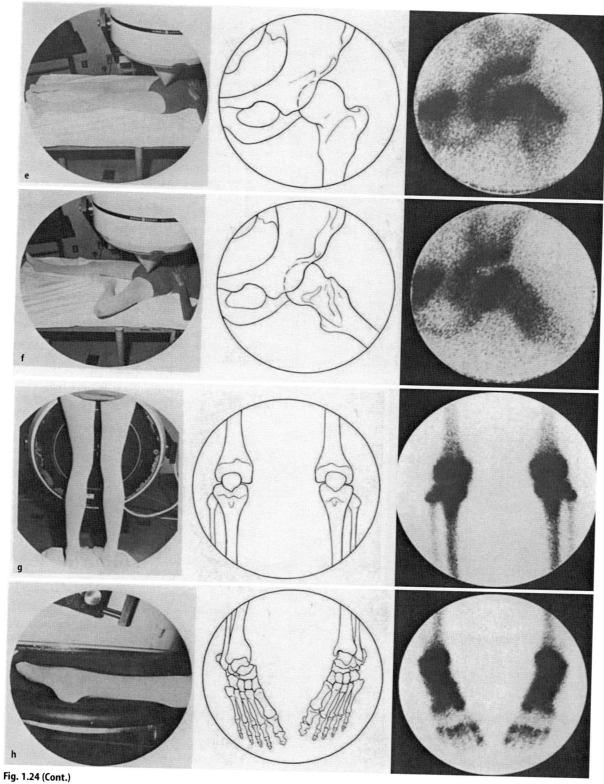

Fig. 1.24 (Cont.)

1.8.2.2
Positioning

Poor patient positioning can easily cause the appearance of false lesions (due to asymmetry), or artificially overlap bony structures which may obscure lesions. The general rules for positioning patients for bone scanning are well known [29]. Additionally, technicians and physicians should be familiar with optional positions, which can be used for specific objectives. The choice of position is determined by clearly defining the clinical question that needs to be answered [30]. Figure 1.24 shows the proper positioning for certain regions and the optional positions. Although whole body imaging is routinely utilized by the vast majority of practices, it is worth considering certain basic optional positions since they can be valuable in resolving diagnostic dilemmas and help to alleviate confusion and uncertainty in interpretation. Such positions include the pelvic oblique and lateral views; the pelvic caudal view can be particularly useful in separating bladder and other soft tissue activity from that of the bones (Fig. 1.25).

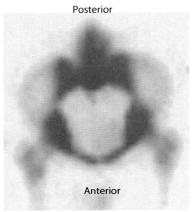

Posterior

Anterior

Fig. 1.25 Caudal view of the pelvis showing clearly the pelvic bones with no possible overlap with the bladder or soft tissues

1.8.2.3
Acquisition

A dynamic flow study (radionuclide angiography) is acquired for 1-s frames for 60 s after the injection of the radiopharmaceutical. The region of interest should be within the camera's field of view (Fig. 1.26). This study should be done if there is a focal radiographic lesion, regional sign or symptom or a site of prior surgery. Immediate static images (blood pool) follow for either 500–1000 kilocount (k) for spot images for the region(s) of interest, or for 5 min for the whole body image (Fig. 1.27). Flow studies show the vascular supply ('vascularity'), while blood pool images show the level of angiogenesis if present and the vascular status of the extravascular tissue. Delayed images (Figs. 1.28, 1.29) are acquired for spot imaging (750 k over chest); all other images for the remainder of the skeleton are acquired for the same time. Whole body imaging should be optimally performed at 2 million counts/whole body view (20 min with a high resolution collimator). The matrix size is usually 256 × 256 for spot images while it is 1024 × 256 or 2048 × 512 for whole body images. To obtain the best resolution for a specific system and collimator, the matrix size should be chosen so that the pixel size is $1/3$ to $1/2$ of the system resolution determined by the full width at half maximum (FWHM). If the pixel size is too small it causes noisy images, while if it is too large it will cause a resolution worse than the system resolution. The pixel size is calculated as follows:

$$\text{Pixel size} = \frac{\text{Long axis of a rectangular detector or diameter of a circular detector}}{\text{Matrix size}}$$

Since the dimensions of the detector and system resolution are fixed, the matrix size is the parameter that can be changed to obtain an optimal pixel size and hence good image quality. With the use of the appropriate matrix, magnifying the images during acquisition, or

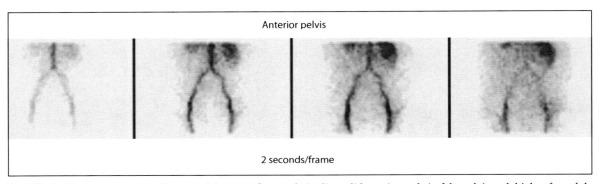

Anterior pelvis

2 seconds/frame

Fig. 1.26. An illustrative example of a normal dynamic-flow study (radionuclide angiography) of the pelvis and thighs of an adult. Note the symmetrical pattern. It is helpful for interpretation to remember that the level of the bifurcation of the aorta corresponds roughly to the level of L4–5 and the bifurcation of common iliac artery to the level of the lesser trochanter

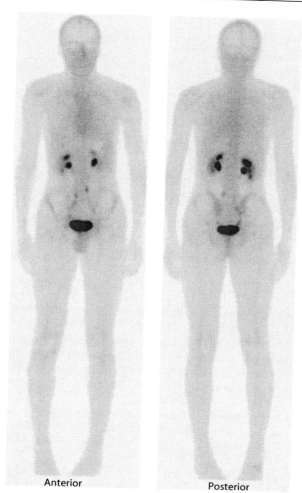

Anterior   Posterior

Fig. 1.27. Normal early static (blood pool) image. Note the activity in the heart, kidneys, ureters, bladder, and narrow containing bones as pelvis and spine

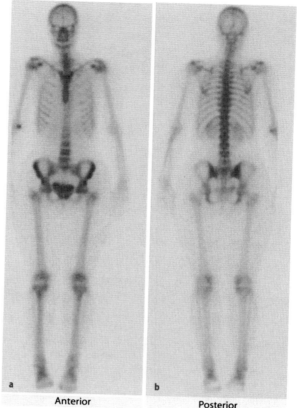

a   Anterior   b   Posterior

Fig. 1.28a, b. Normal bone scan of the entire skeleton in an adult. Note higher uptake in certain areas such as the sacroiliac joints, iliac spine, vertebrae, sternum and ends of long bones reflecting the metabolic activity, thickness, and the presence of bone marrow

processing, will have no effect on the resolution [31]. A four-phase bone scan is performed for the detection of certain disease processes with better specificity. The four-phase bone scan utilizes the fact that while radio-nuclide uptake ceases in normal bone after approximately 4 h following injection, the accumulation continues in woven bone for several hours more [32]. In this way, in cases of osteomyelitis and metastatic tumors [33, 34] a higher lesion-to-background ratio is obtained at 24 h than at 3–4 h. This technique can help improve specificity although it may cause some loss of sensitivity. Additional spot images are often required for a variety of reasons. One should remember to obtain orthogonal (90 degree) images, or oblique images, for the localization of abnormalities when these are noted in the initial images. Body contouring should be considered, and the use of a camera that is equipped with automatic or semi-automatic body contouring is

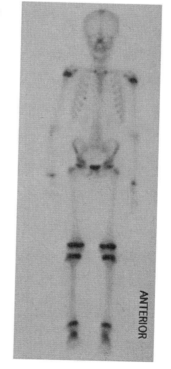

Fig. 1.29. Normal bone scan in a child. Note the activity in the growth plates and the higher relative uptake in the extremities compared to adults. This reflects the higher bone activity in the young

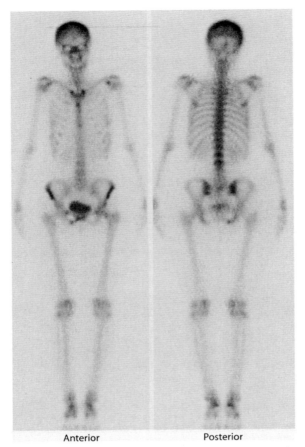

Anterior   Posterior

Fig. 1.30. A whole-body scan of an obese patient showing the decreased uptake in the lower lumbar spine due to the attenuation of fat in the buttocks (steatopygia)

helpful; otherwise, additional spot images should be obtained (with the collimator close to the body part of interest, such as the extremities or skull).

When a SPECT study is required, 25- to 30-s frames are acquired using a high-resolution collimator and a 128 × 128 matrix. If a general purpose collimator is to be used 20-s frames using a 64 × 64 matrix are used. In either case, 64 frames are obtained through 360 deg.

1.8.3
Post-imaging Considerations

It is important to use a proper portrayal of the image on proper film, or computer, as well as adequate image processing to insure accurate interpretation. The technologists as well as the interpreting physician should assess possible pitfalls and artifacts. If hard-copy films are used, the computer image should add useful information. Finally, knowledge of the detailed clinical history and review of other imaging modalities is mandatory at the time of reading, keeping in mind the possible causes of diagnostic errors.

1.8.4
Sources of Diagnostic Errors

Factors Related to History and Physical Examination: Lack of adequate clinical assessment by physicians, including imaging specialists, leads to errors. It is crucial for adequate interpretation of bone scintigraphy to have a detailed patient history and to examine them. Many studies have shown the value of clinical information in improving the accuracy of the interpretation [28, 35] as stated earlier. Prior pathology such as fractures or inflammation cause diagnostic errors if not known to the interpreting physician.

Factors Related to the Patient: Errors can occur in imaging due to patient-related factors, including age, body habitus, underlying diseases, medications, hydration status and lack of cooperation during the study (e.g. patient motion). Full knowledge of the patient's medical background and proper patient-physician communication are needed with a clear explanation of the required preparation and procedure to ensure the patient's cooperation during the procedure. Imaging at the standard time for a patient with a debilitating disease will result in a scan with suboptimal quality; examination should be further delayed. Knowledge of the patient's condition can avoid subsequent errors and problems by planning a longer time to obtain the images. Another interesting issue is the steatopygia that can cause decreased uptake in the lower lumbar spine (Fig. 1.30) of patients with prominent fat in the buttock region [36]. This could also cause an appearance of abnormally increased uptake at the edge of a fat crease (Fig. 1.31) as well as errors in the interpretation of bone densitometry studies with an underestimation of the bone density value due to attenuation.

Factors Related to Radiopharmaceuticals: The presence of aluminum in the generator eluate, injection of the tracer into an unintended compartment such as the arterial circulation or an interstitial space (Fig. 1.32) or introduction of air into the vial during preparation can significantly affect the quality of scan. Etidronate inhibits bone turnover and dramatically shows little uptake by bone coupled with a major distribution in the interstitial tissue [37–41]. Introduction of oxygen to the kit during preparation will cause oxidation and consequently increases the free technetium. Use of a solution several hours after preparation, particularly later than 6 h, will also cause the same problems, since the free technetium will be increased in the preparation. In both situations, uptake by the thyroid and gastric mucosa, and consequently bowel

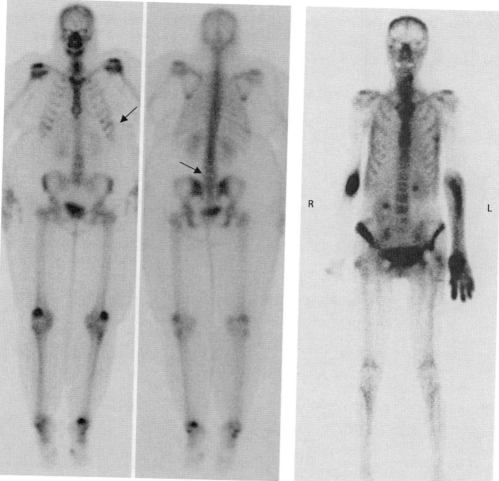

Fig. 1.31. A whole-body bone scan in an obese patient illustrating the effect of body habitus on the images. Note the attenuation in the regions of the breast and buttocks. The activity used for such patients should be increased and the duration between injection and imaging may be increased for better clearance of soft tissue activity and better target to non-target ratios for better images

Fig. 1.32. A 3-h image of the hand of a patient who was injected intra-arterially illustrating retention of activity in the hand and forearm. Patient was difficult to inject in an attempt in the right arm before the activity was injected intra-arterially in the left arm

activity and other soft tissues (Fig. 1.33), will be seen, and will make the scan quality inadequate, and free pertechnetate uptake will simulate or hide lesions. Table 1.22 lists causes of soft tissue uptake seen on bone scan secondary to technical and pathological technologies.

Factors Related to Technique: Problems related to injection technique may cause variable hot spots that can mimic, or mask, lesions. Inadequate count collection provides suboptimal images that leads to diagnostic errors such as missing abnormalities. Faulty positioning can lead to asymmetry, for example with subsequent false diagnoses. A full bladder, as well as bladder diver-

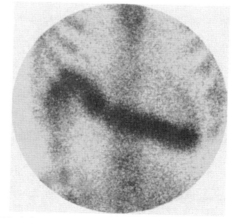

Fig. 1.33. Colon activity of delayed Tc99m MDP images due to bad tagging of the radiopharmaceutical

Table 1.22. Frequent technical and pathologic causes of extra-osseous activity on bone scintigraphy (Data from [44–48])

Generalized
  Faulty radiopharmaceutical preparation
  Poor hydration
  Renal failure
  Chronic iron overload
Localized
  Injection site
  Arterial injection
  Contamination
    Patient contamination
      Urine
      Blood (with injection)
    Instrument contamination
  Hematoma
  Hyperparathyroidism
Sites of intramuscular injections particularly after iron and calcium injection extravasation
Lactation (breasts)
Steroid use (breasts)
Polymyositis
Free pertechnetate (thyroid, stomach)
Hyperthermia (liver)
Obstructed kidney or ureter
Chemotherapy (kidney)
Hemoglobinopathies (kidney)
Enthesopathies
Fat creases and skin folds
Uterine uptake: menstruation, pregnancy
Increased circulating aluminum (liver and kidney uptake)
Frost bite
Malignant effusions
Malignant ascites
Dystrophic and metastatic calcification[a] including
  Abscesses
  Fibrocystic disease
  Amyloidosis
  Cerebral ischemic infarction
  Tumors (primary and/or metastatic)
    Breast
    Neuroblastoma
    Hepatoblastoma
    Gastrointestinal tumors, particularly colon
    Lung
    Endometrial carcinoma
    Uterine fibroids
    Ovarian (particularly mucinous)
    Liver metastases
    Metastatic osteogenic sarcoma
Heterotopic ossification (including myositis ossificans and tumoral calcinosis)
Radiotherapy treatment ports

[a] Refer to Table 7.1 for more details

ticula, may again mask, or simulate, a lesion and negatively affect the quality of the study. This makes the visualization of the pelvic and hip regions difficult. (Fig. 1.34a, b). This is a common source of diagnostic error and should always be dealt with through voiding, catheterization, delayed imaging and special positioning such as caudal and oblique views of the pelvis.

Factors Related to Interpretation: Non-familiarity with various normal and pathological findings can lead to misinterpretation due to lack of pattern recognition. In addition to pathological patterns of various diseases, recognition of normal patterns and those associated with normal variants is particularly important. Normal scans should generally show symmetry. In general, symmetry should be considered normal, and any asymmetry should be considered abnormal, until proven otherwise. Certain areas are normally known to show a relative increased uptake in both the pediatric and adult age groups due to higher bone turnover. These include

1. Acromioclavicular joints
2. Sternoclavicular joints
3. Scapular tips
4. Costochondral junctions
5. Sacroiliac joints
6. Sternum
7. Frontal parasagittal areas
8. Lumbar and cervical spines anteriorly

Additionally, in the pediatric age group certain other areas of normally increased uptake are seen. These include:

1. Growth plates which should have clearly demarcated margins. Any irregularity or asymmetry should be viewed with suspicion. This is specially important since growth plate injuries, which are frequently overlooked, cause irregularities and these areas have a predilection to osteomyelitis and neuroblastoma metastases.
2. Ischiopubic regions or the areas between distal ends of inferior pubic and ischial rami. The mass of cartilage in these areas ossifies between the ages of 4 and 12 years and may show uptake that can be confused with abnormal uptake.

In the normal whole body scan there will be some variation in the uptake due to normal variants. There may be a variety of reasons:

1. Effects of normal muscle stress:
   - The deltoid tuberosity (site of deltoid insertion) shows increased uptake in about 7% of patients and may be asymmetrical.
   - Insertions of the iliocostalis thoracis portion of the erector spinae muscles may cause linear uptake along posterior ribs vertically. This occurs in about 7% of individuals [42]. A similar pattern may be observed in the child because of 'shine-through' from the increased uptake in the costochondral junctions occurring normally at these growth sites.

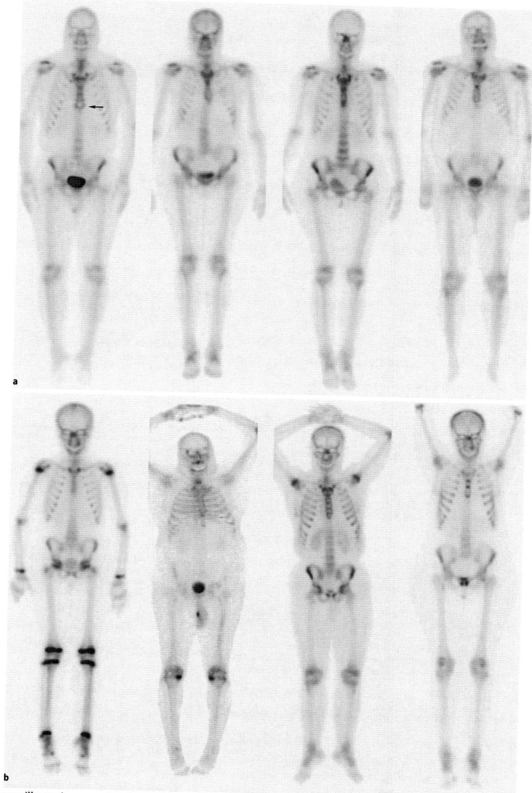

Fig. 1.34. Bone scans illustrating normal variants of the sternum. These include a variant showing a cold area that can be confused with cold metastases (*arrow*) (Courtesy of Dr. Shah Sayed with thanks)

2. The lower anterior part of the neck may show increased uptake which may be due to normal cervical lordosis and/or uptake in the thyroid cartilage.
3. An altered gait resulting from pain is frequently associated with diffuse increased accumulation in the asymptomatic lower extremity, particularly the foot.
4. The sternum shows many variations, including transverse lines of increased uptake and prominent uptake at the junction of the xiphoid and the body of the sternum and at the junction of the manubrium and the body. Diffuse increased uptake may be seen as well as an oval-shaped cold area above the xiphoid process. This latter normal variant is most likely due to localized incomplete fusion and occurs in 2–31% of individuals [43].
5. Postpartal changes: Studies obtained following pregnancy may show alterations from the normal distribution resulting from the effects of pelvic diastasis, especially in the symphysis pubis, which may show increased uptake. Uni- or bilateral increased uptake in the sacroiliac joints is also seen.

References

1. Resnick D, Manolagas SC, Fallon MD (1996) Histogenesis, anatomy and physiology of bone. In: Resnick D (ed) Bone and joint imaging. Saunders, Philadelphia, pp 1–11
2. McCarthy EF (1998) Pathophysiology of bone and joint disorders with clinical and radiographic correlation. Saunders, Philadelphia, pp 1–50
3. Williams PL, Warwick R, Dyson M, Bannister LH (1989) Gray's Anatomy: the anatomical basis of medicine and surgery. 31th edn. Churchill Livingstone, New York, pp 300–304
4. El-Khoury G (1998) University of Iowa Virtual Hospital
5. Mourad LA (1998) Structure and function of the musculoskeletal system. In: McCane KL, Huether SE (eds) Pathophysiology, 3rd edn. Mosby, Philadelphia, pp 1405–1434
6. Suzuki R, Domon T, Wakita M (2000) Some osteocytes released from their lacunae are embedded again in the bone and not regulated by osteoclasts during remodeling. Anat Embryol (Berl) 202:119–128
7. Gillespy T 3rd, Gillespy MP (1991) Osteoporosis. Radiol Clin North Am 29:77–84
8. Boskey AL (1981) Current concepts of the physiology and biochemistry of calcification. Clin orthop and biochemistry of calcification. Clin Orthop 157:225
9. Tondevold E, Eliasen P (1982) Blood flow rates in canine cortical and cancellous bone measured with Tc 99m, labeled human albumin microspheres. Acta Orthop Scand 53:7–11
10. Hughes DE, Brendan FB (1997) Apoptosis in bone physiology and disease. J Clin Pathol Mol Pathol 50:132–137
11. Raisz LG (1999) Physiology and pathophysiology of bone remodeling. Clin Chem 45:1353–1358
12. Manologas SC, Jilka RL (1995) Bone marrow, cytokines, and bone remodeling: emerging insights into pathophysiology of osteoporosis. N Engl J Med 332:305–311
13. McCarthy EF (1997) Histopathologic correlates of a positive bone scan. Semin Nucl Med 27:309–320
14. Russel WJ, Koshinagah AS, Mizuno M (1966) Active bone marrow distribution in adults. Br J Radiol 39:735–739
15. Kricun M (1985) Red-yellow marrow conversion: its effects on the location of solitary bone lesions. Skeletal Radiol 14:10–19
16. Dalinka MK, Aronchick JM, Haddad JG (1983) Paget's disease. Orthop Clin North Am 4:3–19
17. Vogler JB, Murphy WA (1988) Bone marrow imaging. Radiology 168:679–693
18. Seabold JE, Nepola JV, Marsh JL et al (1991) Post operative bone marrow alterations: Potential pitfalls in the diagnosis of osteomyelitis with In-111-labeled leukocyte scintigraphy. Radiology 180:741–747
19. Oswald SG, VanNostrand D, Savory CG, Anderson JH, Callghan JJ (1990) The acetabulum: a prospective study of three-phase bone and indium white blood cell scintigraphy following porous coated hip arthroplasty. J Nucl Med 31:274–280
20. Mourad LA (1998) Alterations of musculoskeletal function. In: McCane KL, Huether SE (eds) Pathophysiology, 3rd edn. Mosby, Philadelphia, pp 1435–1485
21. Resnick D (1998) Articular anatomy and histology. In: Resnick D (ed) Bone and joint imaging. Saunders, Philadelphia, pp 12–18
22. Galakso CSB (1982) Bone metastases studies in experimental animals. Clin Orthop Relat Res 169:269–285
23. Galakso CSB (1980) Mechanism of uptake of bone imaging isotopes by skeletal metastases. Clin Nucl Med 5:565–568
24. Wiliams C (1984) Radiophamaceuticals. In: Silberstein EB (ed) Bone scintigraphy. Futura, Mount Kisco NY, pp 13–20
25. Francis MD, Horn PA, Tofe AJ (1981) Controversial mechanism of technetium 99m deposition on bone (abstract). J Nucl Med 22:72
26. Francis MD, Slough CL, Tofe AJ, Silberstein EB (1976) Factors affecting uptake and retention of technetium-99m-diphosphonate and technetium 99m pertechnetate in osseous, connective and soft tissues. Calcif Tissue Res 20:303–311
27. Brenner W, Sieweke N, Bohuslavizki KH, Kampen WU, Zuhayra M, Clausen M, Henze E (2000) Age- and sex-related bone uptake of Tc-99m-HDP measured by whole-body bone scanning. Nucl Med 39:127–132
28. Sundberg SB, Savage JP, Foster BK (1989) Technetium phosphate bone scanning in the diagnosis of septic arthritis in childhood. J Pediatr Orthop 9:579–585
29. Hughes J (1984) Techniques of bone imaging. In: Silberstein EB (ed) Bone scintigraphy. Futura, Mount Kisco, NY, pp 39–76
30. Van der Wall H, Storey G, Frater C, Murray P (2001) Importance of positioning and technical factors in anatomic localization of sporting injuries in scintigraphic imaging. Semin Nucl Med 26:17–27
31. Ketly NL, Coa ZJ, Holder LH (1997) Technical considerations for optimal orthopedic imaging. Semin Nucl Med 27:328–333
32. Arnold JS (1980) Mechanism of fixation of bone imaging radiopharmaceuticals. In: Billinghurst ME (ed) Studies of cellular function using radiotracers. CRC Press, Boca Raton, Florida, pp 115–144
33. Alazraki N, Dries D, Daz F, Lawrence P, Greensberg E, Taylor A (1985) Value of a 24-hour image (four-phase bone scan) in assessing osteomyelitis in patients with peripheral vascular disease. JNM 26:711–717
34. Israel O, Dov F, Frankel A, Kleinhaus Y (1985) 24hour/4hour ratio of Technetium-99m methylene diphosphonate uptake in patients with bone metastases and degenerative bone changes. J Nucl Med 26:237–240
35. Vanderwall H, Storey G, Frater C, Murray IPC (2001) Importance of positioning and technical factors in anatomic localization of sporting injuries in scintigraphic imaging. Seminars in Nuclear Medicine 31:17–27

36. Embry RL, Delaplain CB(1992) Scintigraphic pitfall in a patient with steatopygia. Clin Nucl Med 17:824–826

37. Dogan AS, Rezai K (1993) Incidental lymph node visualization on bone scan due to subcutaneous infiltration of Tc-99m MDP: a potential for false positive interpretation. Clin Nucl Med 18:208–209

38. Choy D, Murray IPC, Hoschl R (1982) The effect of iron on the biodistribution of bone scanning agents in humans. Radiology 140:197–202

39. Hommeyer SH, Eary JF (1992) Skeletal nonvisualization in a bone scan secondary to intravenous editronate therapy. J Nucl Med 33:748–750

40. Krasnow AZ, Collier BD, Isitman AT et al (1988) False-negative bone imaging due to editronate disodium therapy. Clin Nucl Med 13:264–267

41. Karimeddini MK, Spencer RP (1993) Bone agent and radiogallium deposition around infiltrated calcium gluconate. Clin Nucl Med 18:797–798

42. Datz FU (1988) Handbooks in radiology, nuclear medicine. Yearbook Medical, Chicago, pp 72–106

43. Han JK, Shih WJ, Stipp V, Magoun S (1999) Normal variants of a photon-deficient area in the lower sternum demonstrated by bone SPECT. Clin Nucl Med 24:248–251

44. Silberstein EB, McAfee JG, Spasoff AP (1998) Diagnosis patterns in nuclear medicine. Society of Nuclear Medicine, Reston, Virginia, pp 223–230

45. Heck LL (1981) Gamuts: extraosseous localization of phosphate bone agents. Semin Nucl Med 10:311–312

46. Elgazzar AH, Jahan S, Motawei S (1989) Tc99m MDP uptake in Hepatoblastoma. Clin Nucl Med 14:143

47. Owunwanne A, Patel M, Sadek S (1995) The handbook of radiopharmaceuticals. Chapman and Hall Medical, London

48. Pauwels EKJ, Stokkel MPM (2001) Radiopharmaceuticals for bone lesions. Imaging and therapy in clinical practice. Q J Nucl Med 45:18–26

49. Connolly LP, Treves ST, Daveis RT, Zimmerman TE (1999) Pediatric application of pinhole magnification imaging. J Nucl Med 40:1896–1901

50. Shipman P, Walker A, Bichell C (1985) Human skeleton. Harvard University Press, Cambridge, Massachusetts

Diagnosis of Inflammatory Bone Diseases

2

For the early diagnosis of skeletal infections, the combined and coordinated efforts of the clinician and imaging specialist are crucial. Successful early diagnosis results in prompt treatment, which in turn may reduce morbidity. This chapter focuses on the complexities surrounding this clinical question. Knowledge of the pathophysiology of skeletal infection, as well as of the strengths and limitations of the multitude of imaging modalities available, aids clinicians in making a timely diagnosis. Information regarding the location of a suspected infection, the patient's age, and the history of other conditions such as diabetes, arthritis, trauma, and prior surgery needs to be available to nuclear medicine physicians and radiologists. These factors will affect the choice of optimal imaging modality. For any suspected skeletal infection the initial modality is the standard radiograph. If this simple and inexpensive diagnostic test is not conclusive, other modalities should be considered particularly bone scan. Currently, magnetic resonance imaging (MRI) or a combination of bone and gallium scanning are the modalities of choice for spondylodiscitis. Infection of the diabetic foot is best imaged with combined (preferably simultaneous) bone and white blood cell-labeled scintigraphy. MRI is comparable in accuracy, but more experience is needed in diagnosing skeletal infections. Bone scans for suspected neonatal osteomyelitis has recently been found to be sensitive and specific for diagnosis. Advances in imaging technology, such as positron emission tomography (PET) and antibody labeling, provide other options, which improve the speed and accuracy with which osteomyelitis can be diagnosed. Utilizing the techniques widely used currently, an algorithm for the diagnosis of skeletal infection which incorporates the above-mentioned variables and complicating conditions is presented.

2.1
Introduction

Despite the continuous advancement in prevention and treatment (particularly with antibiotics), infection remains a widespread problem. In fact, infection was first described in an Egyptian papyrus around 3000 BC [1]. Skeletal infection is a challenge to both clinicians and imaging specialists. Accurate and prompt diagnosis is very important to minimize complications such as sepsis, severe bone destruction, deformity, and growth arrest in children. Bone infections are complex processes that can manifest in various ways and mimic many other diseases. They are common in adults and children, and occur both in immunologically competent and incompetent patients. The onset can be seen in individuals with no comorbidities; in those with a history of trauma and post-operative joint replacements; or among patients with diseases such as diabetes, hemoglobinopathies and arthritis.

The dilemma that faces the medical community is reaching an early and accurate diagnosis of these infections. Although physical examination, laboratory tests such as white blood cell count and blood cultures, and standard radiographs are often positive in the later stages of osteomyelitis, these parameters are not adequate for diagnosis in the early stages. Modern imaging plays a crucial role in aiding clinicians in the early diagnosis. For this reason, physicians should be aware of the many imaging techniques suitable for skeletal infections. When this is combined with the patient's clinical background and an understanding of the pathophysiological basis behind skeletal infections, effective decision making can be made to choose an optimal imaging examination.

2.2
Pathophysiology

2.2.1
Inflammation

2.2.1.1
Definition

Inflammation is the complex non-specific tissue reaction to injury, which can be due to pathogenic agents as bacteria and viruses (leading to infection), or agents such as chemical, physical, immunological or radiation. Inflammation can be viewed as a protective reaction to the cause of cell injury as well as the consequences of such injury and can be life-saving in certain situations. However, it may be potentially harmful and even life-threatening [2].

2.2.1.2
Classification

Inflammation is predominantly classified into acute and chronic. Acute inflammation is the immediate and early response to injury that has a relatively short duration lasting for minutes, hours or a few days. Its main characteristics are exudation of fluid and proteins and immigration of leukocytes (predominantly neutrophils). On the other hand, chronic inflammation may last for weeks or years [3].

2.2.1.3
General Pathophysiological Features

Acute inflammation has the following local pathophysiological features:

Vascular Changes

1. Vasodilation first involves the arterioles and then results in the local opening of new capillary beds and lasts for a variable period depending on the stimulus (Fig. 2.1).
2. Increased vascular permeability permits the escape of the protein rich fluid and leukocytes (Fig. 2.1) into the extravascular space (exudate) [3]. This occurs due to the contraction of endothelial cells leading to a subsequent widening of the inter-cellular gaps; direct endothelial injury (resulting in endothelial cell necrosis and detachment) and leukocyte-mediated endothelial injury due to the release of toxic oxygen species and proteolytic enzymes by activated leukocytes. Endothelial cells may proliferate and form new blood vessels (angiogenesis), which remain leaky until they differentiate. Thus, angiogenesis also contributes to increased permeability.
3. Slowing of circulation (stasis): Increased permeability and extravasation of fluid results in the concen-

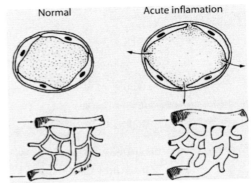

Fig. 2.1. A dilated vessel showing the opening of the intercellular gaps that occur in inflammation compared to a normal vessel

tration of red cells (which become packed in small vessels) and an increased viscosity of the blood. This leads to stasis.

Cellular Changes

With stasis, leukocytes – predominantly neutrophils – are peripherally oriented along the vascular endothelium (leukocytic margination). Leukocytes then emigrate from the microcirculation across the endothelium and accumulate at the site of injury. Cells also migrate in the interstitial tissue towards a chemotactic stimulus, leading to aggregation at the site of inflammation (Figs. 2.2, 2.3).

Chronic inflammation on the other hand, is characterized by a proliferative (fibroblastic) rather than an

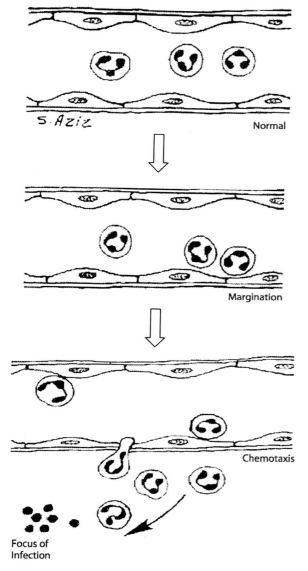

Fig. 2.2. Cellular changes occurring during inflammation

exudative response with predominantly mononuclear-cell infiltration (macrophages, lymphocytes and plasma cells) (Fig. 2.4). Vascular permeability is also abnormal.

2.2.1.4
Healing

Healing of tissue in general is linked closely to inflammation since it starts with acute inflammation, which is considered the defensive phase of healing. The process consists of two overlapping phases, reconstruction and maturation, which includes remodeling.

2.2.1.5
Inflammation in Cancer Patients

Patients with cancer can become immunocompromised due to the underlying malignancy, or as a result of cytotoxic chemotherapy, radiation and other forms of therapeutic intervention. Some malignancies are associated with immune deficiency, which predisposes the patient to certain pathogens. For example Hodgkin's and non-Hodgkin's lymphomas are associated with abnormalities of the cellular immune system that increase the risk to certain viral infections such as herpes simplex and varicella zoster and fungal infections such as cryptococcus. On the other hand patients with acute leukemias are highly susceptible to severe gram-negative bacterial infection due to quantitative, or functional, granulocytopenia. Patients with chronic lymphocytic leukemia and multiple myeloma are prone to infections with staphylococci and streptococci particularly pneumococcus. Therapeutic interventions including cytotoxic chemotherapy, corticosteroids, irradiation and bone marrow transplantation produce deficiencies of the host's defense (e.g. neutropenia after cytotoxic chemotherapy, suppression of T cell defenses after bone marrow transplantation, disruption of natural skin and mucosal barriers). Furthermore, reduced food intake leads to poor nutrition and an increasing risk of infection, including skeletal infections [4].

2.2.2
Skeletal Infections
2.2.2.1
Definitions

The term osteomyelitis is not synonymous with skeletal infection. „Osteomyelitis" should be used to describe an infection that include bone marrow involvement. When infection starts in the periosteum, such as in cases of direct extension bone infection, it produces periosteitis. At this stage, infection may not yet involve the cortex or marrow and is called infectious periostei-

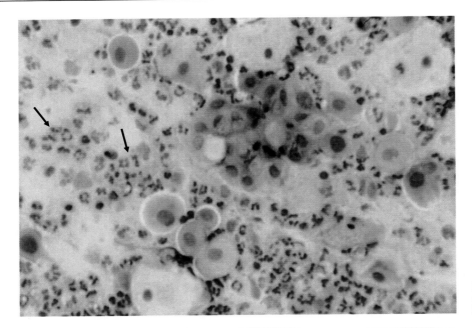

Fig. 2.3. Acute inflammation with polymorphonuclear leukocytes (*arrows*)

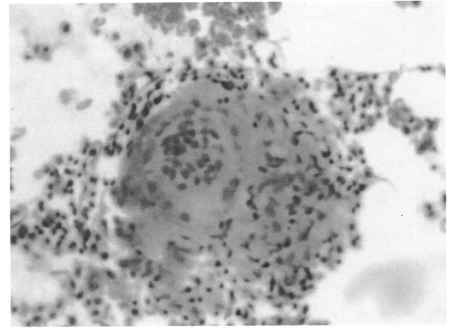

Fig. 2.4. Chronic inflammation. Note the mononuclear cells compared to polymorphonuclear cells in acute inflammation

tis. When infection involves the cortex, the term infectious osteitis is used. When marrow is involved as well, the term osteomyelitis is applicable (Fig. 2.5).

2.2.2.2
Classification

Osteomyelitis may be classified into many types (Table 2.1) based on the route of infection, the patient's age and physiology, the etiology, date of onset and other

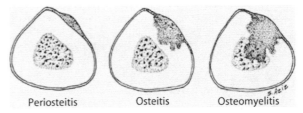

Periosteitis   Osteitis   Osteomyelitis

Fig. 2.5. A comparison of the extent of infection in osteomyelitis compared with the extent of infection in periosteitis and osteitis

Table 2.1. Various classifications of osteomyelitis

Basis of classification	Forms of osteomyelitis
Presentation	I. Acute II. Chronic
Route of infection	I. Hematogenous II. Direct extension (non-hematogenous)
Age	I. Infantile (including neonatal) II. Juvenile III. Adult
Causative organism	I. Pyogenic II. Nonpyogenic
Location of infection	I. Appendicular skeleton osteomyelitis: Metaphyseal Epiphyseal Diaphyseal II. Axial skeleton osteomyelitis (examples: vertebral and bony pelvis osteomyelitis)
Prior pathology	I. Violated bone (complicated) osteomyelitis II. Non-violated bone osteomyelitis
Multifactorial (Waldvogel classification)	I. Hematogenous osteomyelitis. II. Osteomyelitis secondary to contiguous infection III. Osteomyelitis associated with vascular insufficiency.
Anatomy of disease and host physiology (Cierny-Mader classification of adult type)	Anatomic types: I. Medullary II. Superficial III. Localized IV. Diffuse Physiologic class: A. Normal host B. Compromised host: Systemic compromise Local compromise Local and systemic compromise C. Prohibitive: Treatment worse than disease

factors [5–9]. Osteomyelitis may be classified as acute or chronic according to the onset of symptoms and signs. It can also be classified as hematogenous or non-hematogenous according to the route of infection. In hematogenous osteomyelitis, the metaphyses of long bones are the most common site affected. Non-hematogenous osteomyelitis occurs as a result of the spread of a contiguous soft tissue infection, penetrating trauma, or inoculation (e.g. drug addicts). In these situations infection may occur in any part of the bone. Osteomyelitis is also classified into infantile, juvenile, or adult types depending on the age of the patient, and into pyogenic and non-pyogenic depending on the etiology. Infantile osteomyelitis occurs in the first year of life, while the juvenile type occurs between the age of 1 year and the age of closure of the physes; the adult type oc-

curs after the closure of the physes. Cierny and Mader more recently [7] introduced a clinical classification and staging based on the anatomy of the disease and the host physiology. Waldvogel also introduced another clinical classification based on the route of infection and whether vascular insufficiency is present [8]. Finally, it is important to consider the classification of osteomyelitis based on whether the affected bone has been violated by prior pathological conditions, since this is crucial for planning the imaging strategy [9].

2.2.2.3
General Pathophysiological Features

Acute hematogenous osteomyelitis occurs when organisms settling in the bone marrow initiate an acute inflammatory response by neutrophils. This is accompanied by local edema, vasospasm, ischemia, and thrombosis. These features are applicable to other types of acute skeletal infections. Thirty percent of such acute infections may progress to chronic osteomyelitis. Chronic osteomyelitis may follow a clinically obvious acute osteomyelitis, or be the initial presentation. The immune response includes chronic inflammatory cells (such as lymphocytes and plasma cells) and increased osteoclastic-osteoblastic reaction. If the normal blood supply to the bone is interrupted by the edema and thrombi produced by the inflammation, segmental bone necrosis or sequestrum will develop (Fig. 2.6). The body's response can also stimulate the formation of a new layer of bone around the infection, creating an involucrum (Fig. 2.7). This osteogenesis may occasionally continue long enough to give rise to a densely sclerotic pattern of osteomyelitis called a sclerosing osteomyelitis. If the periosteum becomes interrupted by the infectious process, a draining sinus will form [8]. A Brodie's abscess is an intraosseous abscess in the cortex that becomes walled off by reactive bone (Fig. 2.8). It is an active infection that becomes isolated due to decreased organism virulence. Brodie's abscess, sequestrum, and involucrum can re-activate presenting as chronic active osteomyelitis.

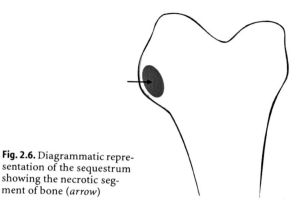

Fig. 2.6. Diagrammatic representation of the sequestrum showing the necrotic segment of bone (*arrow*)

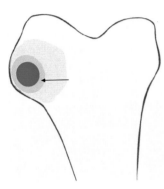

Fig. 2.7. A diagram showing the involucrum. Note the layer of new bone formation (*arrow*) surrounding the focal infection

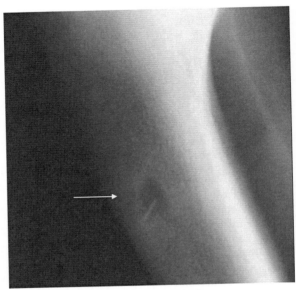

Fig. 2.8. Radiograph showing a Brodie's abscess

Table 2.2. Organisms associated with osteomyelitis in different clinical settings

Clinical situation	Most likely associated microorganisms
All types of osteomyelitis	*Staphylococcus aureus*
Infantile osteomyelitis	*S. aureus* and Group B streptococci
Diabetic foot osteomyelitis	*S. aureus, Enterococcus,* Enterobacteriaceae
Vertebral osteomyelitis	*S. aureus, Pseudomonas aeruginosa, Escherichia coli, Streptococcus*
Sickle-cell disease	*Salmonella, S. aureus*
Intravenous drug abusers	*Pseudomonas aeruginosa, Klebsiella*
Immunosuppressed patients	*Salmonella, Aspergillus, Mycobacterium avium* complex, *Candida albicans*
Hospital acquired infections	*Pseudomonas aeruginosa, Klebsiella*
Drinking raw milk in brucellosis-endemic areas	*Brucella*
Cat and human bites	*Pasteurella multocida, Eikenella corrodens*
Sharp object passing into foot	*Pseudomonas aeruginosa*
Contamination of open wound by soil	*Clostridia, Nocardia*
Bone infections due to infected catheters	*Escherichia coli, Candida albicans*

Osteomyelitis, and in particular the hematogenous form, is usually caused by gram-positive organisms, the most common being *Staphylococcus aureus* [8, 10, 11]. Group B streptococci are also common in infantile osteomyelitis. Gram-negative organisms such as *Pseudomonas aeruginosa* and *Klebsiella pneumonia* have also been encountered as the causative organisms in osteomyelitis, particularly in intravenous drug abusers, in vertebral osteomyelitis, and in hospital-acquired infection. *Escherichia coli* may be the cause of vertebral osteomyelitis following urological surgery (Table 2.2).

Acute hematogenous osteomyelitis is the most common type and occurs most frequently in children, affecting males approximately twice as often as females [12]. It has a predilection for the metaphyses of long bones, where the blood flow is rich and relatively sluggish since blood flows through the typically large intramedullary venous sinusoids in this region. This represents a good medium for bacterial lodgement and proliferation [6]. As mentioned earlier, the process starts by implantation of organisms in the bone marrow, and as the infection becomes established in the marrow, it provokes acute suppurative neutrophilic infiltrates and edema and is accompanied by vasospasm, thrombosis and local ischemia. Subsequently infection may spread first to the subperiosteal space in the metaphyseal area. This is the path of least resistance, because the cortex of this area is porous and because the inflammatory response limits spread down the medullary cavity. In children between 1 and approximately 16 years of age, the blood supply to the medullary space of bone enters through the nutrient artery, then passes through the smaller vessels toward the growth plate. Once these vessels reach the metaphyseal side of the growth plate, they turn back upon themselves in loops (Fig. 2.9) to empty into large sinusoidal veins with a slower blood flow. The epiphyseal plate separating the epiphyseal and metaphyseal blood supplies acts as a barrier to the spread of infection (Fig. 2.10), making joint involvement less common in this age group [11] except when the infection is severe. In this situation, the infection may break through the bone and produce joint infection (Fig. 2.11). This occurs in the locations where the metaphysis is within the joint capsule [proximal femur

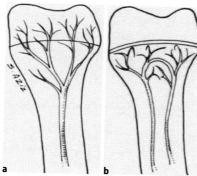

Fig. 2.9a, b. a The vascular communication between the metaphysis and epiphysis. **b** When the growth plate is present it acts as a barrier and the vessels turn on themselves, forming loops

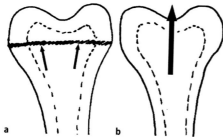

Fig. 2.10a, b. a The growth plate acting as a barrier for the extension of infection from the epiphysis, making the involvement of the joint less likely than the case when the growth plate does not constitute a barrier (**b**) in neonates and also after closure of the growth plate when the infection extends more easily to the joint

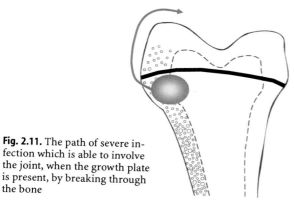

Fig. 2.11. The path of severe infection which is able to involve the joint, when the growth plate is present, by breaking through the bone

in the hip joint, proximal humerus in the shoulder joint, distal tibia in the ankle joint, and proximal radius in the elbow joint (which is rarely involved)]. On the other hand, in infants and adults, the terminal branches of the nutrient artery extend into the epiphysis as there is no growth-plate barrier. This vascular communication between the epiphyses and metaphyses facilitates the spread of infection to adjacent joints (Fig. 2.9). In flat bones acute hematogenous osteomyelitis is mainly found at locations with a vascular anato-

my which is similar to that of the metaphyses such as the bony pelvis, vertebrae, and calcaneus [13].

2.2.2.4
Features of Specific Forms

Chronic Osteomyelitis: It is difficult to clearly differentiate between acute and chronic osteomyelitis. However, it should be noted that cases of obvious chronic osteomyelitis need special diagnostic handling and management. Chronic osteomyelitis has variously been defined as symptomatic osteomyelitis with a duration ranging from 5 days to 6 weeks [14]. Since the pathology of osteomyelitis varies with age, micro-organisms, prior therapy, underlying diseases and other factors, it is somewhat inappropriate to depend only on duration of the disease to define chronicity. Chronic osteomyelitis has a less marked inflammatory cell reaction and may occur without preceding acute inflammation. Microscopically, chronic osteomyelitis predominantly shows lymphocytes and plasma cells rather than polymorphonuclear cells. There is a variable amount of necrotic tissue, and sequestra may form in some cases. The presence of necrotic tissue may also lead to draining sinuses or the organization in the medullary cavity forming Brodie's abscess. Because these abscesses and necrotic foci are avascular, levels of antibiotics sufficient to eradicate the bacteria may not be achieved during treatment. Accordingly, bacteria may remain indolent for a long time (inactive disease). Reactivation of the disease may occur much later (even years) after the initial episode of active disease. It is important to evaluate patients for possible chronic disease and to either exclude, or confirm, the presence of chronic active infection since continuation of intravenous antibiotic therapy and/or surgical intervention to eradicate infection will depend on that determination [15].

Vertebral Osteomyelitis (Spondylodiscitis): This is a specific form of osteomyelitis that has some unique features. The most commonly affected site is the lumbar region, followed by the thoracic and cervical spine. Several factors predispose an individual to vertebral osteomyelitis (Table 2.3). The disease occurs most frequently in adults with a mean age of 60–70 years although it also occurs at all other ages including children. The pyogenic form is most often caused by staphylococcus aureus, but streptococci and gram-negative bacteria are also involved [16–18]. Infection usually originates at a distant site with hematogenous extension to contiguous vertebral bodies and the intervening space via the ascending and descending branches of the posterior spinal artery. Extension to the posterior elements (pedicles, transverse processes, posterior spinous processes and laminae) has been noted in 3% to

Table 2.3. Predisposing factors for vertebral osteomyelitis (spondylodiscitis)

1. Old age
2. Diabetes mellitus
3. Drug addiction
4. Oral steroid therapy
5. Dialysis
6. Urinary tract infection
7. Genitourinary instrumentation
8. Prior back surgery
9. Bacteremia secondary to intravenous cannulation
10. Spinal trauma

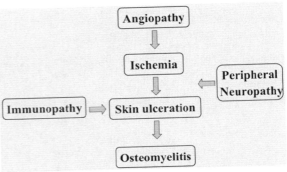

Fig. 2.13. The changes associated with diabetes leading to osteomyelitis of the foot

12% of cases. However, involvement of posterior elements only is exceedingly rare since only 15 cases have been reported to date. Other causes include extension of the infection from adjacent structures and complications following spinal surgery and trauma.

In adults, the causative organism generally settles in the richly vascularized subchondral vertebral endplates with an eventual progression of the infection into the adjacent intervertebral disk (which is relatively avascular) and the infection may progress to adjacent soft tissue structures (Fig. 2.12). In childhood, the infection often starts at the disks, which are nourished, by small perforating vessels. In either case, the local spread of infection eventually occurs and causes endplate destruction, disk-space narrowing, and collapse. These changes may take weeks to be seen on radiographs [18, 19]. It typically affects older children with fever and back pain in the lumbar, thoracic or cervical region [20, 21]. Since the disk is almost invariably involved in vertebral infections, the term spondylodiscitis is preferred [17, 18, 20]. Discitis, however, often occurs separately without involving the bony structures of the vertebrae. In children under the age of 5 years it almost exclusively affects the lumbar spine with no, or low-grade, fever. The child usually is unable to walk or has progressive limping [21].

Diabetic Foot Osteomyelitis: Approximately 15% of diabetics develop foot osteomyelitis, which is most common in the metatarsal bones and proximal phalanges. The differentiation from neuropathic foot can be clinically and radiographically difficult. Diabetics are prone to infections which are secondary to the effects of their

hyperglycemic state which leads to impaired leukocyte function. This immunopathy, along with diabetes-associated vascular disease (angiopathy) and peripheral nerve changes (neuropathy), may lead to skin ulceration and predispose the patient to pedal osteomyelitis (Fig. 2.13). Ulceration of the foot is 50 times more common in diabetics [22]. More than 90% of osteomyelitis of the foot of diabetic patients occurs as a result of the spread of infection from adjacent foot ulcers. If infection is present, prompt treatment is crucial to avoid amputation [23]. The incidence of amputation of the lower extremities is 25 times greater in diabetics than in the general population [22].

Neuroarthropathy is characterized by destructive joint changes. A combination of factors are involved. Loss of protective pain and proprioceptive sensation along with hyperemia (which is secondary to the loss of vasoconstrictive neural impulses) are thought to result in atrophic neuropathy most frequently occurring in the forefoot [24]. On the other hand, sensory fiber involvement only, without involvement of the sympathetic fibers, tends to result in hypertrophic neuroarthropathy, which occurs most frequently in the mid- and hind-foot (Fig. 2.14). Since the patient continues to walk and traumatize the foot, disuse osteoporosis is usually absent. Unnoticed trauma may also result in rapidly progressive destruction (Fig. 2.15), sometimes with disintegration of one or more tarsal bones within a period of only a few weeks. In this rapidly progressive form of neuroarthropathy more inflammatory reaction is present [24–26].

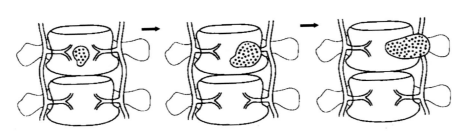

Fig. 2.12. The development and extension of infection in vertebral osteomyelitis

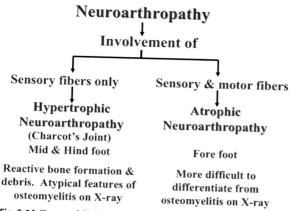

Fig. 2.14. Types of diabetic neuropathy and their characteristics (modified from Giurini et al [216] with permission)

Sickle Cell Disease Osteomyelitis: Since hemoglobin S is sensitive to hypoxemia, erythrocytes become viscous and abruptly sickle-shaped when exposed to hypoxia. This may compromise the microvascular flow and may cause infarction, the most common skeletal complication of sickle-cell disease. Although less common than infarctions, osteomyelitis is the second most common bacterial infection in children with sickle-cell disease after pneumonia. For symptomatic sickle-cell patients, distinguishing infarction from osteomyelitis is critical [14]. Osteomyelitis may occur as a primary event or may be superimposed on infarcts. This occurs because necrotic bone is a fertile site for such secondary infections. *Staphylococcus aureus* and *Salmonella* are the frequent causative organisms.

Periprosthetic Infections: Hip and knee arthroplasties are two of the most common orthopedic procedures, exceeding 600,000 per year in the USA alone [27–29]. Between 10% and 25% of patients experience discomfort within 5 years after hip or knee replacement [30]. This can be due to loosening with or without infection.

Although the incidence of infection was reported previously to be as high as 4% after the primary surgery and 32% after revision of hip arthroplasty, the currently reported rate of infection after total hip or knee arthroplasties is only 0.5–2%, and is less than 3% following revision surgery, the infection occurring mostly within 4 months of operation [31, 32]

The cementless porous coated prosthesis depends on bone in-growth for fixation and induces more reactive bone formation than the cemented prosthesis. Differences between cemented and porous coated hip prostheses largely explain the scintigraphic patterns noted after hip arthroplasty. Depending on the location of the finding and type of prosthesis, 'normal' activity may remain present for years. After knee replacements, on the other hand, the most common complications are fracture, dislocation, and avascular necrosis followed by loosening of the tibial component, with infection occurring less frequently than in the case of hip replacement [33].

Infectious (Septic) Arthritis: The term refers to the invasion of the synovial space by micro-organisms. The synovial space contains synovial fluid, which is produced by the rich capillary network of the synovial membrane. This fluid is viscous and serves to lubricate, nourish and cushion the avascular joint cartilage. When the synovial space is infected, bacterial hyaluronidase causes a decrease of the viscosity of the synovial fluid and pain is then felt with stress on the joint capsule.

Acute infectious arthritis is commonly caused by bacteria, while fungal and mycobacterial pathogens are seen more commonly in chronic arthritis. Acute septic arthritis is a medical emergency. Delay in diagnosis and treatment may result in the destruction of the articular cartilage and permanent disability. The lytic enzymes in the purulent articular fluid destroy the articular and epiphyseal cartilages. Additionally, pus in the joint space increases the intracapsular pressure, which

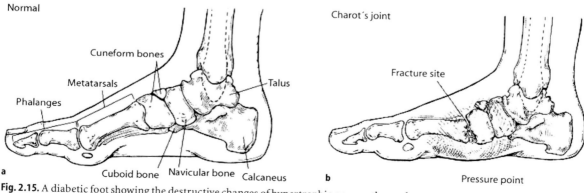

Fig. 2.15. A diabetic foot showing the destructive changes of hypertrophic neuroarthropathy. A normal foot is shown for comparison. (From [216], with permission)

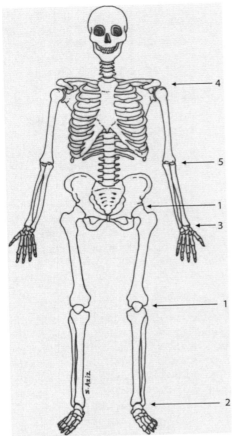

Fig. 2.16. The joints commonly affected by infectious arthritis (*1* indicates highest incidence)

may lead to epiphyseal ischemia. Other sequelae include dislocation, deformity and destruction of femoral head and neck. Hence drainage and antibiotic therapy must be considered without delay [14, 34].

Micro-organisms reach the joint by a hematogenous route, contagiously from an adjacent osseous infection, or through traumatic/surgical inoculation. The joints most commonly involved in children are the hip (35%),

knee (35%) and ankle (10%) (Fig. 2.16). When the synovium becomes hyperemic in septic arthritis, flow to adjacent extra-articular bone will also increase through the anastomoses from the synovial vascular network to juxta-epiphyseal and epiphyseal vessels supplying the epiphysis and metaphysis. Accordingly, increased uptake of bone-seeking radiopharmaceuticals on delayed images typically is seen around affected joints [34–36] (Fig. 2.17).

2.3
Imaging Skeletal Infections

2.3.1
The Need for Diagnostic Imaging

Clinical diagnosis in the late stages of infection is easily achieved in most instances. However, detecting early infection when complete resolution is still possible is a challenge to both physicians and radiologists. In early infection, the clinical picture may be confusing. Furthermore, laboratory findings, including elevated erythrocyte sedimentation rate and leukocytosis, are not specific for bone infection in the early stage. Serial blood cultures are positive in only 50–60% of cases [8, 37, 38]. Cultures of both blood and material obtained by needle aspiration of the involved bone yield a positive result in no more than 80% of cases. Delay in the treatment of osteomyelitis significantly diminishes the cure rate and increases the rate of complications and morbidity [39, 40]. Accordingly, imaging is needed in many cases to establish an early diagnosis.

2.3.2
Imaging Modalities for Skeletal Infections

When confronted with the potential diagnosis of an early skeletal infection, both morphological and functional (scintigraphic) imaging modalities are frequently employed. Morphological modalities such as standard radiographs, ultrasonography, computed tomog-

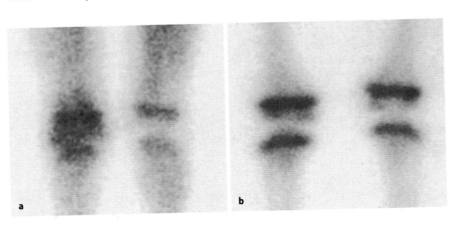

Fig. 2.17a, b. Bone scan of infectious arthritis showing the increased blood pool activity in the region of the knee joint (**a**). Delayed image (**b**) shows minimally increased uptake around the joint

raphy (CT) and magnetic resonance imaging (MRI) depend mainly on structural changes, variations in the density and differences in proton content in tissues. Functional modalities or nuclear medicine procedures, on the other hand, depend on physiological changes. No single modality is ideal in all situations and imaging should be tailored on an individual basis.

The choice of imaging modality often depends mainly on whether or not the bone has been violated (previously affected by other pathological conditions) and on the site of the suspected infection. Over the years major changes and modifications have been introduced to improve the diagnostic accuracy of osteomyelitis imaging. Many of these changes were based on better understanding of the pathophysiological basis of bone infection, which led to an increased recognition of the challenges and limitations which confront current imaging technology.

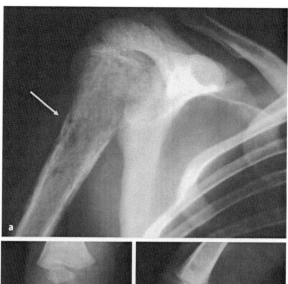
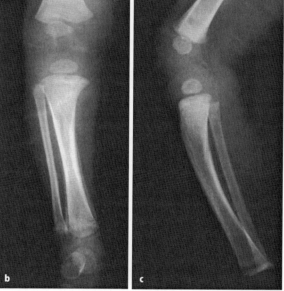

Fig. 2.18a–c. a A radiograph of an adult patient with osteomyelitis showing the typical changes of bone demineralization, bone lysis and cortical lucency (*arrow*). **b, c** Radiographs of a neonate with osteomyelitis demonstrating periosteal reaction

2.4
Diagnosis of Skeletal Infection by Imaging
2.4.1
Diagnosis Using Morphologic Imaging Modalities
2.4.1.1
Standard Radiographs

Standard radiographs, although useful if they show the classic findings of bone destruction and periosteal reaction (Fig. 2.18), may not show abnormalities until 10–21 days after the onset of infection. A 30–50% loss of bone density must occur before radiographs show any abnormalities, and radiographs are therefore relatively insensitive to the presence of acute bone infections [8, 11]. Additionally, radiological findings are unreliable in establishing the diagnosis of osteomyelitis among patients with violated bone. In these situations radiographic findings are non-specific, being diagnostic in as low as 3–5% of culture-positive cases. Nevertheless, radiography should be the initial modality for the work-up of skeletal infection. Standard radiographs are relatively inexpensive, are easily obtained, may determine that another underlying pathological condition exists, and frequently aid physicians in deciding what sort of additional imaging studies are required. From cumulative data in the literature, the overall sensitivity for standard radiograph for skeletal infections is 28–94% and the specificity is 3–92% [41].

2.4.1.2
Ultrasonography

Osteomyelitis in infants and children predominantly affects the growth-intensive end regions of the long bones. This is because the inflammatory process commonly affects the articular regions adjacent to the me-

taphyseal and epiphyseal sites. Ultrasound accordingly may be of benefit in this group of patients and can be helpful in planning the management [42–44]. In a recent study, ultrasonography was found to be a very useful tool both in detecting osteomyelitis in infants and children and in reducing the need for additional imaging modalities [42]. The common ultrasonography findings of osteomyelitis are intra-articular fluid collection and subperiosteal abscess formation. These findings were found to precede any radiological changes by several days. Ultrasonography is also helpful in guiding aspiration for immediate microscopic and later bacteriological examinations. The most helpful role of ultrasonography, however, is in the diagnosis and management of septic arthritis. In particular, ultrasonography is very sensitive in detecting joint effusions and may clearly define the extent of septic arthritis, differentiate septic arthritis from soft tissue abscesses, or tenosynovitis, and help avoid unnecessary joint aspirations. This was illustrated by Jien et al. [45], who reported 31 patients with joint effusion detected by ultrasonography with 22 proven septic arthritis cases of the hip and knee joints; three patients with concurrent osteomyelitis were detected as well using ultrasonography, resulting in a sensitivity of 100 % for septic arthritis. The nine patients without effusion had no proven septic arthritis, resulting in 100 % specificity [45]. Although the number of patients in this recent study is small, it is in agreement with other reports indicating a generally high sensitivity and specificity of ultrasonography for detecting septic arthritis [46, 47].

2.4.1.3
Computed Tomography

Following the highly successful introduction of MRI, CT has no major role in the diagnosis of osteomyelitis. However, it is a complementary procedure that is useful in sensitively detecting sequestra and can be useful in chronic osteomyelitis, in particular when determining the presence, or absence, of the sequestra is important for decision-making (regarding possible surgical intervention) [48].

2.4.1.4
Magnetic Resonance Imaging

MRI offers excellent depiction of both bone and soft tissue infection. Accordingly, MRI is often used instead of CT for the diagnosis of osteomyelitis. The results indicate that MRI is excellent in vertebral osteomyelitis and encouraging in diabetic foot osteomyelitis. The advantages of MRI over CT include improved soft-tissue contrast resolution, absence of beam-hardening artifacts from bone, and multi-planar capabilities [49]. The sensitivity and specificity of MRI for osteomyelitis range from 60 % to 100 % and from 50 % to 95 % respectively [49–53]. Although the average overall accuracy of MRI for the diagnosis of osteomyelitis is approximately similar to that of multi-phase bone scans, it is not used routinely as it is more expensive and less available. It is used on an individual basis particularly when vertebral involvement is suspected; in complicated cases of chronic osteomyelitis when it is important to determine the extent of infection; in suspected diabetic foot osteomyelitis; and in situations when anatomical details are necessary for planning surgical intervention.

2.4.2
Diagnosis by Scintigraphic Methods
2.4.2.1
Radiopharmaceuticals for Infection Imaging

Many radioisotopes have been used to detect and localize infection (Table 2.4). Several mechanisms explain the accumulation of different radiotracers at the site of infection (Table 2.5). Since there are limitations of the available radiopharmaceuticals for infection, the search continues for better agents with ideal properties

Table 2.4. Radiopharmaceuticals for infection [78, 205–207]

1. Tc-99m Diphosphonates
2. Gallium-67 citrate
3. Labeled white blood cells using In-111 oxime or Tc-99m HMPAO (Tc-99m hexamethyl propyleneamine oxime)
4. Labeled particles
   1. Nanocolloid
   2. Liposomes
5. Labeled large protein
   1. Non-specific immunoglobulins
   2. Specific immunoglobulins: polyclonal and monoclonal
      a) Antigranulocyte monoclonal antibodies
      b) Anti E-selectin antibodies
6. Labeled receptor-specific small proteins and peptides
   1. Chemotactic peptides
   2. Interleukins
7. Labeled antibiotics: ciprofloxacin
8. Positron emission radiotracers

Table 2.5. Mechanisms of uptake of radiotracers for infection [78, 205–207]

I.	Increased vascular permeability and capillary leakage
	In-111 and Tc-99m human polyclonal IgG
	In-111 monoclonal IgM antibody
	In-111 and Tc-99m liposomes
	In-111 biotin and streptavidin
	Tc-99m nanocolloids
	In-111 chloride
	Gallium-67 citrate
II.	Migration of white blood cells to the site of infection
	In-111 and Tc-99m labeled leukocytes
	Tc-99m anti-white blood cell antibodies
III.	Binding to protein receptors at site of infection
	Ga-67 citrate (iron-containing proteins)
VI.	Binding to white blood cells at the site of infection
	Chemotactic peptides
	Interleukins
V.	Binding to bacteria
	Tc-99m-labeled ciprofloxacin antibiotic
	Ga-67 citrate
VI.	Metabolic trapping
	F-18 fluorodeoxyglucose
VII.	Uptake by infection-induced osteogenesis
	Tc-99m Diphosphonates

Table 2.6. Ideal properties of radiotracers for infection localization

1. Easy to prepare
2. Low cost and wide availability
3. Rapid detection and localization of infections (< 3 h)
4. Low toxicity and no immune response
5. Rapid clearance from blood with no significant uptake in liver spleen, GI tract, bone, kidneys, bone marrow or muscle
6. Rapid clearance from the background
7. High sensitivity and specificity
8. Ability to differentiate infection from other inflammatory and neoplastic conditions
9. Ability to differentiate acute from chronic infection
10. Ability to monitor therapeutic response

(Table 2.6) for infection imaging. Labeled white blood cells and gallium-67 are the most widely used agents. Sfakianekis et al. [54] found Indium-111 leukocyte imaging to be the most accurate for relatively acute infections (less than 2 weeks) with 27% false negatives among patients with prolonged infections. On the other hand, gallium-67 imaging had its highest sensitivity in long-standing infections with a false-negative rate of 19% in acute infections of less than 1 week's duration. Bitar et al. [55], in a comparative study using rabbits with experimental abscesses, found that indium-111 leukocytes were clearly superior to gallium for imaging early abscesses. Furthermore, the authors found that the accumulation of indium-111 leukocytes in experimental subcutaneous abscesses was inversely proportional to the age of the abscess. In abscesses 1–2 h old, 6–8 h old, 24 h old and 7 days old, 10.4%, 5.2%, 3% and 0.73% of the injected dose, respectively, was accumulated in the abscesses. Gallium uptake, on the other hand, was not significantly affected by infection age (Table 2.7). In abscesses 7 days old, Ga-67 accumulated to a greater extent than did indium-111-labeled leukocytes. Thus Bitar et al. and Sfakianakis et al. came to similar conclusions, namely that labeled white blood cells are more suitable for infections of short duration while Ga-67 is a better agent for infections of a longer duration (Fig. 2.19).

Table 2.7. Relation of percent infection uptake of In-111 WBC and Ga-67 citrate and abscess age

Abscess age	Percent uptake In-111 white blood cells	Ga-67 citrate
1–2 hours	10.4%	1.5%
6–8 hours	5.2%	1.5%
24 hours	3%	1.4%
7 days	0.73%	1.1%

Data from Bitar et al. [55]

Experimentally, McAfee et al. [56] showed that as many as 10% of circulating neutrophils accumulate daily at focal sites of inflammation. This high percentage of white blood cells migrating to the site of infection facilitates identification of the abscess on a scintigraphic image (Table 2.8). The authors also showed abscess:muscle uptake ratios of 3,000:1 with In-111 white blood cells at 24 h compared to 72:1 with Ga-67 and 7:1 with In-111 chloride. Accordingly a small dose of only 500 μCi of In-111 leukocytes is sufficient for positive identification and localization of abscesses on an image. In Ga-67 imaging, a higher dose of approximately 5 mCi is needed, which may be higher if SPECT is used. There is higher radiation dose to the spleen from 500 μCi of In-111-labeled white blood cells but radiation doses to gonads, marrow and whole body are higher with 5 mCi of Ga-67 [56]. Overall, labeled leukocytes with In-111 or Tc-99m hexamethylpropyleneamine oxime (HMPAO) have a higher sensitivity and specificity than Ga-67 for acute infections [57, 58]. Several labeled antibodies have been used in recent years to diagnose bone and soft-tissue infection. Tc-99m or I-123 monoclonal antigranulocyte antibodies and In-111 or Tc-99m labeled human non-specific polyclonal immunoglobulin G (IgG) have been used in humans [59–70]. Human non-specific polyclonal immunoglobulin (hIgG) is prepared commercially for intravenous therapeutic use and conjugated with diethylenetriamine penta-acetic acid (DTPA) carboxycarbonic anhydride [71]. In contrast to the labeled leukocyte technique, which is complicated and time consuming, IgG is readily available for convenient one-step labeling that is ready for injection within 30 min. Acquisition of gamma camera images at 6, 24, and 48 h post-injection is the standard method. The accumulation of IgG at injection sites has been shown to be due to non-specific ac-

Table 2.8. Correlation of imaging findings and pathophysiological features of infection

Pathological change at the site of infection	Imaging pattern
Vasodilation of blood vessels	Increased flow and blood pool activity on bone scan, increased Ga-67 and Tc-9m nanocolloid accumulation
Chemotaxis	Increased accumulation of In-111 or Tc-99m labeled white blood cells
Increased secretion of iron containing globulin by injured and stimulated white blood cells	Increased accumulation of Ga-67
Formation of woven bone	Increased uptake of Tc-99m MDP on delayed images with continuing accumulation beyond 3–4 h

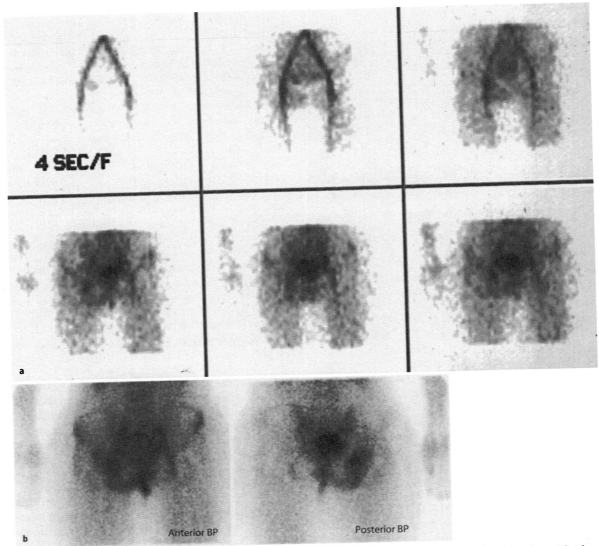

Fig. 2.19a–f. A three-phase bone scan and Tc-99m HMPAO labeled leukocyte scans for a 81-year-old female patient with a long history of pain in the right groin region. Flow (**a**) and blood pool (**b**) images reveal increased activity in the right hip and groin regions.

cumulation of the protein secondary to increased vascular permeability [72]. In-111, and more recently Tc-99m monoclonal antibody against granulocytes, have also been used for detecting infections including those affecting the skeleton [71, 73, 74].

Recently In-111 and Tc-99m-labeled chemotactic peptide analogs have been shown to be useful for detecting and localizing infections. These agents have a potentially important advantage over other radionuclide agents in that imaging can be performed less than 3 h post-injection, compared to the 18–24 h or more needed for most other agents [75–78]. Labeled liposomes have been used for scintigraphic imaging of infection [79] and inflammation [80–82]. Boerman et al. [83] used In-111 labeled sterically stabilized liposomes (long circulating) in rats and showed that the clearance of this agent is similar to that of In-111 IgG. The uptake in abscesses was twice as high as that of IgG, and the abscesses could be visualized as early as 1 h post-injection. Fluorodeoxyglucose (FDG) has been recently used in the diagnosis of osteomyelitis, particularly its chronic active form. It has a potential role in other situations such as vertebral osteomyelitis. A recently reported use of early and delayed imaging using FDG may prove useful in differentiating infections from tumors, increasing its specificity [84].

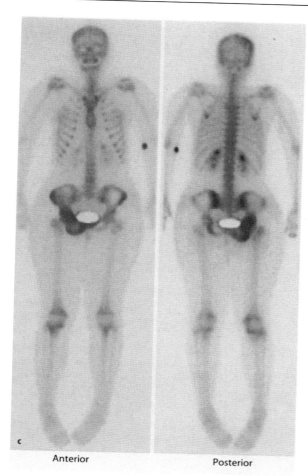

Anterior   Posterior

2.4.2.2
Bone Scanning

Multi-phase bone scanning is the imaging modality of first choice for suspected osteomyelitis. These studies become positive within 24–48 h after the onset of symptoms [85]. The three-phase bone scan consists of a flow phase, a blood pool phase, and a delayed phase. Twenty-four hour (fourth phase) imaging may be added and has been reported to improve accuracy in the detection of osteomyelitis by increasing the ratio between the lesion and normal bone due both to prolonged uptake of Tc-99m methylene diphosphonate (MDP) by the woven bone of osteomyelitis compared with normal lamellar bone and to reduction in background tracer activity with time [86, 87].

The classic findings of osteomyelitis in the multiphase bone scan are increased regional perfusion as seen in flow and blood pool images and a correspondingly increased uptake on delayed images (Figs. 2.20). Pinhole imaging can be of value in small children for better characterization of the delayed focal uptake (Fig. 2.21). This is different from cellulitis, which shows regional, or diffusely, increased perfusion in the area involved with either no corresponding increase of uptake on delayed images or only mildly increased uptake secondary to the hyperemia of adjacent or surrounding soft tissue infection (Fig. 2.22). It should be noted, however, that in some cases, osteomyelitis affects the entire bone or more than one bone, particularly in infants.

(Fig. 2.19 Contin.)
Delayed planar images (**c, d**) reveal focally increased uptake in the right acetabulum, ischium and pubic bones. The subsequently obtained Tc-99m-labeled leukocyte scan (**e–f**) shows no significant accumulation of labeled leukocytes at the site of the above-mentioned abnormalities seen on bone scan. Only a focus of accumulation at a site of recent intramuscular injection is noted in the soft tissue of the left buttock region. Pathologically, tuberculous osteomyelitis was proven. This case illustrates how chronic forms of skeletal infection, even when active, may show false-negative leukocyte studies due to the nature of the pathologic changes compared to acute infections

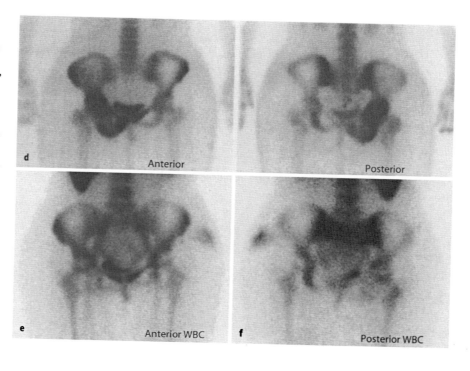

Anterior   Posterior

Anterior WBC   Posterior WBC

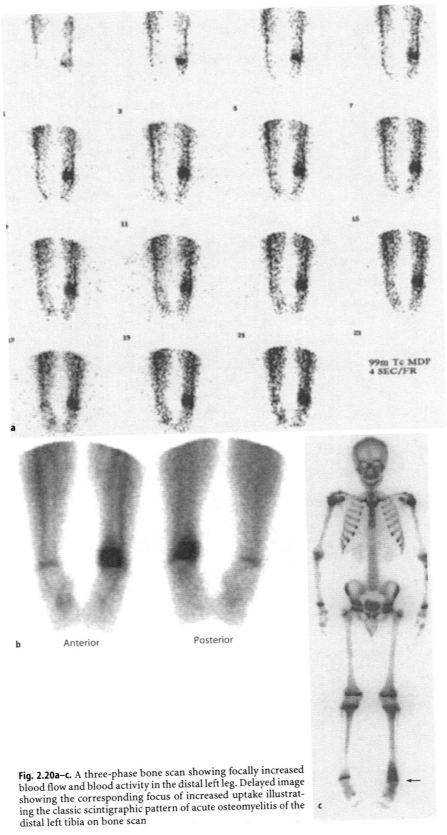

Fig. 2.20a–c. A three-phase bone scan showing focally increased blood flow and blood activity in the distal left leg. Delayed image showing the corresponding focus of increased uptake illustrating the classic scintigraphic pattern of acute osteomyelitis of the distal left tibia on bone scan

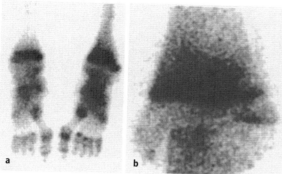

Fig. 2.21a, b. Images from a case of acute hematogenous osteo-myelitis illustrating the value of pinhole collimator. **a** High resolution image shows the increased tracer uptake in the left distal metaphysis. **b** Pinhole magnification image confirms increased uptake extending beyond physis into metaphysis. (From Connolly et al. [208] with permission)

The clearance of blood pool activity despite persistent bone uptake on delayed images may help differentiate such cases from cellulitis, which shows bone hyperemic changes on delayed images but with concomitant residual blood pool activity (Fig. 2.23). Four-phase bone scans can be of help in difficult cases to differentiate cellulitis from osteomyelitis.

Bone scintigraphy is very sensitive in the early diagnosis of osteomyelitis [85, 88]. When the bone is not previously affected by other pathological conditions (non-violated), the bone scan has a high specificity as well [89–95] and is an efficient and cost-effective modality in the diagnosis of osteomyelitis. The overall sensitivity and specificity of bone scans for osteomyelitis in non-violated bone is 90–95%. However, there have been some reports of false negative studies of cases with proven early acute osteomyelitis demonstrating either reduced, or normal, accumulation of the radiopharmaceutical, particularly in neonates. However, these reports were based on the use of earlier gamma

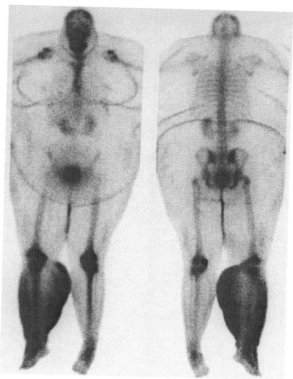

Fig. 2.22. Cellulitis with residual hyperemic changes in the right leg on delayed images

instrumentation. With the use of modern technology, more recent reports show high accuracy of bone scan in the diagnosis of neonatal osteomyelitis [96–98]. Tuson et al. [97] found that the positive predictive value of reduced uptake (a 'cold' scan) in a selected group of patients was higher (100%) than that of a typical 'hot' scan (82%), confirming an earlier report [99] that a 'cold' scan (Fig. 2.24) indicates a more virulent disease. Cold lesions in this report [97] had an average shorter

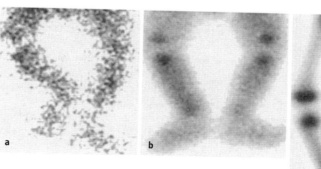
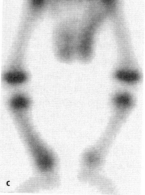

Fig. 2.23. Neonatal osteomyelitis involving right tibia. There is increased flow (**a**) blood pool (**b**) tibia and delayed (**c**) activity in the area of involved bone

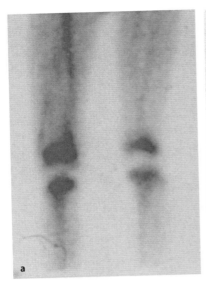

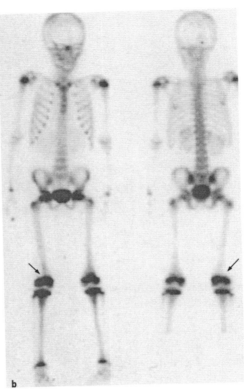

Fig. 2.24a, b. A two-phase bone scan of a 7-year-old boy with fever, pain and swelling in the region of the right knee. **a** There is increased vascular activity in the region. **b** A photon-deficient area on delayed images in the lateral aspect of the right distal femoral metaphysis (*arrows*) illustrating an example of cold osteomyelitis

history (4 days) than did hot scans (7 days). Cold foci on bone scan in cases of osteomyelitis are thought to be secondary to an increased intraosseous and subperiosteal pressure. A more recent report of seven cases with cold scan osteomyelitis also supported the earlier data [regarding the more aggressive nature of this infection that was also associated with elevated erythrocyte sedimentation rate (ESR), significantly elevated temperature, and resting pulse, longer hospital stay and higher rate of surgical interventions] [100]. When the bone scan is normal but the clinical picture strongly suggests osteomyelitis, a repeat bone scan within 24–48 h, Ga-67 citrate, or indium-111 leukocyte imaging may be helpful [50, 97, 101–105]. The normal appearance of bone scans at regions of osteomyelitis may be due to their being obtained during the transition from cold to hot phases [97].

When bone is violated the bone scan remains generally sensitive (90–95%) [106–121] but is non-specific (30%) [119]. Four-phase bone scans improve the specificity. This was demonstrated by Alazraki et al. [86], who reported that the specificity improved from 73% to 87% for three-phase bone scans in a selected group of patients, but the sensitivity dropped from 100% to 80%. Accordingly, when the bone has been violated, the bone scan alone may not establish the diagnosis, requiring a complementary radionuclide modality, such as In-111 leukocyte or Ga-67; this improves the specificity. In this

situation, the main benefit of the bone scan is to exclude the presence of osteomyelitis if it is unequivocally negative and to localize the abnormality better than other studies such as labeled leukocytes or gallium-67.

An attempt to improve the specificity of the three-phase bone scan was reported by Seldin et al. [122] among patients with diabetes. These authors classified hyperemia according to the time of its appearance compared to the surrounding soft tissue. Hyperemia that was apparent before, or at the same time as, the appearance of activity in the surrounding soft tissue was considered to be arterial, and hyperemia which became evident only after the activity appeared in the tissue was considered venous. Bone scans accordingly were interpreted as showing acute osteomyelitis only when focal arterial hyperemia, and increased activity on blood pool and delayed images, were evident. Scans showing venous hyperemia were interpreted as soft tissue pathology or non-osteomyelitis conditions such as neuroarthropathy. Using these parameters, the authors reported a sensitivity of 94% and a specificity of 79%. This method, along with adding the fourth phase, may help decrease the number of additional diagnostic modalities needed, particularly when resources are limited.

Although the bone scan becomes positive very early in the course of the disease, it may not be useful in evaluating the response to treatment as it may remain positive for months after clinical resolution of the disease [123].

2.4.2.3
Gallium-67 Citrate Imaging

The gallium-67 scan also becomes positive in osteomyelitis 24–48 h after the onset of symptoms [124]. Unlike a bone scan, Ga-67 activity generally returns to baseline approximately 6 weeks after successful treatment and can be used to monitor the clinical course of osteomyelitis [85, 123]. In the clinical setting of acute osteomyelitis, gallium-67 scans are 80–85% sensitive. On the other hand, positive gallium-67 scans are seen also with primary and metastatic neoplasms [86], chronic infections [125], and aseptic inflammatory and traumatic lesions [126]. Specificity accordingly is approximately 70% [15]. To improve specificity, Tumeh et al. [127] suggested that osteomyelitis is more likely to be present when Ga-67 uptake exceeds that of Tc-99m MDP or differs in distribution. If Ga-67 localization is less than Tc-99m MDP localization, infection is unlikely. If the two uptake patterns are equivalent, the findings may be indeterminate. These equivalent patterns can occur in up to 72% of patients with pre-existing focal abnormalities and accordingly in complicated cases, such as diabetic or post-traumatic osteomyelitis, Ga-67 may not be able to differentiate osteomyelitis from neuroarthropathy or healing fractures [128]. Seabald et al. [129] studied 49 patients with fracture non-unions 4–48 months after injury using Tc-99m MDP on day 1, combined Tc-99m MDP and indium-111 labeled leukocytes on day 2, and gallium-67 on day 3. Gallium-67 studies were interpreted as non-diagnostic if localization of the tracer at fracture sites was equal to that of Tc-99m MDP, positive if Ga-67 localization was greater than that of Tc-99m MDP, and negative if it was less than that of Tc-99m MDP. A total of 52% of culture positive fracture sites showed a non-diagnostic pattern. Lewin et al. [111] using Tc-99m MDP and Ga-67 had a poor specificity for osteomyelitis in a highly selected group of patients, although combined Tc-99m MDP/Ga-67 yielded higher specificity than Tc-99m MDP alone in the group of patients with violated bone: the specificity for Tc-99m MDP bone scan was 25% but, when combined with Ga-67, it was 63%. Causes of Ga-67 false positives in this group included fractures and juvenile rheumatoid arthritis. Ga-67 combined with Tc-99m MDP, however, is particularly useful in the diagnosis of chronic active and vertebral osteomyelitis and has an accuracy similar to that of MRI [127, 130]. Recently, Love found, in a small number of patients, that SPECT gallium-67 and bone scans were more sensitive and specific than planar gallium-67 and bone scintigraphy (91% and 92% vs 64% and 85% respectively). The authors found that gallium SPECT alone has identical accuracy to combined Ga-67 and bone SPECT and suggested the use of Ga-67 SPECT alone in the diagnosis of vertebral osteomyelitis since it was also sensitive and slightly more specific than MRI in their series [131].

2.4.2.4
Labeled Leukocyte Imaging

Indium-111 oxine and Tc-99m HMPAO leukocyte studies are widely used in the diagnosis of osteomyelitis as specific agents for infection (Fig. 2.25). Overall, In-111 leukocyte studies are sensitive (88%) as well as specific (91%) for osteomyelitis [132] and are particularly useful in excluding infection in a previously violated site of bone such as post-traumatic, diabetic, and post-surgical conditions [133] and in some patients with pressure sores [134]. False-positive scans, however, have been reported with recent trauma and following arthroplasty, and, accordingly, in these situations culture confirmation of positive scans, or the addition of a bone marrow scan, may be needed [135, 136]. Bone scintigraphy

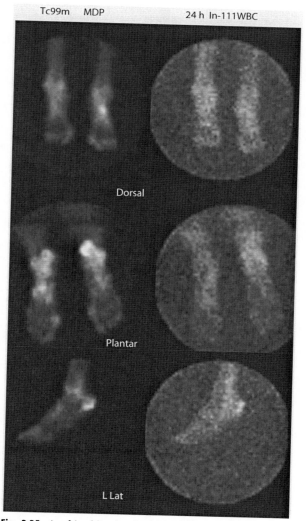

Fig. 2.25. A white blood cell scan showing abnormally increased accumulation of labeled leukocytes at the site of infection (left calcaneus)

should be performed in conjunction with labeled leukocyte imaging for anatomical localization, although separating bone from any adjacent soft tissue infection may still be difficult. Toward this end, the simultaneous acquisition of 24 h In-111 leukocyte and 3 h or 24 h Tc-99m MDP imaging has been employed. Schauwecker [137] studied 453 patients with bone and In-111 WBC scanning (173 sequentially and 280 simultaneously). It was possible by superimposing images to separate osteomyelitis from simple non-infectious bone turnover, or the adjacent soft tissue, particularly in the extremities. The overall sensitivity of this technique in locating infection in proven cases was 90 % and the specificity was 91 %. Determining that the infection was present in the bone rather than the adjacent soft tissue was more difficult, with a sensitivity of 84 % and a specificity of 90 % for proven osteomyelitis cases. Comparing sequential to simultaneous scanning shows that the simultaneous scans were able to separate bone from soft tissue infection 96 % of the time, which is significantly higher than the 86 % for sequential studies. Ezuddin et al. compared planar and SPECT simultaneous dual imaging of these agents and found that SPECT is superior in differentiating osteomyelitis from cellulitis. These authors reported 85 % sensitivity and 100 % specificity using SPECT and 85 % sensitivity and 57 % specificity with planar imaging in diagnosing osteomyelitis [138].

Tc-99m HMPAO labeled leukocytes have been reported to yield an accuracy similar to that of In-111 leukocyte studies in the diagnosis of osteomyelitis but have the additional benefit of providing results on the same day [108, 139 – 142]. This technique may be particularly useful in children as the radiation dose is much lower than that of In-111 leukocyte technique. Its disadvantage, however, is the inability to acquire dual Tc-99m-MDP and labeled WBC simultaneously.

Indium-111 labeled leukocyte scans are not generally useful in the diagnosis of vertebral osteomyelitis as the images may show normal or decreased uptake and their accuracy is low [59, 60].

2.4.2.5
Immunoscintigraphy

Results of IgG immunoscintigraphy are encouraging in both acute and chronic osteomyelitis, including those cases associated with orthopedic appliances, with an average sensitivity of 95 % and a specificity of 83 %. It has been found to be as useful as labeled leukocytes in diagnosing infections and when it was compared directly to Ga-67 citrate it was found to be more sensitive and specific for infection than Ga-67 [59, 60, 73, 143, 144]. On the other hand, Tc-99m antigranulocyte antibody which is reactive against NCA-90 antigen present on the surface of leukocytes was found to be 84 – 93 % sensitive and 72 % specific for non-vertebral osteomye-

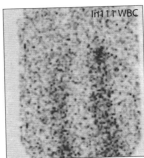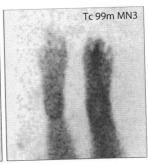

Fig. 2.26. Osteomyelitis in a case of diabetic foot showing positive Tc-99m anti-granulocyte antibody pattern (courtesy of Dr. C. Palestro with thanks)

litis (Fig. 2.26). This agent is not useful in the diagnosis of vertebral osteomyelitis and hip replacement [74, 145]. In a manner similar to the patterns of labeled white blood cells, this agent also showed cold lesions in vertebral osteomyelitis [145].

2.4.2.6
Tc-99m Nanocolloid Scintigraphy

A number of studies have evaluated the efficacy of Tc-99m nanocolloid imaging of infections including osteomyelitis. The mechanism of nanocolloid uptake by infection is believed to be due to 'spillage' secondary to increased permeability of blood vessels and increased size of intercellular spaces associated with particularly acute infections. Accordingly there will be increased nanocolloid concentration at sites of infection because of leakage into the extravascular space. The sensitivity of this method ranges from 87 % to 95 % and specificity ranges from 77 % to 100 % [142, 146 – 148]. Two studies [147, 148] compared this method to that using In-111-labeled leukocytes and found Tc-99m nanocolloid to be of at least equivalent accuracy to the In-111 leukocyte method. Additionally, Tc-99m nanocolloid has been found to be helpful in chronic osteomyelitis, since indium-111-labeled leukocytes consist primarily of granulocytes which, while attracted to sites of acute inflammation, are much less involved in chronic osteomyelitis, often resulting in false-negative studies. However, we have seen a case of proven soft tissue and bone infection that showed photon deficiency on a Tc-99m nanocolloid study at the site of infection, probably secondary to edema, which subsequently showed an increased gallium-67 uptake. The technique has not gained popularity although it can be useful when labeled leukocyte techniques are not available as the case in certain departments and even certain countries.

Table 2.9. Summary of commonly used imaging modalities for skeletal infection

Modality	Advantages	Disadvantages	Typical findings and overall accuracy
Standard radiograph	Cost effectiveness: no additional imaging needed if positive Identify other cause of symptoms and signs (ex. fracture) Assess co-morbidities such as fractures and arthritis	Low sensitivity: findings take up to 2–3 weeks to appear, delaying diagnosis Low specificity to identify infection in violated bone	Cortical destruction (very sensitive finding) Soft tissue swelling with obliteration of fat planes Endosteal scalloping; cortical tunneling Ill-defined radiolucent lesions Osteopenia Sensitivity: 28–94% (average of 56%) Specificity: 3–92% (average 75%)
Computed tomography	Excellent visualization of the cortex Multi-planar and thin-slice reconstructions enhance ability to evaluate infection and identify sequestra	Less resolution than plain radiography Beam-hardening artifact	Increased attenuation of bone marrow Periosteal reaction and new bone formation Sequestrum Intraosseous and/or soft tissue gas
MRI	Excellent delineation of soft tissue versus bone infections Evaluation of bone marrow edema Excellent for suspected vertebral osteomyelitis Very useful in neonatal pelvic osteomyelitis to identify associated soft tissue abscesses	Bone marrow edema is non-specific – can be seen in osteonecrosis, fractures, and metabolic bone disease Specificity is lower with small bones and in complicated cases of infection	Cortical destruction. Increased T2 signal (particularly on STIR); Decreased T1 signal and post gadolinium enhancement Sensitivity: 60–100% (Average: 90%) Specificity: 50–95% (Average: 86%)
Multiphase bone scan	Earlier detection (24–48 h after infection) than radiographs Very high sensitivity for infections even in the presence of other co-morbidities Whole body imaging permits detection of infection at other unsuspected sites	Specificity decreases when other pathologies are present Scans will stay positive for a long time after infection heals, therefore is not ideal for monitoring response to treatment	Focal increased activity on blood flow, blood pool and delayed images Sensitivity: 90–95% Specificity: Non-violated bone 92% Violated bone 0–76% (average of 30%)
White blood cell scan alone or with bone scan	High specificity for infection. Improves bone scan specificity in the setting of violated bone Scans normalize as early as a few days, and so may be used to monitor response to therapy	If used alone, difficult to differentiate bone versus soft tissue infections A tedious procedure	Focal increased uptake Average specificity: 84% Average sensitivity: 88% Dual imaging will show concordant uptake with bone scan in positive studies. Combined imaging increases sensitivity to 86–90% and specificity to 91–94% in violated bone cases
Gallium-67 scintigraphy alone or with bone scan	Early detection of infection Scans return to normal in 6 weeks with successful therapy, allowing use for monitoring treatment Useful for chronic active and vertebral osteomyelitis	Positive findings can be non-specific, and may be positive in other settings such as tumor and inflammation	Combined scanning is considered positive when they are spatially incongruent or spatially congruent with greater Ga-67 intensity than bone scan Average sensitivity: 89% Average specificity: 70%
Bone marrow scan as an addition to white blood cell scan only or along with bone scan	Improves specificity for infection in complicated cases, such as post-arthroplasty infections	Adds time and cost to the diagnostic imaging	Infection is confirmed when no bone marrow activity corresponding to the positive area on labeled white blood cell scan. If activity is present, it indicates physiologic bone marrow as a cause of WBC uptake

(Table 2.9. Cont.)

Modality	Advantages	Disadvantages	Typical findings and overall accuracy
Ultrasound	Excellent for rapid and accurate detection of joint effusions in the setting of septic arthritis Identifies soft tissue and sub-periosteal abscesses No radiation	Poor modality to visualize bone Slightly less sensitive in effusion detection than MRI	Fluid collection adjacent to the cortex of infected bone with communication to the medullary cavity. Occasionally, superficial local defects and periosteal reactions in advanced cases Absence of joint effusion will rule out septic arthritis
PET	Useful in chronic active osteomyelitis and periprosthetic infections as a single modality Useful in early assessment of the response to therapy	Availability; expense	Focally increased uptake with moderate to high SUV Sensitivity: 95–100% (chronic osteomyelitis) 90% (Periprosthetic infection) Specificity: 86%-100% (chronic osteomyelitis), 89% hip periprosthetic infection, 72% knee periprosthetic infection

2.4.2.7
Positron Emission Tomography Imaging

Positron emission tracers are known to concentrate in some inflammatory lesions including bone infections [149–151]. Positron emission tomography (PET) has been found to be useful in assessing the activity of chronic osteomyelitis [152, 153] and peri-prosthetic infections [154, 155]. In a small series of patients, accuracy of FDG SPECT coincidence imaging of chronic infections has been comparable to that of dedicated PET imaging [156].

2.4.3
Imaging Using Combined Modalities

Since no single morphological or scintigraphic modality is adequate in many cases with suspected skeletal infections when bone is affected by a prior pathologic condition, different combinations of these modalities have been used to improve the diagnostic accuracy of imaging. Combined modality approaches have particularly emerged in recent years to face the diagnostic challenges of complicated skeletal infections. Examples of these combinations are as follows:

a. Ga-67 and bone scans
b. Labeled white blood cell and bone scans
c. Labeled white blood cell, bone and bone-marrow scans
d. Labeled white blood cell and bone-marrow scans
e. Bone and immunoscintigraphy scans
f. MRI, bone and immunoscintigraphy studies
g. MRI, labeled white blood cell and bone studies

This approach is commonly used in diabetic foot osteomyelitis, vertebral osteomyelitis, post-arthroplasty infections, sickle-cell disease infections, post-traumatic osteomyelitis and chronic active osteomyelitis when a single modality cannot provide a diagnosis [14, 127, 157–163]. The use of these techniques and their accuracies are detailed throughout the chapter under the various, specific, forms of osteomyelitis. Table 2.9 shows the major morphological and scintigraphic modalities currently used for the diagnosis of skeletal infections.

2.5
Diagnosis of Specific Forms of Skeletal Infections

2.5.1
Diabetic Foot Osteomyelitis

As expected, bone scanning is very sensitive, but not specific, for the detection of infection in diabetes. This is because it is positive in cases of neuroarthropathy as well as infection, with a specificity ranging from 0 to 70% (average of 27%) [15]. Accordingly, three-phase bone scanning cannot reliably separate infection from neuroarthropathy. The four-phase bone scan (using arterial hyperemia in flow studies for scan interpretation along with increased activity on blood pool and delayed images for diagnosing osteomyelitis) may improve the specificity. Ga-67 is not able to discriminate between osteomyelitis in the diabetic foot and non-infected neuroarthropathy. Indium-111 leukocyte imaging is both sensitive and specific for diabetic foot infections. However, sensitivities range from 50–100% and specificities from 29–100% [16]. All ulcers which expose bone were found to be associated with osteomyelitis (Fig. 2.27), and patients therefore may be treated

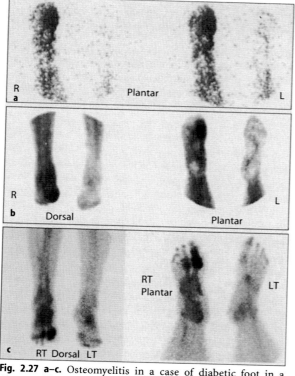

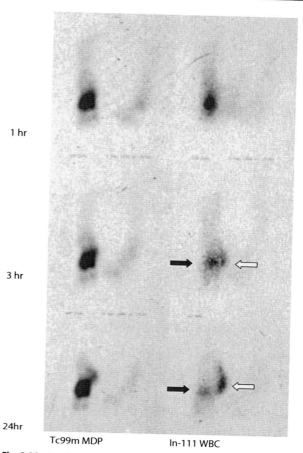

Fig. 2.27 a–c. Osteomyelitis in a case of diabetic foot in a 49-year-old woman with a 19-year history of diabetes mellitus and a recent history of an ulcer on the plantar surface of the right foot which exposed bone. **a** Blood flow, **b** blood pool and **c** delayed images show focally increased activity in the first metatarsal and proximal phalanx and second metatarsal bones. Since the overlaying pedal ulcer is exposing bone, this positive bone scan is diagnostic of osteomyelitis

Fig. 2.28. Combined bone and In-111-labeled white blood cell scan acquired simultaneously showing osteomyelitis with an increasing uptake of labeled leukocytes (open arrow) and neuroarthropathy. There was a decreasing uptake pattern over time (block arrow)

without the need for imaging. However, patients with ulcers which did not expose bone are recommended to have indium-111 leukocyte studies in order to detect the osteomyelitis [113]. False-positive results have been reported in several conditions, including rapidly progressive neuroarthropathy. The vast majority of neuroarthropathies are not rapidly progressive and show no abnormal accumulation of labeled leukocytes. Only in the minority of cases of the rapidly progressive variant does indium-111 white blood cell imaging show an increased uptake. Combined bone-labeled leukocyte imaging improves the accuracy of the diagnosis of foot osteomyelitis, and its differentiation from soft tissue infection. Grerand [164] reported a sensitivity of 93% and a specificity of 83% for this dual-isotope technique and concluded that it can reliably determine the site and extent of osteomyelitis of diabetic foot. In a small number of patients Vesco et al. reported a sensitivity of 85% and a specificity of 82% of the dual-isotope technique using Tc-99m HMPAO-labeled leukocytes [158]. False-positive results, however, can still occur in some cases of non-infected neuroarthropathy [159]. A de-

creasing lesion:background ratio of labeled white blood cells between 4 h and 24 h helps differentiate the condition from osteomyelitis, which does not show a decreasing ratio (Fig. 2.28). Because of the poor spatial resolution of labeled leukocyte studies, uptake in soft tissues could be incorrectly attributed to bone uptake and vice versa. Dual-isotope studies for diabetic foot permit better localization of white blood cell activity and consequently help increase the accuracy in differentiating osteomyelitis from cellulitis [157]. Collective studies have shown an average sensitivity of 83% for labeled leukocyte and combined bone-leukocyte scintigraphy. The average specificity, however, improved only from 64% for leukocyte scan alone to 80% when combined with bone scintigraphy [164].

Combined In-111-labeled leukocyte and Tc-99m sulfur colloid marrow scans (Fig. 2.29) have also been reported to further improve the specificity since they differentiate marrow uptake of labeled leukocyte from

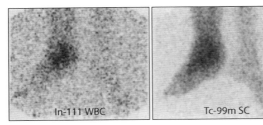

Fig. 2.29. White blood cell and bone marrow scans in a patient with diabetes and suspected osteomyelitis. The images reveal an increased accumulation of labeled leukocytes in the right mid-foot with corresponding uptake on sulfur colloid bone marrow scan indicating no osteomyelitis. The patient had Charcot joint (Courtesy of Dr. Christopher Palestro with thanks)

uptake by actual bone infection. Palestro recently found that this approach is superior to combined bone-leukocyte scintigraphy [159].

MRI can differentiate between soft tissue and bone infections [50]. This is particularly important in diabetics and has been found useful in the diagnosis of diabetic foot osteomyelitis. Several investigators have found that MRI is clearly superior to standard radiographs and bone scintigraphy with a sensitivity and specificity approaching 100%. These studies, however, involved mostly severe infections with significant pathological changes. Newman et al. [165] reported a sensitivity of only 29% for relatively low-grade osteomyelitis compared to 100% for labeled leukocyte scanning of the same patients. The specificity was similar for both modalities. Cook et al. also reported a sensitivity of 91% and a specificity of only 69% for MRI [166]. Morrison et al. reported a lower accuracy of MRI for diabetic than for to non-diabetic cases with a sensitivity and specificity of 82% and 80% respectively for diabetic osteomyelitis compared to 89% and 94% for non-diabetic bone infections [167]. Recently MRI was compared to combined Tc-99m HDP bone scan and Tc-99m HMPAO-labeled scintigraphy in a small number of diabetic patients. MRI was 100% sensitive compared to 77% for the combined scintigraphic technique. The specificity was identical at 82% [158]. Beltran [49] reported the characteristic pattern of osteomyelitis as a high signal intensity from the marrow space on T2-weighted images. However, this finding itself is not specific for osteomyelitis and can be seen with other conditions including rapidly progressive neuroarthropathy; which may be indistinguishable from that of osteomyelitis. Finally, some authors suggested treating all patients with antibiotics when diabetic foot infection is suspected clinically as they are most cost effective [168].

2.5.2
Vertebral Osteomyelitis (Spondylodiscitis)

Spinal osteomyelitis accounts for approximately 2–7% of all cases of osteomyelitis and occurs more often in the elderly [131]. Standard radiographs are neither sensitive, nor specific, for the diagnosis of the relatively common condition. Bone scanning is sensitive but is not specific. Labeled leukocyte scanning using both indium-111 and Tc-99m-HMPAO is also neither sensitive nor specific. This low sensitivity is due to the different patterns of uptake in cases of proven vertebral osteomyelitis including normal uptake, decreased uptake or increased uptake [169, 170]. This was demonstrated by Palestro et al., who studied 71 patients with suspected vertebral osteomyelitis [170], and found that In-111 leukocyte scintigraphy showed increased, or decreased, uptake in 28 patients with proven osteomyelitis. Increased uptake (Fig. 2.30) was associated with a high specificity of 98%, but was only 39% sensitive for the condition. The photopenic pattern was neither sensitive (54%) nor specific (52%) for osteomyelitis. Whalen et al. [169], in a study of 91 patients with suspected vertebral osteomyelitis, also reported a sensitivity of 17%, a specificity of 100% and an accuracy of 31% for indium-111 leukocyte imaging. The authors found photon-deficient areas at the sites of proven osteomyelitis in 50% of 18 patients with proven osteomyelitis, and these were considered to be false-negative scans. Because the diagnosis of vertebral osteomyelitis is often delayed, most infections are chronic in nature, which can in part explain the low sensitivity of indium-111 leukocytes in their diagnosis. Photopenic areas on In-111 leukocyte imaging in proven vertebral osteomyelitis could be secondary to the secretion of anti-chemotactic factors by some causative organisms such as *Pseudomonas aeruginosa* and *Klebsiella pneumoniae*, which prevents enough accumulation of labeled cells at

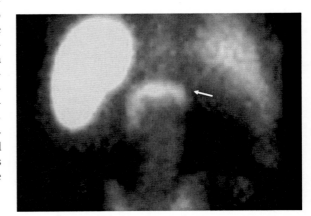

Fig. 2.30. In-111-labeled white blood cell studies for proven vertebral osteomyelitis showing a pattern of increased uptake

the site of infection [171]. Using Tc-99m-HMPAO-labeled leukocytes, Ruther reported five cases of proven vertebral osteomyelitis that were all missed [117]. Hovi also reported three cases of proven infection detected by MRI but none by Tc-99m HMPAO-labeled leukocyte studies [172].

Gallium-67, on the other hand, has a sensitivity of 88% and a specificity of 100% when combined with Tc-99m MDP for the diagnosis of osteomyelitis [167], comparable to that of MRI, which is an excellent modality for the diagnosis of vertebral pathology including infection (Fig. 2.31). For scan interpretation, the degree of bone uptake is compared to that of gallium-67; this allows the high specificity of this combined approach (Figs. 2.32, 2.33). Vertebral osteomyelitis and accompanying soft tissue infection have been reported more recently to be diagnosed accurately with a single rather than combined radionuclide procedure. SPECT Ga-67 was as accurate as SPECT bone and Ga-67 and as sensitive as MRI (91%); the radionuclide study was slightly but not significantly more specific (92% vs 77%) than MRI (Table 2.10). This procedure can be used as a reliable alternative when MRI cannot be performed and as an adjunct in patients in whom the diagnosis is uncertain [131]. Gratz et al. [173] used Ga-67 to identify vertebral osteomyelitis and determine the severity of infection and, potentially, the response to therapy. Although MRI was able to identify all the lesions, it failed to differentiate between mild infections and concurrent degenerative processes and in these cases, Ga-67-citrate SPECT was instrumental in reaching the correct diagnosis. In a study of vertebral osteomyelitis and discitis in children, Fernandez and associates found that the age of children with discitis alone is younger than those with vertebral osteomyelitis and the duration of symptoms is shorter [21]. The authors also found that MRI detected 90% of discitis cases and 100% of osteomyelitis cases and concluded that MRI is the modality of choice for pediatric patients with suspected vertebral osteomyelitis [21].

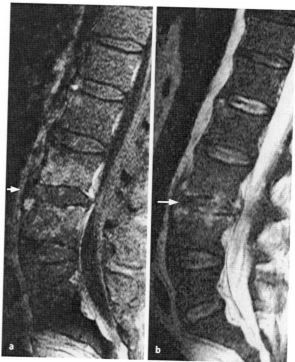

Fig. 2.31. MRI in vertebral osteomyelitis. Note increase signal on T2 W1 image (**a**), end plate destruction (*arrow*) and contrast enhancement (**b**)

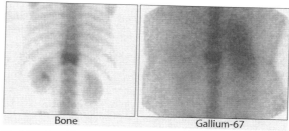

Fig. 2.32. Combined Ga-67 and bone scan in vertebral osteomyelitis showing an increased uptake on Ga-67 scan which is more intense than that on bone scan, illustrating the pattern of osteomyelitis (Courtesy of Dr. C. Palestro with thanks)

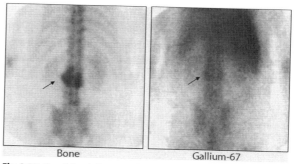

Fig. 2.33. Combined Ga-67 and bone scan in a case of suspected vertebral osteomyelitis showing less intense Ga-67 uptake than that of the bone scan (*arrows*) indicating no infection (Courtesy of Dr. C. Palestro with thanks).

Table 2.10. Accuracy of imaging modalities in the diagnosis of vertebral osteomyelitis (combined literature data)

Modality	Sensitivity	Specificity
Standard radiograph	50%	57%
CT	76%	No information available
MRI	97%	95%
Bone scan	79%	73%
Ga-67 (planar)	85%	77%
Ga-67 SPECT	91%	92%
Combined bone/Ga-67 (planar)	92%	94%
In-111 WBC	30%	98%
Combined bone/Ga-67 SPECT	95%	96%

2.5.3
Chronic Active Osteomyelitis

Non-invasive diagnosis of chronic active skeletal infections remains a challenge. The radiological diagnosis of chronic active osteomyelitis is neither sensitive nor specific, while bone scintigraphy is sensitive but not specific. This low specificity is due to the chronic bone repair that is associated with increased bone metabolism and increased uptake on bone scan in the absence of active infection. It is therefore difficult to differentiate bone turnover due to healing from chronic active disease, although increased activity in all phases of the bone scan is suggestive of chronic active disease. The bone scan accordingly cannot confirm the presence of active disease, but a negative scan accurately excludes it.

Gallium-67 citrate imaging is more specific than bone scanning for chronic osteomyelitis, although false positives commonly occur in conditions such as healing fractures, tumors, and non-infected prostheses. Combined Tc-99m MDP and gallium-67 scans can be helpful in making the diagnosis of active disease. As Tumeh et al. suggested, when gallium uptake exceeds Tc-99m MDP uptake in intensity or differs in spatial distribution, active osteomyelitis is present [127].

A controversy exists regarding the role of indium-111 leukocytes in the diagnosis of chronic osteomyelitis. Since the majority of labeled cells are polymorphonuclear cells, the test may be normal in true chronic active osteomyelitis. and the results are variable and may be confusing. Tumeh and Tahmeh reported no advantage in using indium-111 leukocytes over Ga-67 as there was no significant difference between them in the sensitivity and specificity for chronic active osteomyelitis [174]. Determining the presence, or absence, of sequestra is important, as they need to be resected for the treatment of chronic active osteomyelitis to be useful [175]. CT is a sensitive modality for the detection of sequestra. MRI was found in limited numbers of patients to be useful in detecting sequestra and was also useful in identifying the presence and sites of active chronic infection [176]. It was recently reported to be sensitive in detecting low-grade infections [160]. Sciuk et al. [177] used Tc-99m IgG and Tc-99m monoclonal antigranulocyte antibodies in 25 patients with suspected chronic osteomyelitis. Three-phase bone scanning was 71% sensitive and 50% specific. IgG was 71% sensitive and 100% specific while monoclonal antibodies had 40% sensitivity and 100% specificity. Both agents were sensitive in peripheral lesions (5/6 for IgG and 6/6 for monoclonal antibodies) while in the central skeleton with active bone marrow IgG was able to detect 5 of 8 lesions while monoclonal antibodies detected none of the eight lesions. This study also confirmed the lack of specificity of multi-phase bone scans for chronic osteo-

myelitis and suggested a possible role for labeled IgG as a more specific agent in both central and peripheral chronic bone infections. In this way the combination of bone and Ga-67 scanning is highly recommended for detecting chronic active osteomyelitis. MRI should be seen as a complementary procedure which is useful in equivocal bone and gallium scans. Combined MRI and bone/Tc-99m anti-granulocyte antibody scintigraphy was found more sensitive and specific than MRI or bone/antigranulocyte antibody imaging. MRI was found to be 100% sensitive and 60% specific for chronic infection, while bone-antigranulocyte antibody imaging was 77% sensitive and 50% specific, but 100% sensitive and 80% specific when combined with MRI [160].

PET has been found useful in assessing the activity of chronic osteomyelitis [152–156]. Recently de Winter et al. reported 60 patients with suspected chronic musculoskeletal infection studied with F-18 FDG PET. Twenty-five patients had proven infection while 35 did not (based on histopathology, microbiologic culture or clinical findings). All 25 infections were correctly identified by two readers with a sensitivity of 100%. There were four false-positive cases and the overall specificity was 88% (90% for central skeleton and 86% for peripheral skeleton). The authors concluded that this single technique is accurate, simple and has a potential to become a standard technique for the diagnosis of chronic musculoskeletal infections [156]. Overall this technique has a sensitivity of 95% to 100% and a specificity of 86% to 100% [152–156].

2.5.4
Periprosthetic Infection

Making the distinction between a mechanical failure of a prosthesis and infection is not easy. Symptoms and signs of early infection are not specific and may be similar to those of the normal healing process. The erythrocyte sedimentation rate and leukocyte count are not sensitive, and the standard radiographic appearance of infection can mimic that of mechanical loosening. Standard radiographs demonstrate signs of loosening only in relatively advanced cases, and the technique is much less sensitive than bone scintigraphy, which detects signs of prosthetic loosening but is not very useful for differentiating loosening from infection [178]. Intense periprosthetic uptake suggests loosening and/or infection and there is no scintigraphic pattern that is highly specific for the presence of infection. Furthermore, the pattern of normal post-operative increased uptake of bone remodeling varies considerably depending on the type of prosthesis used. Aspiration arthrograms are more specific, but again the sensitivity as reported by Johnson [33] is only 67%. Joint aspiration and culture results in up to 15% false negatives [31, 32].

The late stages of infection can be detected easier on the basis of clinical findings. It is crucial, however, to initiate treatment in the early stage as a progression to a serious infection may occur rapidly [73].

In the case of hip replacements, knowledge of the type of implant is important to plan a diagnostic strategy. In cemented total hip replacements, most asymptomatic individuals show no significant increase in bone remodeling adjacent to the stem after 6 months; however, mild to moderate uptake may seen up to 12 months after the joint replacement. However, the distal tip, greater trochanter, and the acetabular component show increased bone repair for at least a year or more after the procedure [178]. Bone scintigraphy of cemented hip replacement shows focal uptake at the tip of the femoral component is more typical of loosening, while diffuse uptake around the shaft is more typical of infection. These patterns, however, are not highly specific in discriminating loosening from infection [178]. In cementless porous coated hip arthroplasty (which depends on bony in-growth for fixation instead of cement) postoperative periprosthetic uptake on bone scintigraphy continues for 2 years or longer in asymptomatic patients and is more variable than the case with cemented prostheses [179, 180].

In knee replacement, postoperative increased uptake are also seen on bone scintigraphy in more than 60% of femoral components and 75–90% of tibial components for a long time of at least 1 year in asymptomatic patients [181]. Accordingly, for both cemented and porous coated hip and knee replacements bone scanning is more useful in excluding infections when it is clearly negative.

Combined bone and gallium-67 scans have better specificity than either scans alone (Table 2.11). However, indium-111 leukocyte imaging has proved more accurate than a combined Ga-67-bone scan. Still, false-positive indium-111 leukocyte results occur as a result of physiological uptake by cellular bone marrow. Oswald et al. [180] found focal or diffuse accumulation of In-111 leukocytes around the prostheses for up to 2 years in 48% of uncomplicated cases. Combined bone-white blood cell scans are more accurate than white blood cell scanning alone and improve localization of abnormalities (Fig. 2.34). Although this technique has been described as highly accurate (Table 2.12), false

Table 2.11. Combined bone/gallium-67 scans for the diagnosis of hip peri-prosthetic infection

Author	Year	Sensitivity	Specificity
Lyons [209]	1985	67%	100%
Tehranzadeh [175]	1988	80%	100%
Merckel [210]	1985	57%	89%
McKillop [211]	1987	83%	79%
Alibadi [212]	1989	37%	100%

Table 2.12. Combined bone and in-111 white blood cell scans for the diagnosis of hip peri-prosthetic infection

Author	Year	Sensitivity	Specificity
Mulamba [213]	1983	92%	100%
Merckel [210]	1985	86%	100%
Pring [214]	1986	100%	66%
Palestro [182]	1991	87%	94%
Cuckler [215]	1991	60%	73%

positives have been reported. Again, this is due to physiological marrow uptake. Addition of Tc-99m sulfur colloid bone marrow to indium-111 leukocyte scanning helps further improve the specificity (Fig. 2.35). Palestro reported an improvement in specificity from 12–94% with the addition of sulfur colloid bone marrow scanning, while Seabald showed specificity improved from 59% to 92% [40, 182]. A study is considered to be positive for infection when the indium-111 leukocyte uptake exceeds Tc-99m colloid activity on bone marrow scanning in extent and/or focal intensity (discordant pattern). If the relative intensity and distribution of indium-111-labeled leukocyte localization is equal to that of Tc-99m colloid (concordant pattern) the study should be considered negative for infection [40, 183]. Accordingly the procedure of choice for diagnosing the infection of joint replacements is combined labeled leukocyte-marrow scintigraphy, which has a diagnostic accuracy of more than 90% [40–42, 178, 181].

In some cases of early or low-grade infection there may not be sufficient alteration in the marrow to show a definite discordant or incongruent pattern on planar Tc-99m sulfur colloid scan compared to the indium-111 leukocyte finding. The use of combined In-111 white blood cell-bone and bone marrow SPECT imaging has further improved the diagnostic accuracy for detection of an infected hip prosthesis and is recommended by Seabald et al. [30, 184]. Logistically, bone marrow and bone SPECT images can be obtained first while the leukocytes are being labeled, and simultaneous combined In-111 WBC/bone SPECT images can be obtained the next day 16–24 h after injection of the labeled leukocytes [30, 184]. Furthermore, Magnuson et al. [112] suggested a grading system which compares the intensity of labeled leukocyte localization along the prosthesis to that of marrow uptake at the same location which can further improve the accuracy of this technique. It adds additional specificity in difficult cases, since the intensity and patterns of leukocyte and Tc-99m colloid marrow may vary with the type of prosthesis used (cemented vs cementless), the time interval after surgery and the number of revisions [30].

Antibody imaging has also been used to diagnose infections in patients with hip and knee prostheses,

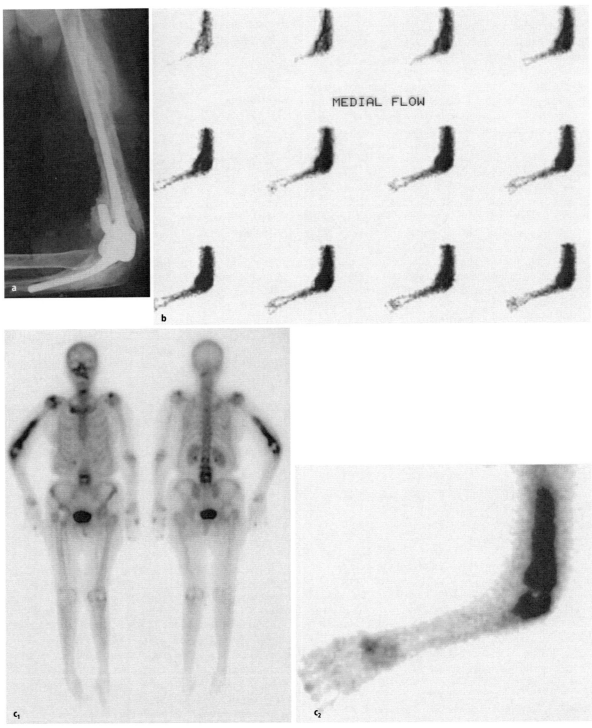

Fig. 2.34a–c. Combined bone and WBC scans for a case of infected elbow prosthesis as illustrated on the standard radiograph (**a**). **b** Flow study reveals significantly increased flow in the region of the right elbow and arm. **c** Delayed whole body scan reveals corresponding increased uptake. In-111 labeled white blood cell scan reveals intense accumulation of leukocytes at the same area in a case with proven infection (courtesy of Dr. Nikpoor with thanks)

Fig. 2.35. a In-111 WBC and **b** Tc-99m sulfur colloid arteria images for a patient with bilateral hip replacement and suspected infection. Images reveal increased accumulation of labeled white blood cells in the right hip prostheses and to a lesser extent in the left. On Tc-99m SC imaging there are discongruent patterns on the right (*arrows*) and a congruent pattern on the left indicating infected right prosthesis and no infection on the left side

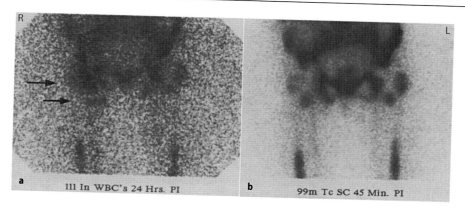

with sensitivity of 70–100% and specificity of 83–100% for Tc-99m anti-granulocyte antibodies [73] and sensitivity of 92% and specificity of 88% for In-111-labeled IgG [71].

FDG-PET has recently been shown to be able to detect both infections and loosening and also to be able to differentiate between both conditions in patients with hip and knee prostheses. The results are promising and appear to be more accurate for hip than for knee prostheses [185, 186]. The sensitivity and specificity for detecting infection are 90% and 89% for hip and 90% and 72% for knee peri-arthroplasty infections respectively [186]. Although the intensity of FDG uptake as determined by standardized uptake value (SUV) is important in making the diagnosis of malignancy, this is not the case with periprosthetic infections. Infected prostheses often show a moderately increased uptake which is not higher than that noted with aseptic loosening [185]. Accordingly, using the uptake intensity as the sole criterion for infection will lead to false-positive results for infection [185]. The location of the increased uptake is more important in discriminating infection from loosening since infection is characterized by the uptake along the interface between bone and the prostheses, while in loosening the uptake is around the neck and head.

2.5.5
Osteomyelitis Following Fractures

The incidence of osteomyelitis secondary to open fracture is reported to be 2–16%, with a rate of 1–10% after open reduction with internal fixation of closed fractures [187]. Osteomyelitis is behind 5% and 10% of fracture non-unions, and almost all infected non-united fractures are associated with a previously open fracture, or open operative reduction, since fractures that are treated in a closed manner rarely become infected [8, 30]. Simultaneous In-111-white blood cell-Tc-99m MDP bone imaging is more accurate than Ga-67-Tc-99m MDP bone imaging for the detection of osteomye-

litis at fracture non-union sites. Seabald found that the accuracy of Ga-67-Tc-99m MDP for detecting osteomyelitis at fracture sites is 39% compared with 88% for combined Tc-99m MDP-In-111 white blood cell imaging [129]. Bone marrow scanning may further improve the specificity of white blood cell findings when physiological marrow uptake of labeled white blood cells is suspected as a cause of their accumulation.

2.5.6
Osteomyelitis in Patients with Sickle-Cell Disease

Differentiating bone infarcts from osteomyelitis is clinically difficult. Initial radiographs are either normal or show non-specific changes. On bone scintigraphy the findings vary. If bone scintigraphy is performed a week after the onset of symptoms, healing of the infarct may cause increased uptake rather than the typical pattern of a cold defect. To add more difficulty, osteomyelitis may also cause cold defects rather than increased uptake [17, 30, 161, 188]. Addition of gallium-67 or Tc-99m sulfur colloid imaging to bone scans enhances the specificity and can resolve the majority of diagnostic problems related to osteomyelitis in patients with sickle-cell disease. If the bone scan shows areas of increased uptake, a bone marrow scan could be added. If the marrow scan of the area of interest is normal, it indicates osteomyelitis, while if radiocolloid photon deficiency is seen it suggests a healing infarct. On the other hand, if the bone scan shows a photon-deficient area, Ga-67 may help differentiate osteomyelitis by showing incongruent pattern spatially or if gallium-67 uptake is more than that of bone scan. Infarcts will show a congruent pattern [161].

Labeled leukocytes have also been used, although we encountered technical difficulties in labeling cells of sickle-cell patients with failed scans. MRI and contrast enhanced CT scans have also been reported to be of help in patients with non diagnostic radiographs and bone scan.

2.5.7
Chronic Recurrent Multifocal Osteomyelitis

Chronic recurrent multifocal osteomyelitis, or Giedion's osteomyelitis, is a rare variant of osteomyelitis that primarily affects children and young adults and may be related to SAPHO syndrome (synovitis, acne, pustulosis, hyperostosis, osteitis). Clinically, it is characterized by an insidious, or acute, onset of pain, tenderness and local swelling, mimicking acute osteomyelitis but usually without fever, leukocytosis or elevated ESR [189]. Pain resolves spontaneously but may recur at the same site or at a different location. The disease mainly affects the metaphyses of the long tubular bones.

Sometimes, it has a symmetric distribution; that is, similar sites in both extremities are involved. The most commonly involved skeletal sites are the tibia, femur, clavicle, and fibula. Other bones involved are the pubic bones, calcaneus and phalanges [190]. On radiographs the lesion presents with lytic foci and associated sclerosis. Bone scan reveals multi-focal areas of increased uptake that may be subtle in some cases.

The etiology of this disorder is unknown. Infectious and autoimmune causes have been suggested. Bone and blood cultures have always been reported to be negative. Early lesions contain polymorphonuclear (neutrophilic) leukocytic infiltrate in the marrow. Long-standing lesions show fibrosis with predominantly lymphocytic infiltrates. Prominent formation of new reactive bone can be a dominant feature in later phases of the disease [191], and in the majority of those cases the erythrocyte sedimentation rate is elevated. Some authors have reported a high incidence of prior throat infections and elevation of the anti-streptolysin O titers. The number of relapse episodes ranges from 1 to 6 [190].

In the differential diagnosis it is helpful to consider the entire clinical picture and radiographic presentation of the lesion. Lymphoma of the bone almost never occurs in young patients whose disease presents with multi-focal involvement of the metaphyseal regions.

2.5.8
Neonatal Osteomyelitis

In neonates, the ability of infection to violate the growth plate predisposes them to an increased risk of joint involvement and extension into adjacent bone. The periosteum is less approximated to the cortex in infants and children. The degree of periosteal reaction is increased and subperiosteal abscesses are more likely to occur in neonatal and juvenile osteomyelitis. Scintigraphy has generally been thought to play a limited role in neonatal skeletal infections due to reported high false-negative rates. A recent publication by Connolly et al. [96] reported 99% sensitivity and specificity for neonatal osteomyelitis using bone scintigraphy utilizing today's modern gamma cameras. In their study no single case was diagnosed only by MRI. However, the authors recommended MRI for pelvic osteomyelitis since it detects the drainable abscesses which commonly (20%) occur at this site [96].

2.5.9
Epiphyseal Osteomyelitis

In children osteomyelitis confined to the epiphysis is an entity seen particularly below the age of 4 years. The most frequently affected sites are the epiphyses of the distal femur and proximal tibia. The pinhole images are particularly valuable for correctly localizing the findings on bone scan, where isolated epiphyseal focally increased uptake is seen in delayed images corresponding to regional hyperemia seen on flow and blood pool images [192, 193].

2.6
Follow-up of Response to Therapy

Since many therapies for infection are relatively toxic, shortening the duration of therapy to the minimum required to control the infection is desirable. Monitoring the response to infection therapy in cancer patients is complicated by the slow response in many patients.

Bone scanning is not a suitable modality for determining the response to therapy when treating skeletal infections because it may remain positive for years in the absence of active infection. Several nuclear medicine studies are generally useful to achieve the evaluation of the response to therapy, including Ga-67; labeled white blood cells; and polyclonal and monoclonal radiolabeled antibodies. Understandably, FDG PET has potential in this area but no data are yet available.

2.7
Differentiating Osteomyelitis from Infectious Arthritis

Although it is sometimes difficult scintigraphically to differentiate osteomyelitis from septic arthritis, it has been established that bone scans can identify joint involvement and distinguish bone from joint infection in up to 90% of cases [89, 97, 194]. Detailed clinical information is crucial in making the correct diagnosis. Sundberg et al. [194] studied 106 children suspected of having septic arthritis and showed that the bone scan interpretation was correct in 13% when read without clinical information, while the sensitivity improved to 70% when a clinical history was available. It is our experience that if we follow the criteria for the differentiation, it is possible in the vast majority of cases to make the distinction between infectious arthritis and osteomyelitis. In septic arthritis there is peri-articular distribution of the abnormal uptake, which is largely limited to the joint capsule and has a uniform pattern. On the other hand, osteomyelitis shows abnormal uptake beyond the confines of the joint capsule or shows uptake within the joint capsule that is non-uniform [89, 97]. Combined bone and gallium-67, or labeled leukocyte scintigraphy can provide more precise information in equivocal cases on bone scanning alone.

2.8
Differentiating Tumors from Infection

In certain situations it is clinically difficult to differentiate between infection and tumors due to their similar manifestations. Labeled leukocyte scans can be useful in excluding infection if the study is negative. However, if the study is positive, it is more likely to be secondary to infection, although some false-positive studies resulting from tumor uptake have been reported [195]. MRI can also be useful, although differentiating tumors from infection in certain locations can be difficult [196, 197]. Thallium-201 imaging using recent modifications [198] can be useful in differentiating infection from the tumor. Early (20 min) and delayed (3 h) imaging, with or without SPECT, depending on the location, are useful in differentiating infection from a viable tumor. Absence of uptake will make a viable tumor unlikely. Decreasing the uptake ratio between early and delayed imaging is also suggestive of infection rather than a viable tumor, while a stable or rising ratio is more suggestive of a tumor [197] than infection. Matthies reported the use of early FDG PET (70 min post-injection) and delayed (2 h) imaging in differentiating tumor from benign conditions including inflammatory conditions [85].

It is clear that the imaging strategy for osteomyelitis is rather complicated given the many forms of the condition. The co-morbidities complicate the issue, together with specific pathological aspects at different locations, as well as the strengths and limitations of the modalities. An algorithm is proposed in order to help choose the appropriate modality for the diagnosis in different clinical settings (Fig. 2.36).

2.9
Non-Infectious Inflammatory Conditions
2.9.1
Osteitis Condensans Ilii

Osteitis condensans ilii is a non-specific inflammatory condition of the iliac bone that is self-limiting. It pre-

dominantly affects women of child-bearing age, particularly the multiparous. Although the cause of the condition is not clear, the predominant theory suggests abnormal mechanical stress across the sacroiliac joints coupled with an increased vascularity during pregnancy and delivery [199, 200]. The condition is rare in men. Scintigraphically, an increased uptake is seen in the iliac bone at the region of sacroiliac joints that is usually bilateral and symmetric but can be asymmetrical and unilateral.

2.9.2
Osteitis Pubis

Osteitis pubis represents a non-specific inflammation of the pubic bones which follows delivery and pelvic operations. In men, it is particularly frequent after prostate or bladder surgery. Low-grade infection, trauma, venous congestion due to injury or inflammation are proposed etiologies [199]. Scintigraphically, there is intense uptake in the para-articular regions of the pubic bones.

2.9.3
Infantile Cortical Hyperostosis (Caffey's Disease)

Infantile cortical hyperostosis is a rare inflammatory condition of early infancy described first by Caffey in 1946. The etiology is unknown with a tendency to be familial [201]. It is thought to be due to a genetic defect that is autosomally dominant. It presents during the first few weeks of life and usually before the age of 6 months. It most commonly affects the mandible (Fig. 2.37) followed by the clavicles, ribs, ulna, radius, tibia, fibula and can affect any other bone but not usually the vertebrae, pelvis and phalanges. There is extensive periosteal new bone formation which appears on bone scans as areas of irregularly increased uptake described by Bahk as 'pumpy' [200]. The course is usually benign and the lesions resolve spontaneously in less than a year. Non-steroidal anti-inflammatory drugs or steroids may be needed.

2.9.4
Sternoclavicular Hyperostosis

This chronic inflammatory process affecting predominantly adult men involves the sternum, clavicle and upper ribs and the adjacent soft tissue [202]. Increased uptake in the involved areas, which are usually bilateral and symmetrical, is the typical scintigraphic feature [203, 204].

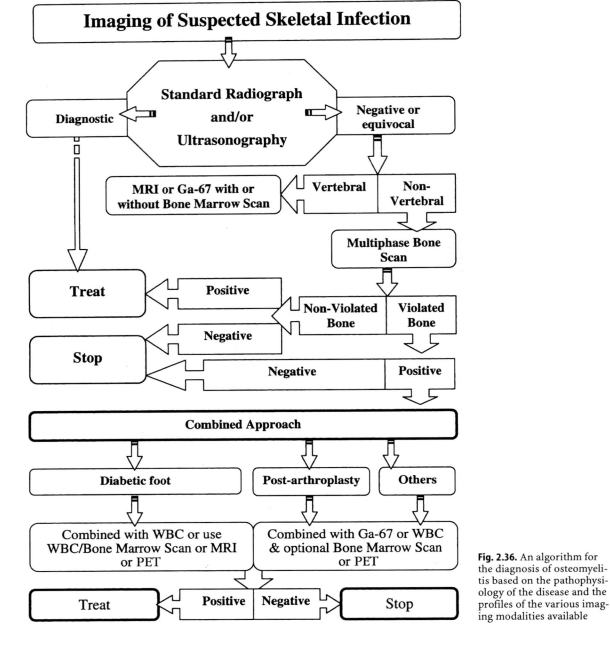

Fig. 2.36. An algorithm for the diagnosis of osteomyelitis based on the pathophysiology of the disease and the profiles of the various imaging modalities available

2.9.5
Osteitis Condensans of the Clavicle

This condition is also called condensing osteitis of the clavicle and occurs among women with an average age of 40 years with a history of stress to the sternoclavicular joint region [199]. It causes pain that is commonly referred to the shoulder and there is intense unilateral focal uptake in the medial end of the clavicle and the sternoclavicular joint which is clearly seen on pinhole imaging [200] (Fig. 2.38).

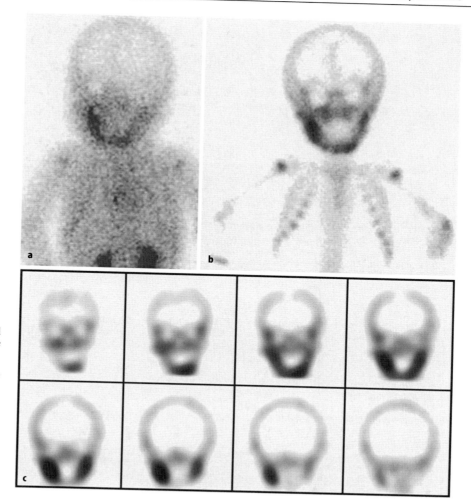

Fig. 2.37a–c. Infantile cortical hyperostosis of the mandible in a 5-month-old boy with a history of fever, irritability and swelling of the region of the right mandible. **a** Blood pool image shows the significantly increased level of activity in the right-hand side mandible with a corresponding increased uptake on the delayed image (**b**). This is also seen clearly on the SPECT study (**c**)

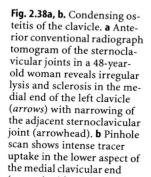

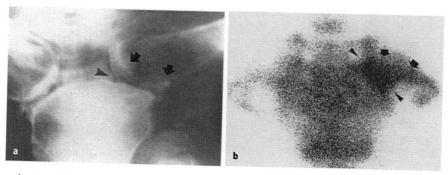

Fig. 2.38a, b. Condensing osteitis of the clavicle. **a** Anterior conventional radiograph tomogram of the sternoclavicular joints in a 48-year-old woman reveals irregular lysis and sclerosis in the medial end of the left clavicle (*arrows*) with narrowing of the adjacent sternoclavicular joint (arrowhead). **b** Pinhole scan shows intense tracer uptake in the lower aspect of the medial clavicular end (*arrows*) with relatively more prominent uptake (specifically in the sternoclavicular joint) that is involved secondarily (*arrowheads*) (From Bahk [200 p. 64], with permission)

References

1. Weissman G (1990) Inflammation: historical perspectives. In: Gallin JI Goldstein IM, Snyderman R (eds) Inflammation: basic principles and clinical correlates, 2nd edn. Raven press, New York, pp 5–13
2. Rote NSV (1998) Inflammation. In: McCance KL, Huether SE (eds) Pathophysiology, 3rd edn. Mosby, St Louis, pp 205–236
3. Cotran RS, Kumar V, Robins SL (1999) Inflammation and repair. In: Cotran RS, Kumar V, Robins SL (eds) Robbins pathologic basis of disease, 6th edn. Saunders Philadelphia, pp 50–88
4. Freifeld AG, Pizzo PA, Walsh TJ (1997) Infections in the cancer patient. In: Devita VT, Hellman S, Rosenberg SA (eds) Principles and practice of oncology, 5th edn. Lippincott Raven, Philadelphia, pp 2659–2704
5. Trueta J (1957) The normal vascular anatomy of the human femoral head during growth. J Bone Joint Surg 39B:358–394
6. Trueta J (1959) The three types of acute hematogenous osteomyelitis: a clinical and vascular study. J Bone Joint Surg 41B:671–680
7. Cierny G, Mader JT, Pennick HA (1985) Clinical staging system of adult osteomyelitis. Contemp Orthop 10:17–37
8. Waldvogel FA, Medoff G. Swartz MM (1970) Osteomyelitis: a review of clinical features, therapeutic considerations and unusual aspects. N Engl J Med 282:198–206
9. Elgazzar AH, Shehab D, Malki A, Abdulla M (2001) Musculoskeletal system. In: Elgazzar AH (ed) The pathophysiologic basis of nuclear medicine. Springer, Berlin Heidelberg New York, pp 88–102
10. Kahn DS, Pritzker KPH (1973) The pathophysiology of bone infection. Clin Orthop Rel Res 96:12
11. Bonakdar-Pour A, Gaines VD (1983) The radiology of osteomyelitis. Orthop Clin North Am 14:21–37
12. Nixon GW (1976) Acute hematogenous osteomyelitis. Pediatr Ann 5:64–81
13. Kasser JR (1984) Hematogenous osteomyelitis: untangling the diagnostic confusion. Postgrad Med 76:79–86
14. Elgazzar AH, Abdel-Dayem HM (1999) Imaging skeletal infections: evolving considerations. In: Freeman LM (ed) Nuclear medicine annual. Lippincott Williams and Wilkins, Philadelphia, pp 157–191
15. Elgazzar AH, Abdel-Dayem HM, Clark J, Maxon HR (1995) Multimodality imaging of osteomyelitis. Eur J Nucl Med 22:1043–1063
16. Torda AJ, Gottlieb T, Bradbury R (1995) Pyogenic vertebral osteomyelitis: analysis of 20 cases and review. Clin Infect Dis 20:320–328
17. Song KS, Ogden JA, Ganey T, Guidera KT (1997) Contiguous discitis and osteomyelitis in children. J Pediatr Orthop 17:470–477
18. Ring D, Wenger DR, Johnson C (1994) Infectious spondylitis in children. The convergence of discitis and vertebral osteomyelitis. Orthop Trans 18:97–98
19. Waldvogel FA, Vasey H (1980) Osteomyelitis: the past decade. N Engl J Med 303:360–370
20. Perrone C, Saba J, Behloul Z, Salmon-Ceron D, Leport C, Vilde JL, Kahn MF (1994) Pyogenic and tuberculous spondylodiskitis (vertebral osteomyelitis) in 80 adult patients. Clin Infect Dis 19:746–750
21. Fernandez M, Carrol CL, Baker CJ (2000) Discitis and vertebral osteomyelitis in children: an 18 year review. Pediatrics 15:1299–1304
22. Forrest RD, Jacobson CA, Yudkin JS (1986) Glucose intolerance and hypertension in north London: the Islington diabetes survey. Diabet Med 3:338–342
23. Forrest RD, Jacobson CA, Yudkin JS, Bamberger DM, Daus GP, Gerding DN (1987) Osteomyelitis in the feet of diabetic patients: long term results, prognostic factors, and the role of antimicrobial and surgical therapy. Am J Med 83:653–660
24. Schwartz GS, Berenyi MR, Siegel MW (1969) Atrophic arthropathy and diabetic neuritis. AJR 106:523–529
25. Horwitz SH (1993) Diabetic neuropathy. Clin Orthop 296:78–85
26. Gold RH, Tang DTF, Crim JR, Seeger LL (1995) Imaging the diabetic foot. Skeletal Radiol 24:563–557
27. Rand JA (1995) Preoperative planning for total knee arthroplasty. In: Callaghan JJ, Dennis DA, Paprosky WG, Rosenberg AG (eds) Orthopedic knowledge update. Hip and knee reconstruction. Rosenmont. American Academy of Orthopedic Surgeons
28. Anonymous (1995) Proceedings of the American Academy of Orthopaedic Surgeons, Rosemont, IL, pp 255–263
29. Griffiths HJ (1995) Orthopedic complications. Radiol Clin North Am 33:401–410
30. Seabald JE, Nepola JV (1999) Imaging techniques for evaluation of postoperative orthopedic infections. Quart J Nucl Med 43:21–28
31. Harris WH, Sledge CB (1990) Total hip and total knee replacement, part I. NEJM 323:725–731
32. Harris WH, Sledge CB (1990) Total hip and total knee replacement, part II. NEJM 323:801–807
33. Johnson JA, Christle MJ, Sandler MP, Parks PF Jr, Horma L, Kayle JJ (1988) Detection of occult infection following total joint arthroplasty using sequential technetium-99m HDP bone scintigraphy and Indium-111 WBC imaging. J Nucl Med 29:1347–1353
34. Barton LL, Dunkle LM, Habib FH (1987) Septic arthritis in childhood: a 13 year review. Am J Dis Child 141:898–900
35. Welkon CJ, Long SS, Fisher MC, Alburger PD (1986) Pyogenic arthritis in infants and children: a review of 95 cases. Pediatr Infect Dis 5:669–676
36. Silberstein EB, Elgazzar AH, Fernandez-Uloa M, Nishiyama H (1996) Skeletal scintigraphy in non-neoplastic osseous disorders. In: Henkin RE, Bles MA, Dillehay GL, Halama JR, Karesh SM, Wagner PH, Zimmer AM (eds) Textbook of nuclear medicine. Mosby, New York, pp 1141–1197
37. Nixon GW (1978) Hematogenous osteomyelitis of metaphyseal equivalent locations. AJR 130:123–129
38. Cole WG, Dalziel RE, Leitl S (1982) Treatment of acute osteomyelitis in childhood. J Bone Joint Surg (Br) 64:208–213
39. Harris NH (1960) Some problems in the diagnosis and treatment of acute osteomyelitis. J Bone Joint Surg (Br) 42:535–541
40. Seabald JE, Nepola JV, Marsh JL et al (1991) Post operative bone marrow alterations: Potential pitfalls in the diagnosis of osteomyelitis with In-111-labeled leukocyte scintigraphy. Radiology 180:741–747
41. Bayoun C, Elgazzar AH (2002) Skeletal infections. Presented at Radiologic society of North America annual meeting
42. Riebel T, Nasir R, Nazarenko O (1996) The value of sonography in the detection of osteomyelitis. Pediatr Radiol 26:291–297
43. Howard CB, Einhorn M, DaganR, Nyaska M (1993) Ultrasound in diagnosis and management of acute hamatogenous osteomyelitis in children. J Bone Gurs (Br) 75:79–82
44. Abernethy LJ, Lee YC, Cole WG (1993) Ultrasound localization of subperiosteal abscess in children with late acute osteomuelitis. J Pediatr Orthop 13:766–768
45. Jien Y, Chih H, Lin G, Hsien S, Lin S (1999) Clinical application of ultrasonography for detection of septic arthritis in children. Kaohsiung J Med Sci 15:542–549

46. Mah et, LeQuesne GW, Gent RJ, Paterson DC (1994) Ultrasonic features of acute osteomyelitis in children. J Bone Joint Surg (Br) 76:969–974
47. Cardinol E, Bureau NJ, Aubin B, Chhem RK (2001) Role of ultrasound in musculoskeletal infections. Radiol Clin North Am 39:191–200
48. Tumeh SS, Aliabadi P, Seltzer SE et al (1988) Chronic osteomyelitis: the relative role of plain radiographs and transmission computed tomography. Clin Nucl Med 13:710
49. Beltran J, Campanini DS, Knight C et al (1990) The diabetic foot: Magnetic Resonance Imaging evaluation. Skeletal Radiol 19:37–41
50. Mason MD, Zlatkin MB, Esterhai JL et al (1989) Chronic complicated osteomyelitis of the lower extremity: evaluation with MR imaging. Radiology 173:355–359
51. Meyers P, Wiener S (1991) Diagnosis of hematogenous pyogenic vertebral osteomyelitis by magnetic resonance imaging. Arch Intern Med 151:683–687
52. Moore JE, Yuh WTC, Kathol MH et al (1991) Abnormalities of the foot in patients with diabetes mellitus: findings on MR imaging. AJR 157:813–816
53. Tang JSH, Gold RH, Bassett LW et al (1988) Musculoskeletal infection of the extremities: evaluation with MR imaging. Radiology 166:205–209
54. Sfakianakis GN, Al-Sheikh W, Heal A et al (1982) Comparison of scintigraphy with In-111 leukocytes and Ga-67 in the diagnosis of occult sepsis. J Nucl Med 23:618–626
55. Bitar RA, Scheffel U, Murphy PA, Bartlett JG (1986) Accumulation of In-111 labeled neutrophils and gallium-67 citrate in rabbit abscesses. J Nucl Med 27:1883–1889
56. McAfee JG, Subramanian G, Gagne G (1984) Technique of leukocyte harvesting and labeling: Problems and prospectives. Semin Nucl Med 14:83–106
57. Peters AM (1994) The utility of Tc-99m HMPAO leukocytes for imaging infection. Semin Nucl Med 24:110–127
58. Datz FL (1994) Indium-111 labeled leukocytes for the detection of infection: current status. Semin Nucl Med 24:92–109
59. Schauwecker DS (1992) The scintigraphic diagnosis of osteomyelitis. AJR 158:9–18
60. Rubin RH, Fischman AJ, Callahan JR et al (1989) Indium-111 labeled non-specific immunoglobulin scanning in the detection of focal infection. N Engl J Med 321:935–940
61. Buscombe JR, Lui D, Ensing G et al (1990) Tc-99m-human immunoglobulin (HIG) – first results of a new agent for the localization of infection and inflammation. Eur J Nucl Med 16:649–655
62. Dominguez-Gadea L, Martin-Curto LM, Diez L et al (1993) Scintigraphic findings in Tc-99m antigranulocyte monoclonal antibody imaging of vertebral osteomyelitis. Eur J Nucl Med 20:940 (abstract)
63. Fischman AJ, Rubin RH, Khaw BA et al (1988) Detection of acute inflammation with In-111 labeled non-specific polyclonal IgG. Semin Nucl Med 18:335–344
64. Glaubitt D, Függe K, Witt U, Schäfer E (1993) Clinical value of delayed images in immunoscintigraphy using I-123 labeled monoclonal antigranulocyte antibodies in infection. Eur J Nucl Med 20:941 (abstract)
65. Lind P, Langsteger W, Koltringer P et al (1990) Immunoscintigraphy of inflammatory processes wtih a technetium-99m labeled monoclonal antigranulocyte antibody (MAb BW 250tl83). J Nucl Med 31:417-423
66. Oyen WJG, Claessens RAMJ, VanHorn JR et al (1990) Scintigraphic detection of bone and joint infections with indium-111 labeled nonspecific polyclonal human immunoglobulin G. J Nucl Med 31:403–412
67. Oyen WJG, Netten PM, Lemmens JAM et al (1992) Evaluation of infectious diabetic foot complications with indium-111 labeled human nonspecific immunoglobulin G. J Nucl Med 33:1330–1336
68. Rubin RH, Young LS, Hansen WP et al (1988) Specific and non-specific imaging of localized Fisher immunotype 1 and Pseudomonas Aeruginosa infection with radiolabeled monoclonal antibody. J Nucl Med 29:651–656
69. Serafini A, Alavi A, Tumeh S et al (1993) Multicenter phase II trial of In-DTPA-IgG. Eur J Nucl Med 20:825
70. Sciuk J, Brandau W, Vollet B et al (1991) Comparison of technetium-99m polyclonal human immunoglobulin and technetium-99m monoclonal antibodies for imaging chronic osteomyelitis. Eur J Nucl Med 18:401–407
71. Oyen WJG, VanHorn JR, Claessens RAMJ, Slooff JJH, van der Meer JWM, Corstens HM (1992) Diagnosis of bone, joint and joint prosthesis infections with In-111 labeled nonspecific human immunoglobulin G scintigraphy. Radiology 182:195–199
72. Rubin RH, Fischman AJ, Needleman M et al (1989) Radiolabeled, non-specific polyclonal human immunoglobulin in the detection of focal inflammation by scintigraphy: comparison with gallium-67 citrate and technetium-99m-labeled albumin. J Nucl Med 30:385–389
73. Reuland P, Winker KH, Heuchert T, Ruck P, Muller-Schuenburg W, Weller S, Feine U (1991) Detection of infection in post-operative orthopedic patients with Tc-99m labeled monoclonal antibodies against granulocytes. J Nucl Med 32:2209–2214
74. Kaim A, Maurer T, Ochsner P, Jundt G, kirsch E, Muller-Brand J (1997) Chronic complicated osteomyelitis of the appendicular skeleton: diagnosis with technetium-99m labeled monoclonal antigranulocyte antibody-immunoscintigraphy. Eur J Nucl Med 24:732–738
75. Rubin RH, Fischman AJ (1996) Radionuclide imaging of infection in the immunocompromised host. Clin Infect Dis 22:414–422
76. Van der Laken CJ, Boerman OC, Oyen WJG, van den Ven MTP, Edwards DS, Barrett JA, van der Meer JWM, Corsten FHM (1997) Technetium-99m labeled chemotactic peptides in acute infection and sterile inflammation. J Nucl Med 38:1310–1315
77. Babich JW, Tompkins RG, Graham W, Barrow SA, Fischman AJ (1997) Localization of radiolabeled chemotactic peptide at focal sites of Escherichia coli infection in rabbits: evidence for a receptor specific mechanism. J Nucl Med 38:1316–1322
78. Vallabhajosula S (1997) Tc-99m labeled chemotactic peptides: specific for imaging infection. JNM 38:1322–1326
79. Morgan JR, Williams LA, Howard CB (1985) Technetium labeled liposome imaging for deep seated infection. Br J Radiol 58:35–39
80. O'Sullivan MM, Powell N, French AP, Williams KE, Morgan JR, Williams BD (1988) Inflammatory joint disease: a comparison of liposome scanning, bone scanning and radiography. Ann Rheum Dis 47:485–491
81. Williams BD, O'Sullivan M, Saggu GS, Wiliams KE, Williams LA, Morgan JR (1987) Synovial accumulation of technetium labeled liposomes in rheumatoid arthritis. Ann Rheum Dis 46:314–318
82. Love WG, Amos N, Kellaway IW, Williams BD (1990) Specific accumulation of cholestrol-rich liposomes in the inflammatory tissue in rats with adjuvant arthritis. Ann Rheum Dis 49:611–614
83. Boerman OC, Storm G, Oyen WJG, van Bloois L, van der Meer JM (1995) Sterically stabilized liposmes labeled with In-111 to image focal infection. J Nucl Med 36:1639–1644
84. Matthies A, Hickeson M, Cuchiara A, Alavi A (2002) Dual time point F-18 FDG for the evaluation of pulmonary nodules. J Nucl Med 43:871–875

85. Handmaker H, Leonards R (1976) The bone scan in inflammatory osseous disease. Semin Nucl Med 6:95–105
86. Alazraki N, Dries D, Datz F et al (1985) Value of a 24 hour image (four phase bone scan) in assessing osteomyelitis in patients with peripheral vascular disease. J Nucl Med 26:711–717
87. Israel O, Gips S, Jerushalmi J et al (1987) Osteomyelitis and soft tissue infection: differential diagnosis with 24 hour/4 hour ratio of Tc-99m MDP uptake. Radiology 163:725–726
88. Bihl H, Rossler B, Borr U (1992) Assessment of infectious conditions in the musculoskeletal system: experience with Tc-99m HIG in 120 patients. J Nucl Med 33:839
89. Gilday DL, Paul DJ, Paterson J (1975) Diagnosis of osteomyelitis in children by combined blood pool and bone imaging. Radiology 117:331–335
90. Howie DW, Savage JP, Wilson TG et al (1983) The technetium phosphate bone scan in the diagnosis of osteomyelitis in childhood. J Bone Joint Surg 65A:431–437
91. Kolyvas E, Rosenthall L, Ahronheim GA et al (1978) Serial Ga-67 citrate imaging during treatment of acute osteomyelitis in childhood. Clin Nucl Med 3:461–466
92. Lisbona R, Rosenthall L (1977) Observations on sequential use of Tc-99m phosphate complex and Ga-67 imaging in osteomyelitis, cellulitis and septic arthritis. Radiology 123:123–129
93. Majd M, Frankel RS (1976) Radionuclide imaging in skeletal inflammatory and ischemic disease in children. AJR 126:832–841
94. Maurer AH, Chen DC, Camargo EE et al (1981) Utility of three phase skeletal scintigraphy in suspected osteomyelitis: concise communications. J Nucl Med 22:941–949
95. Schauwecker DS (1992) The scintigraphic diagnosis of osteomyelitis. AJR 158:9–18
96. Connolly LP, Connolly SA, Drubach LA, Jaramillo D, Treves ST (2002) Acute hematogenous osteomyelitis of children: assessment of skeletal scintigraphy-based diagnosis in the era of MRI. J Nucl Med 43:1310–1316
97. Tuson GE, Hoffman EB, Mann MD (1994) Isotope bone scanning for acute osteomyelitis and septic arthritis in children. J Bone Joint Surg (Br) 76B:306–310
98. Handmaker H, Giammona ST (1984) Improved early diagnosis of acute inflammatory skeletal-articular diseases in children: a two radiopharmaceutical approach. Pediatrics 73:661–669
99. Sfakianakis GN, Scoles P, Welch M et al (1978) Evolution of the bone imaging findings in osteomyelitis. J Nucl Med 19:706
100. Pennington WT, Mott MP, Thometz JG, Sty JR, Metz D (1999) Photopenic bone scan soteomyelitis: a clinical perspective. J Pediare Orthop 19:695–698
101. Demopulos GA, Black EE, McDougall R (1988) Role of radionuclide imaging in the diagnosis of acute osteomyelitis. J Pediatr Orthop 8:558–565
102. Fleisher GR, Paradise TE, Plottin SA, Borden S (1980) Falsely normal radionuclide scans for osteomyelitis. Am J Dis Child 134:499–502
103. Rinsky L, Goris ML, Schurman DJ et al (1977) Technetium bone scanning in experimental osteomyelitis. Clin Orthop 128:361–366
104. Sullivan DC, Rosenfield NS, Ogden J et al (1980) Problems in the scintigraphic detection of osteomyelitis in children. Radiology 135:731–736
105. Wald ER, Mirror R, Gartner JC (1980) Pitfalls in the diagnosis of acute osteomyelitis by bone scan. Clin Pediatr 19:597–600
106. Al-Sheikh W, Sfakianakis GN, Mnaymneh W et al (1985) Subacute and chronic bone infections: diagnosis using In-111, Ga-67 and Tc-99m MDP bone scintigraphy and radiography. Radiology 155:501–506
107. Hadjipavlou A, Lisbona R. Rosenthall L (1983) Difficulty of diagnosing infected hypertrophic pseudoarthrosis by radionuclide imaging. Clin Nucl Med 8:45–49
108. Ivanovic V, Dodig D, Livakovic M et al (1990) Comparison of three phase bone scan, three phase Tc-99m HMPAO leukocyte scan and gallium-67 scan in chronic bone infection. Prog Clin Biol Res 355:189–198
109. Keenan AM, Tindel NL, Alavi A (1989) Diagnosis of pedal osteomyelitis in diabetic patients using current scintigraphic techniques. Arch Intern Med 149:2262–2266
110. Larcos G, Brown ML, Sutton RT (1991) Diagnosis of osteomyelitis of the foot in diabetic patients: value of In-111 leukocyte scintigraphy. AJR 157:527–531
111. Lewin JS, Rosenfield NS, Hoffer PB et al (1986) Acute osteomyelitis in children: combined Tc-99m and Ga-67 imaging. Radiology 158:795–804
112. Magnuson JE, Brown ML, Mauser MF et al (1988) In-111 labeled leukocyte scintigraphy in suspected orthopedic prosthesis infection: comparison with other modalities. Radiology 168:235–239
113. Maurer AH, Millmond SH, Knight LC et al (1986) Infection in diabetic osteoarthropathy: use of indium-labeled leukocytes for diagnosis. Radiology 161:221–225
114. Modic MT, Pflanze W, Feiglin DH et al (1986) Magnetic resonance imaging of musculoskeletal infections. Radiol Clin North Am 24:247-258
115. Newman LG, Waller J, Palestro CJ et al (1991) Unsuspected osteomyelitis in diabetic foot ulcers: diagnosis and monitoring by leukocyte scanning with In-111 oxyquinoline. JAMA 266:1246–1251
116. Park HM, Wheat LJ, Siddiqui AR et al (1982) Scintigraphic evaluation of diabetic osteomyelitis: concise communication. J Nucl Med 23:569-573
117. Ruther W, Hotze A, Moller F et al (1990) Diagnosis of bone and joint infection by leukocyte scintigraphy: a comparative study with Tc-99m HMPAO labeled leukocytes, Tc-99m labeled antigranulocyte antibodies and Tc-99m labeled nanocolloid. Arch Orthop Trauma Surg 110:26–32
118. Schauwecker DS, Park HM, Mock BH et al (1984) Evaluation of complicating osteomyelitis with Tc-99m MDP, In-111 granulocytes and Ga-67 citrate. J Nucl Med 25:849–853
119. Splittgerber GF, Spiegelhoff DR, Buggy BP (1989) Combined leukocyte and bone imaging used to evaluate diabetic osteoarthropathy and osteomyelitis. Clin Nucl Med 14:156–160
120. Sugarman B (1987) Pressure sores and underlying bone infection. Arch Intern Med 147:553–555
121. Unger E, Moldofsky P, Gatenby R et al (1988) Diagnosis of osteomyelitis by MR imaging. AJR 150:605–610
122. Seldin DW, Heiken JP, Feldman F et al (1985) Effect of soft tissue pathology on detection of pedal osteomyelitis in diabetics. J Nucl Med 26:988–993
123. Scoles PV, Hilty MD, Sfakianakis GN (1980) Bone scan patterns in acute osteomyelitis. Clin Orthop 153:210–217
124. Namey TC, Halla JT (1978) Radiographic and nucleographic techniques. Clin Rheum Dis 4:95–132
125. Deysine M, Rafkin H, Teicher I et al (1975) The detection of acute experimental osteomyelitis with gallium-67 citrate scanning. Surg Gynecol Obstet 141:40–42
126. Rosenthall L, Kloiber R, Damtew B et al (1982) Sequential use of radiophosphate and radiogallium imaging in the differential diagnosis of bone, joint and soft tissue infection: quantitative analysis. Diagn Imag 51:249–258
127. Tumeh SS, Aliabadi P, Weissman BN et al (1986) Chronic

osteomyelitis: bone and gallium scan patterns associated with active disease. Radiology 158:685–688

128. Knight D, Gary HW, Bessent RG (1988) Imaging for infection: caution required with the Charcot joint. Eur J Nucl Med 13:523–526

129. Seabald JE, Nepola JV, Conrad GR et al (1989) Detection of osteomyelitis at fracture nonunion sites: comparison of two scintigraphic methods. AJR 152:1021–1027

130. Modic M, Feiglin DH, Piraino DW et al (1985) Vertebral osteomyelitis: assessment using MR. Radiology 57:157–166

131. Love C, Petel M, Lonner BS, Tomas MB, Palestro CJ (2000) Diagnosing spinal osteomyelitis: a comparison of bone and Ga-67 scintigraphy and magnetic resonance imaging. Clin Nucl Med 25:963–977

132. Kolindou A, Liu Y, Ozker K, Krasnow A, Isitman AT, Hellman RS, Collier BD (1996) In-11 WBC imaging of osteomyelitis in patients with underlying bone scan abnormalities. Clin Nucl Med 21:183–191

133. McCarthy K, Velchik MG, Alavi A et al (1988) Indium-111-labeled white blood cells in the detection of osteomyelitis complicated by a preexisting condition. J Nucl Med 29:1015–1021

134. Lewis VL, Bailey MH, Pulawski G et al (1988) The diagnosis of osteomyelitis in patients with pressure sores. Plastic Reconstr Surg 81:229–232

135. Borman TR, Johnson RA, Sherman FC (1986) Gallium scintigraphy for the diagnosis of septic arthritis and osteomyelitis in children. J Pediatr Orthop 6:317–325

136. Seabald JE, Ferlic RJ, Marsh JL et al (1993) Periarticular bone sites associated with traumatic injury: false-positive findings with In-111 labeled white blood cells and Tc-99m MDP scintigraphy. Radiology 186:845–849

137. Schauwecker DS (1989) Osteomyelitis: diagnosis with indium-111 labeled leukocytes. Radiology 171:141–146

138. Ezuddin S, Yuille D, Spiegelhoff D (1992) The role of dual bone and WBC scan imaging in the evaluation of osteomyelitis and cellulitis using both planar and SPECT imaging. J Nucl Med 33:839

139. Roddie ME, Peters AM, Danpure HJ et al (1988) Inflammation: imaging with Tc-99m-HMPAO-labeled leukocytes. Radiology 166:767–772

140. Verlooy H, Mortelmans L, Verbruggen A et al (1990) Tc-99m HMPAO labeled leukocyte scanning for detection of infection in orthopedic surgery. Prog Clin Biol Res 355:181–187

141. Vorne M, Lantto S, Paakkinen S, Salo S, Soini I (1989) Clinical comparison of Tc-99m-HMPAO labeled leukocytes and Tc-99m nanocolloid in the detection of inflammation. Acta Radiol 30:633–637

142. Vorne M, Soini I, Lantto T et al (1989) Technetium-99m-HMPAO-labeled leukocytes in detection of inflammatory lesions: comparison with gallium-67-citrate. J Nucl Med 30:633–637

143. Fishman JA, Strauss HW, Fishman AJ et al (1991) Imaging of pneumocystis carinii pneumonia with In-111 labeled non-specific polyclonal IgG: an experimental study. Nucl Med Commun 12:175–178

144. Rubin RH, Fishman AJ (1994) The use of radiolabeled non specific immunoglobulin in the detection of focal inflammation. Semin Nucl Med 24:169–179

145. Gratz S, Braun HG, Behr TM et al (1997) Photopenia in chronic vertebral osteomyelitis with technetium 99m antigranulocyte antibody. J Nucl Med 38:211–216

146. Abramovici J, Rubinstein M (1988) Tc-99m nanocolloids: an alternative approach to diagnosis of inflammatory lesions of bones and joints (abstract). Eur J Nucl Med 24:244

147. Filvik G, Sloth M, Rydholm U et al (1993) Technetium-99m nanocolloid scintigraphy in orthopedic infections: a comparison with indium-111-labeled leukocytes. J Nucl Med 34:1646–1650

148. Streule K, de Schrijver M, Fridrich R (1988) Tc99 labeled HSA-nanocolloid versus In-111 oxine-labeled granulocytes in detecting skeletal septic process. Nucl Med Commun 9:59–67

149. Brudin LH, Valind SO, Rhodes CG et al (1994) Fluorine-18 deoxyglucose uptake in sarcoidosis measured with positron emission tomography. Eur J Nucl Med 21:297–305

150. Sugawara Y, Gutowski TD, Fischer SJ et al (1999) Uptake of positron emission tomography tracers in experimental bacterial infections: a comparative biodistribution study of radiolabeled FDG, thymidine, L-methionine, Ga-67-citrate and I-125 HAS. Eur J Nucl Med 26:333–341

151. Kalicke T, Schmitz A, Risse JH et al (2000) Fluorine-18 fluorodeoxyglucose PET in infectious bone diseases: results of histopathologically confirmed cases. Eur J Nucl Med 27:524–528

152. Guhlmann A, Brecht-Krauss D, Sugar G, Glatting G, Kotzerke J, Kinzi L Reske SN (1998) Chronic osteomyelitis: detection with FDG PET and correlation with histopathologic findings. Radiology 206:749–753

153. Guhlman A, Brecht-Kraus D, Sugar G et al (1998) Fluorine-18-FDG PET and technitium-99m antigranulocyte antibody in chronic osteomyelitis. J Nucl Med 39:2145–2152

154. Zhuang HM, Duarte PS, Poudehnad M et al (2000) The exclusion chronic osteomyelitis with F-18 fluorodeoxyglucose poitron tomography imaging. Clin Nucl Med 25:281–284

155. De Winter F, Dierckx R, de Bondt P et al (2000) FDG PET as a single technique is more accurate than the combination bone scan/white blood cell scan in chronic orthopedic infection (COI). J Nucl Med 41:59 (abstract)

156. De Winter F, Van de Wiele C, Vandenberghe S, de Bondt P, de Clercq D, D'Asseler Y, Dierckx R (2001) Coincidence camera FDG for the diagnosis of chronic orthopedic infections: a feasibility study; J Comput Assist Tomogr 25:184–189

157. Tailji S, Yacoub TY, Abdella N, Albunni A, Mahmoud A, Doza B, Loutfi I, Al-Za'abi K, Heiba S, Elgazzar A (1999) Optimization of simultaneous dual In-111 labeled leukocytes and Tc-99m MDP bone scans in diabetic foot (abstract). Eur J Nucl Med, 26:1201

158. Vesco L, Boulahdour H, Hamissa S, Kretz S, Montazel J, Perlemuter L, Meignan M, Rahmouni A (1999) The value of combined radionuclide and magnetic resonance imaging in the diagnosis and conservative management of minimal or localized osteomyelitis of the foot in diabetes mellitus. Metabolism 48:922–927

159. Palestro CJ, Mehta HH, Patel M, Freeman SJ, Harrington WN, Tomas MB, Marwin SE (1998) Marrow versus infection in Charcot joint: Indium-111 leukocyte and technetium 99m sulfur colloid scintigraphy. JNM 39:349–350

160. Kaim A, Ledermann HP, Bongartz G, Messmer P, Muller-Brand J, Steinbrich W (2000) Chronic post-traumatic osteomyelitis of the lower extremity: comparison of magnetic resonsnce imaging and combined bone scintigraphy/immunoscintigraphy with radiolabelled monoclonal antigranulocyte antibodies. Skeletal Radiol 29:378–386

161. Mandell GA (1996) Imaging in the diagnosis of musculoskeletal infections in children. Curr Probl Pediatr 26:218–237

162. Greenwald L, Fajman W (1982) Utility of gallium scans in differentiating osteomyelitis from infection in sickle cell patients. Clin Nucl Med 7:71 (abstract)

163. Palestro CJ, Torres MA (1997) Radionuclide imaging in orthopedic infections. Semin Nucl Med 27:334–345
164. Grerand S, Dolan M, Laing P, Bird M, Smith ML, Klenerman L (1996) Diagnosis of osteomyelitis in neuropathic foot ulcers. J Bone Joint Surg (Br) 78-B:51–55
165. Newman LG, Waller J, Palestro CJ, Hermann G, Klein MJ, Schwatrz M, Harrington E et al (1992) Leukocyte scanning with 111-In is superior to magnetic resonance imaging in diagnosis of clinically unsuspected osteomyelitis in diabetic foot ulcers. Diabetes Care 15:1527–1530
166. Cook TA, Rahim N, Simpson HC, Galland RB (1996) Magnetic resonance imaging in the management of diabetic foot infection. Br J Surg 83:245–248
167. Morrison W, Schweitzer ME, Wapner KL, Hecht PJ, Gannon FH, Behm WR (1995) Osteomyelitis in diabetics: clinical accuracy, surgical utility and cost effectiveness of MR imaging. Radiology 196:557–564
168. Eckman MH, Greenfield S, Mackey WC, Wong JB, Kaplan S, Sulivan L et al (1995) Foot infections in diabetic patients. JAMA 273:712–720
169. Whalen IL, Brown ML, McLeod R et al (1991) Limitations of indium leukocyte imaging for the diagnosis of spine infections. Spine 16:193–197
170. Palestro Cl, Kim CK, Swyer A et al (1991) Radionuclide diagnosis of vertebral osteomyelitis: indium-111-leukocyte and technetium-99m-methylene diphosphonate bone scintigraphy. J Nucl Med 32:1861–1865
171. Fernandez-Ulloa M, Vasavada Pl, Hanslits MJ et al (1985) Vertebral osteomyelitis imaging with In-111 labeled white blood cells and Tc-99m bone scintigrams. Orthopedics 8:1144–1150
172. Hovi I (1996) Complicated bone and soft tissue infections: imaging with 0.1 MR and Tc99m HMPAO labeled leukocytes. Acta Radiol 37:870–876
173. Gratz S, Dorner J, Oestmann JW, Opitz M, Behr T, Meller J, Grabbe E, Becker W (2000) Ga67-citrate and Tc-99m MDP for estimating the severity of vertebral osteomyelitis. Nucl Med Commun 21:111–120
174. Tumeh SS, Tohmeh AG (1991) Nuclear medicine techniques in septic arthritis and osteomyelitis. Rheum Dis Clin North Am 17:559–583
175. Tehranzadeh J, Wong E, Wang F, Sadighpour M (2001) Imaging of osteomyelitis in the mature skeleton. Radiol Clin North Am 39:223–250
176. Erdman WA, Tamburro F, Jayson HT, Weatherall PT, Ferry KB, Peshoch RM (1991) Osteomyelitis: characteristics and pitfalls of diagnosis with MR imaging. Radiology 180:533–539
177. Sciuk J, Brandau W, Vollet B, Stucker R, Erlemann R, Bartenstein P et al (1991) Comparison of technetium-99m-polyclonal human immunoglobulin and technetium-99m monoclonal antibodies for imaging chronic osteomyelitis. Eur J Nucl Med 18:401–407
178. Utz JA, Lull RJ, Galvin EG (1986) Asymptomatic total hip prosthesis: natural history determined using 99mTc MDP bone scans. Radiology 161:509–512
179. Oswald SG, VanNostrand D, Savory CG, Callaghan JJ (1989) Three phase bone scan and indium white blood cell scintigraphy following porous-coated hip arthroplasty: a prospective study of the prosthetic hip. J Nucl Med 30:1321–1331
180. Oswald SG, VanNostrand D, Savory CG, Anderson JH, Callghan JJ (1990) The acetabulum: a prospective study of three-phase bone and indium white blood cell scintigraphy following porous coated hip arthroplasty. J Nucl Med 31:274–280
181. Rosenthall L, Lepanto L, Raymond F (1987) Radiophosphate uptake in asymptomatic knee arthroplasty. J Nucl Med 28:1546–1549
182. Palestro CJ, Swyer AI, Kim CK et al (1991) Infected knee prosthesis: diagnosis with In-111 leukocyte, Tc-99m sulfur colloid and Tc-99m MDP imaging. Radiology 179:645–648
183. Elgazzar AH, Yeung HW, Webner PJ (1996) Indium-111 leukocyte and Technetium 99m sulfur colloid uptake in Paget's disease. J Nucl Med 37:858–861
184. Seabald JE, Forstrom LA, Schauwecker DS, Brown ML, Datz FL, McAfee JG et al (1997) Procedure guideline for indium-111-leukocyte scintigraphy for suspected infection/inflammation. J Nucl Med 38:997–1001
185. Chacko TK, Zhuang H, Stevenson K, Moussavian B, Alavi A (2002) The influence of the location of fluorodeoxyglucose uptake in periprosthetic infection in painful; hip prostheses. Nucl Med Commun 23:851–855
186. Zhuang H, Durate PS, Pourdehnad M et al (2001) The promising role of F-18-FDG PET in detecting infected lower limb prosthesis implants. J Nucl Med 42:44–48
187. Turpin S, Lambert R (2001) Role of scintigraphy in musculoskeletal and spinal infections. Radiol Clin North Am 39:169–189
188. Epps CH, Bryant DD, Coles M, Castro O (1991) Osteomyelitis in patients who have sickle cell disease: diagnosis and treatment. J Bone Joint Surg 73:1281
189. Mandell GA, Contreras SJ, Conard K et al (1998) Bone scintigraphy in the detection of chronic recurrent multifocal osteomyelitis. J Nucl Med 39:1178
190. Girschick HJ, Huppertz H, Harmsen D, Krauspe R, Muller-Hermelink HK, Papadopoulos T (1999) Chronic recurrent multifocal osteomyelitis in children: diagnostic value of histopathology and microbial testing. Hum Pathol 30:59–65
191. Quelquejay C, Job Deslandre C, Hamidou A et al (1997) Recurrent multifocal chronic osteitis in children. J Radiol 78:115
192. Green NE, Beauchamp RD, Griffin PP (1981) Primary subacute epiphyseal osteomyelitis. J Bone Joint Surg (Am) 63:107–114
193. Rosenbaum DM, Blumhagen JD (1985) acute epiphyseal osteomyelitis in children. Radiology 156:68–92
194. Sundberg SB, Savage JP, Foster BK (1989) Technetium phosphate bone scan in the diagnosis of septic arthritis in childhood. J Pediatr Orthop 9:579–585
195. Fortner A, Datz FL, Taylor A Jr et al (1986) Uptake of In-111-labeled leukocytes by tumor. AJR 146:621
196. Unger E, Moldofsky P, Gatesby R et al (1988) Diagnosis of osteomyelitis by MRI. AJR 150:605–610
197. Marcus CD, Ladam-Marcus VJ, Leone J, Malgrange D, Bonnet-Gausserand FM, Menanteau BP (1996) MR imaging of osteomyelitis and Neuropathic osteoarthropathy in the feet of diabetics. Radiographics 16:1337–1348
198. Elgazzar AH, Fernandez-Ulloa M, Silberstein EB, Gelfand MJ, Abdel-Dayem HM, Maxon HR (1993) Diagnostic value of Tl-201 as a tumor imaging agent. Nucl Med Commun 14:96–103
199. Resnick D (1989) Disorders of other endocrine glands and of pregnancy. In: Resnick (Ed) Bone and joint imaging. Saunders, Philadelphia, pp 572–580
200. Bahk YW (2000) Noninfective osteitides. In: Bahk YW (ed) Combined scintigraphic and radiographic diagnosis of bone and joint diseases, 2nd edn. Springer, Berlin Heidelberg New York, pp 65–67
201. Swischuk LE (1989) Infantile cortical hyperostosis (Caffey's disease). In: Swischuk LE (ed) Imaging of the newborn, infant and young child, 3rd edn. Williams and Wilkins, Baltimore, pp 159–764
202. Sonozaki H, Azuma A, Okai K et al (1979) Clinical features of 22 cases with"inter-sterno-clavicular ossifica-

tion" a new rheumatic syndrome. Arch Orthop Unfall 95:13–22

203. Bahk YW, Chung SK, Kim SH et al (1992) Pinhole scintigraphic menifestations of sternoclavicular hyperostosis: report of a case. Korean J Nucl Med 26:155–159

204. Sarorin DJ, Schreiman JS, Kerr R et al (1986) a review and report of 11 cases. Radiology 158:125–128

205. Vallbhajosula S (2001) Pathophysiology and mechanisms of radiopharmaceutical localization. In: Elgazzar AH (ed) Pathophysiologic basis of nuclear medicine. Springer, Berlin Heidelberg New York, pp 23–40

206. Chianelli M, Mather SJ, Martin-Comin J, Signore A (1997) Radiopharmaceuticals for the study of inflammatory processes. A review. Nucl Med Commun 18:437–455

207. Datz FL, Morton KA (1992) Radionuclide detection of occult infection: current strategies. Cancer Invest 9: 691–698

208. Connolly LP, Treves ST, Davies RT, Zimmerman RE (1999) Pediatric application of pinhole magnification imaging. J Nucl Med 40:1896–1901

209. Lyons CW, Berquist TH, Lyons JC, Rand JA, Brown ML (1985) Evaluation of radiographic findings in painful hip arthroplastics. Clin Orthop Rel Res 195:239–251

210. Merckel KD, Brown ML, Dewanjee MK et al. (1985) Comparison of indium-labeled leukocyte imaging with sequential technetium-gallium scanning in diagnosis of low grade musculoskeletal sepsis: a prospective study. J Bone Joint Surg 67A:465

211. McKillop JH, Gray HW (1987): Sequential technetium-99m HMDP-gallium 61 citrate imaging in the painful prosthesis. J Nucl Med 28:926–927

212. Aliabadi P, Tumeh SS, Weissman BN et al. (1989) Cemented total hip prosthesis: radiographic and scintigraphic evaluation. Radiology 173:203–206

213. Mulamba L, Ferrant A, Leners N, de Nayer P, Rombonts JJ, Vincent A (1983) Indium-III leukocyte scanning in the evaluation of painful hip arthroplasty. Acta Orthopaedica Scandinavia 54:695–697

214. Ring DJ, Henderson RG, Keshavarzian A, Rivett AG, Kwase T, Coombs RR, Lavander T (1986) Indium-granulocyte scanning in the painful prosthetic joint. AJR 147:167–172

215. Cuckler JM, Star AM, Alavi A, Noto RB (1991): Diagnosis and management of the infected total joint arthroplasty. Orthop clin North America 22:523–530

216. Giurini JM, Chizan JS, Gibbons GW et al. (1991) Charcot's Joint in diabetic patients. Postgraduate Med 89:163–169

CHAPTER 3

Diagnosis of Metabolic, Endocrine and Congenital Bone Disease

3

Although metabolic bone diseases are common, they may be difficult to diagnose on the basis of clinical and radiological findings. Understanding their diverse manifestations using different imaging studies allows early and specific diagnosis. In the early stages of the disease, bone scintigraphy shows generalized increased uptake. As the disease progresses, bone scintigraphy has well-recognized features, such as focal and generalized increased uptake in the long bones, axial skeleton and peri-articular areas. Generalized uptake of the skull, mandible and sternum are other patterns. Finally, focal uptake in the costochondral junctions, soft-tissue calcification and faint, or absent, kidney uptake are additional features. Knowledge of these different scintigraphic patterns helps obtain the highest diagnostic value. Important practical applications of bone scan in metabolic bone disease are the detection of focal conditions or focal complications of such generalized disease such as the detection of fractures in osteoporosis, pseudo-fractures in osteomalacia and the evaluation of Paget's disease, particularly disease activity.

3.1 Introduction

The role of nuclear medicine in metabolic bone diseases is expanding. These conditions are not uncommon, and their diagnosis and therapeutic follow up can be enhanced significantly by understanding and utilizing nuclear medicine. The most important advantages of bone scintigraphy in metabolic bone disease are its high sensitivity and its capacity to easily image the whole body. In the early stages of these diseases, bone scintigraphy may face difficulties in the detection of disease varieties because of the usual generalized increased uptake. When the disease progresses, bone scintigraphy has well-recognized patterns (and armed with knowledge of the pathophysiology and different abnormal appearances) and its highest diagnostic value is obtained. Certain congenital diseases such as osteopetrosis, medullary-diaphyseal sclerosis and Gorlin's syndrome are highlighted below as they can be evaluated by scintigraphic methods.

3.2 Paget's Disease (Osteitis Deformans)

Paget's disease is a chronic and focal metabolic bone disease first reported by Sir James Paget in 1877 when he described five cases of a slowly progressive, deforming bone disorder he termed osteitis deformans [1, 2]. The name osteitis deformans suggests that he considered the disease to be a chronic inflammation of bone. However, it is now known that the bone-resorbing osteoclast is primarily affected in Paget's disease, and whether an infectious agent is responsible for the disorder is still uncertain.

It is thought that the disorder affects 1–2% of the population over the age of 45 years [3] and is particularly important in the geriatric population, since it is the second most common metabolic bone disease after osteoporosis among this age group [4].

The incidence of the disease varies because of its distinctive geographic distribution throughout the world. The disease is generally common in temperate countries as North America, UK, Australia, New Zealand,

France and Germany. The incidence is lower in Chile, Venezuela, Malta and Switzerland, and the disease is rare in Africa, Asia and the Middle East [5, 6] although it could be underestimated particularly in Asia [7].

An estimate of the overall prevalence of Paget's disease in the United States was at least 1% and perhaps as high as 2% of the general population. It has a near-equal sex distribution and the highest prevalence is in the northeastern states [8]. The disease increases in frequency with increasing age, affecting 3–4% over 50 years of age and 10% of those surviving to the eighth decade of life [5, 9–12].

The etiology of Paget's disease is not known. Recent progress has focused on environmental as well as genetic etiologies for this disease [13]. Many studies have pro-

posed that a slow virus is the causative agent, specifically paramyxoviruses [14] although direct observation of a virus has not been made [15–18]. The role of genetic factors in Paget's disease has been strengthened recently by the observation that as many as 15–30% of patients may have a positive family history of the disease [19].

Both bone resorption and formation occur at an increased rate in pagetic bone, but the pathology arises in osteoclasts. These primary bone-resorbing cells that are derived from the hemopoietic system; in contrast to the mesenchymal origin of osteoblasts, continuously migrate through and degrade the mineralized extracellular matrix of the bone. Reflecting their increased resorptive activity, osteoclasts in Paget's disease are markedly increased in number and size, have increased

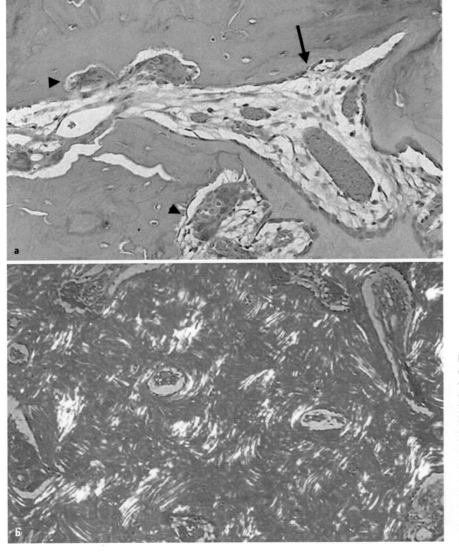

Fig. 3.1. a Photomicrograph of a mixed osteoblastic-osteoclastic stage of Paget's disease. A line of osteoblasts is present at the center-right forming new bone (*arrow*) and lacunae containing multinucleate osteoclasts are seen [center left and lower center (*arrowheads*)]. The result is a patchwork mosaic of bone without an even lamellar structure. **b** Under polarized light, the irregularities of the bony lamellae are apparent

numbers of nuclei per cell (Fig. 3.1), and demonstrate an increased resorption capacity and increased sensitivity to 1,25-(OH)2D3 (the active form of vitamin D). The responsible factor was shown to be the cytokine interleukin-6 (IL-6), a peptide produced by bone cells that increases the differentiation of monocyte-macrophage cells to osteoclasts. The excess IL-6 stimulates bone resorption and activates c-*fos* proto-oncogenes, which interfere with normal bone development. Elevated levels of IL-6 have been demonstrated in bone marrow plasma and peripheral blood in the majority of subjects with Paget's disease but not in controls. Other studies indicate a role of a recently identified candidate gene on chromosome 18q [13].

Normal bone remodeling depends on a coupled metabolic response of bone-forming osteoblasts and bone-resorbing osteoclasts. Paget's disease is characterized by an initial phase of intense osteoclastic resorption followed by an increase in bone formation. Coupling remains intact in Paget's disease, resulting in a greatly excessive, but disordered, bone. This leads to the production of excessive, dense, but structurally deficient skeletal tissue (Fig. 3.1) with enlargement and softening of the bones affected. There is possible development of bony deformities and an increased risk of fracture. When the process affects bones near joints, it promotes the development of osteoarthritic changes in these joints. Hence for many patients, joint pain and limited mobility are major complaints. Although the reasons for the osteoarthritic changes are not clear, growth factors and cytokines produced by pagetic bone cells may promote the erosion of cartilage, leading to the development of osteoarthritis. In addition, sufferers from Paget's disease are also susceptible to the development of inflammatory arthritis: gouty arthritis, rheumatoid arthritis, psoriatic arthritis, and ankylosing spondylitis. However, it is osteoarthritis that is most often the source of chronic joint pain and limited mobility.

The disease is more commonly polyostotic. Approximately one third of Paget's disease patients have monostotic disease; 72% of such cases involve the pelvic bones [14]. The skeletal distribution of Paget's disease (Fig. 3.2) suggests that the disease predominates in bones containing red marrow and may be dependent on the blood supply. Normal hematopoietic bone marrow may be replaced by loose fibrous connective tissue. With time, the increased osteoblastic and osteoclastic activity ceases and marrow abnormalities return to normal and the affected bones become sclerotic [20]. Renier and Audran [21] have reported (in a large series of 200 patients with Paget's disease), 169 (85%) with polyostotic involvement, with data suggesting that the disease process spreads across a joint in some patients, even in the absence of degenerative joint disease. (The authors reported several cases with extensive pagetic lesions seen on one side of a joint and a considerably

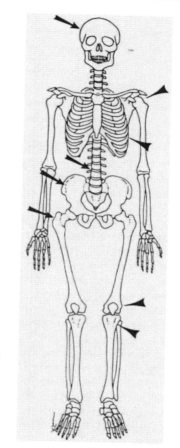

Fig. 3.2. Skeletal distribution of monostotic Paget's disease. Very common (*arrows*) and common (*arrowheads*) sites are indicated. From Resnick D: Resnick bone and joint imaging. Elsevier, 1996 (with permission)

smaller lesion on the other side.) The study also found that Paget's disease may involve paired bones and involvement could be symmetrical [21].

Paget's disease begins with a phase of active and excessive bone resorption (lytic or resorption phase) which may progress rapidly and results in softening of bone. Pathological fractures, particularly of the femur and tibia, frequently occur. During this phase the bone trabeculae are slender and very vascular. Giant osteoclasts are present and have been shown to take up Ga-67 [22]. This is followed by a mixed phase characterized by the accelerated formation as well as resorption of bone. If bone formation predominates in the mixed phase this is sometimes called the osteoblastic phase, and the term 'mixed' can be reserved for those with approximately equal resorption and formation. The final phase (the sclerotic or burned-out phase) is characterized by predominantly new bone formation, more disorganized structure, thick trabeculae and less prominent vascular sinusoids [23]. In the active phases of the disease, the rate of bone remodeling may be up to 10 times greater than normal, which is reflected by both elevated serum levels of alkaline phosphatase (a marker for increased bone formation) and by increased urinary excretion of collagen pyridinoline crosslinks (an index of increased bone resorption) [24].

In the lytic phase of Paget's disease there are increased numbers of large multinucleate osteoclasts that may show bizarre shapes and contain as many as 100 nuclei, compared with 5–10 in normal osteoclasts. In the mixed phase, a profusion of osteoblasts and osteoclasts, evidence of high bone turnover, co-exist in a matrix of highly vascularized fibrous tissue. This may facilitate the development of microfractures in long bones and basilar invagination when the base of the skull is diffusely involved. The late sclerotic phase is characterized by a disordered mosaic pattern of thickened lamellae.

Although asymptomatic in many patients, the disease causes symptoms particularly in older patients. Chronic pain is the most common complaint; it is present in two thirds of patients over 60 years old and is the presenting symptom in 5–30% of patients in general [19, 25, 26]. In contrast to the pain from degenerative joint disease, pagetic pain is typically increased at night (when the limbs are warm) and on weight bearing. Pain in the extremities may be caused by the expansion of bone with the involvement of the periosteum, whereas in the lumbar spine, pain may result from vertebral expansion, or collapse, as a result of micro-fractures [25, 26]. Localized disruption of bone architecture leads to an increased risk of pathological fractures in patients with Paget's disease, and it appears that there is also a significantly increased risk of vertebral fractures in un-involved bones [27].

Calcification of the arterial walls frequently occurs in Paget's disease. Both coronary artery disease and peripheral vascular disease may occur at a relatively young age. Vascular calcification has been observed in as many as 50% of patients and is apparent on radiographs of the pelvis that show calcified femoral vessels [28]. A previous series showed less vascular disease when Paget's disease was detected earlier; this was also found in asymptomatic cases. Cardiac insufficiency occurs in Paget's disease due to lower peripheral vascular resistance and a higher stroke volume (compared with controls). This in turn may lead to progressively increased cardiac output [29]. Paget's disease of bone is associated with an involvement of the central and peripheral nervous system. Neurological syndromes are uncommon but include headache, dementia, brainstem and cerebellar dysfunction, cranial neuropathies, myelopathy, cauda equina syndrome, and radiculopathies. Central neurological symptoms and signs in Paget's disease are caused by pagetic involvement of the skull with a subsequent reduction in the size of neural foramina. This leads to compression of the cranial nerves. Softening of the skull leads to basilar invagination with compression of the brain stem, cerebellum, and lower cranial nerves. The peripheral complications are due to compression by expanded bones [30, 31].

The most serious complication of Paget's disease is sarcomatous degeneration of pagetic bone. The incidence of sarcomatous degeneration varies from 0.1% in patients with limited Paget's disease to as high as 5–10% in those with extensive severe disease [32]. The occurrence of malignancy is more frequent in the presence of severe polyostotic disease [33] and increases with age; the mean age at discovery is 68 years. Multifocal sarcomatous degeneration, although uncommon, occurs mainly in polyostotic Paget's disease [34].

Although Paget disease can be diagnosed economically with standard radiographs, other modalities are needed, particularly scintigraphy, given the limitations of standard radiography. The early radiological lesions of Paget's disease reflect severe localized osteolysis. These are typically 'flame-shaped', or inverted 'V', lesions that most commonly occur proximal to the distal epiphysis of a long bone and then gradually progress to the opposite end of the bone (Fig. 3.3). Osteoporosis circumscripta is the term applied to osteolytic lesions in the skull. In the vertebrae, osteolytic lesions may simulate malignancy. When the disease progresses, the ingrowth of fibrovascular tissue 'mixed stage' and a high rate of bone remodeling may lead to deformities of the skull, enlarged dense vertebral bodies, and slowly progressive deformities of weight-bearing bones. It should be noted that radiologically the pagetic process may be seen to involve subchondral bone but not to cross the joint space.

Magnetic resonance imaging (MRI) can add unique diagnostic information by demonstrating bone marrow changes when they are present and can contribute

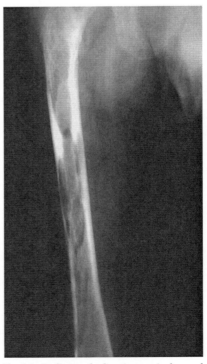

Fig. 3.3. Radiograph showing typical osteolysis pattern of Paget's disease (flame-shaped)

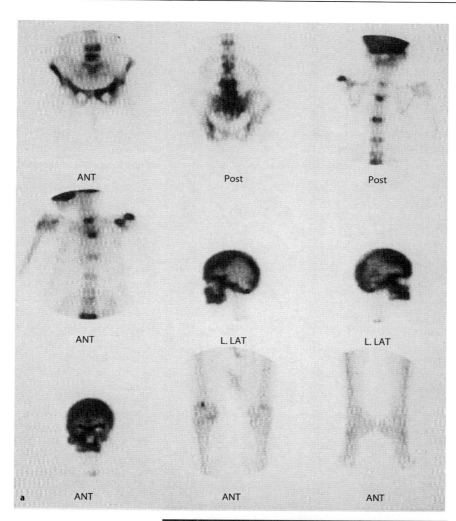

Fig. 3.4a, b. Paget's disease. **a** Bone scan of a patient with polyostotic disease involving the skull, spine, pelvis and right femur. Note the intense uptake in this case with lytic phase. **b** Standard radiograph of the skull of the patient showing the mosaic pattern

to a non-invasive diagnosis of Paget's disease in atypical presentations [35]. It can also demonstrate the presence, and extent, of several characteristic disease complications, including basilar impression, spinal stenosis, and secondary neoplasm [36].

Although bone densitometry studies have little to do with the diagnosis of Paget's disease, the bone density pattern should be known to avoid misinterpretation of density data. Although bone density may be increased in bone that is affected by Paget's disease, density in non-involved bones is unaffected. Osteoporotic vertebrae may be overlooked if the average value of bone mineral density is taken in the lumbar spine without reviewing each vertebra [37].

Using multiphase bone scanning, the dynamic flow and blood pool images, show varying degrees of hyperemia at the sites of involvement, depending on the stage of the disease; the earlier the phase, the higher the degree of hyperemia. On delayed static images, the appearance of Paget's disease depends on the stage of the

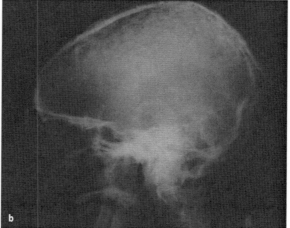

disease. During the active lytic phase involvement of Paget's disease is characteristically seen as intensely increased uptake which is uniformly distributed throughout the region affected (Figs. 3.4, 3.5). An ex-

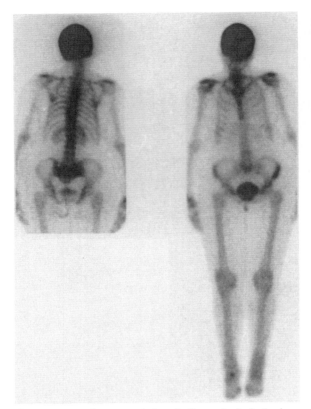

Fig. 3.5. A case of monostotic Paget's disease in the lytic phase illustrating further the regionally diffuse intense uptake in the skull

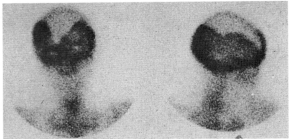

Fig. 3.6. Selected images of the bone scan of a patient with Paget's disease illustrating the cold scintigraphic pattern in the skull: "osteoporosis circumscripta"

ception to this characteristic pattern of the early phase is the pagetic skull lesion, osteoporosis circumscripta, which shows an intense uptake at the periphery of the lesion while the center is cold (Fig. 3.6) [38]. With time, the disease activity gradually decreases towards the sclerotic phase and uptake of the bone imaging agents decrease as well. With time the sclerotic phase may show practically no abnormal uptake of the radiopharmaceuticals and hence the disease can be detected by radiographs and missed by bone scanning. In about 5% of cases, the radiograph may demonstrate diffuse pagetic involvement, for example of the pelvis, whereas the bone scan reveals little uptake of the isotope. In this circumstance, the alkaline phosphatase level may be normal, or only slightly elevated, reflecting lesions that are sclerotic, relatively inactive, or burned-out.

This is in contrast to the early lytic phase, when bone scanning is much more sensitive than radiographs and will identify 15–30% of lesions not visualized on radiographs [33, 38]. Bone scanning also detects abnormalities in bones that are difficult to explore by radiography, such as those in the sternum, ribs and scapula [39].

The disease is often non-uniform within the skeleton. Individual bones can simultaneously contain more than one stage of the disease process, reflecting varia-

tions of the duration of the disease at different sites. Paget's disease may show absent and expanded bone marrow uptake or a mixture of both. This can be explained by the presence of areas of advanced, sclerotic disease with active bone marrow and areas of earlier active disease with replaced bone marrow. Since In-111-labeled white blood cells are taken up by hematopoietic bone marrow, uptake is seen in areas of Paget's disease with active marrow (Fig. 3.7). This can mimic uptake of infection particularly when it is focal [40].

The therapeutic options for treating this disorder have advanced significantly during the past decade through the development of a nasal calcitonin preparation and the newer bisphosphonates [41]. The assessment of disease activity became a key element in caring for the patient with Paget's disease. Assessment of disease activity in Paget's disease can be generally achieved by imaging particularly bone scintigraphy, laboratory parameters reflecting biochemical alterations accompanying the disease and bone biopsy. In one study a scintigraphic visual activity index, together with a quantitative activity index that reflects both the extent and activity of the disease, was obtained and added diagnostic value to the routinely used scintigraphy [42]. The quantitative activity index is calculated as a geometric mean for all the affected bones divided by a reference obtained in non-affected bones.

3.3
Osteoporosis

Osteoporosis is the most common metabolic disorder of the skeletal system. It affects approximately 20 million older Americans, 90% of who are post-menopausal [43]. Osteoporosis is „a condition in which bone tissue is reduced in amount increasing the likelihood of a fracture" [44, 45]. In other words the bone is quantitatively normal but qualitatively abnormal. Understanding the basic pathophysiology of bone density and remodeling is a prerequisite for understanding the disease and its evaluation.

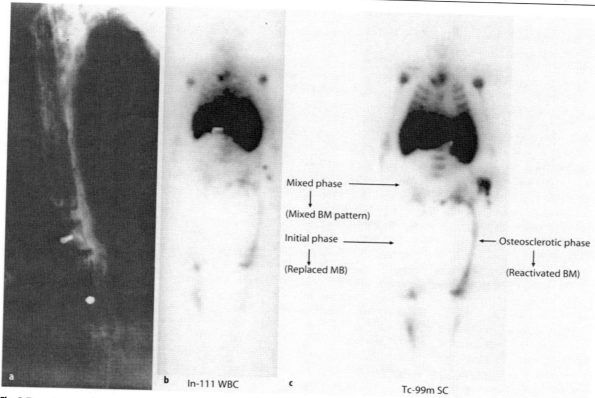

Fig. 3.7a–c. In-111 white blood cell images of pagetic bone mimicking infection in an 83-year-old man. This patient had Paget's disease at various phases who presented with a fracture of his right femur, as seen on the standard radiograph (**a**). The patient was later referred to rule out osteomyelitis at the fracture site. An In-111 white blood cell scan (**b**) showed abnormal uptake at different sites including the right femur. A Tc-99m sulfur colloid bone marrow scan obtained later (**c**) showed a concordant pattern indicating physiologic marrow uptake at the sites of the late-phase disease while it is absent at those at earlier phases (from Elgazzar A et al. [40] with permission)

Bone mass gradually increases during childhood and increases rapidly once the skeleton approaches maturity. The longitudinal skeletal growth slows [46] until it reaches the peak bone mass in the second decade although this is somewhat controversial [47]. At maturity, black men have a denser skeleton than white men and black women (Fig. 3.8) whereas white women have the least dense bones [48]. Generally men

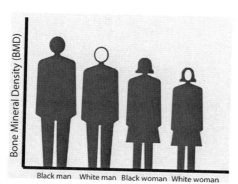

Fig. 3.8. Histogram illustrating peak bone mass density among men and women. Note that white women have the lowest value

have an average 20% greater peak-bone mass than women [49]. Peak-bone mass appears to be a major factor in determination of the risk of developing osteoporosis.

After reaching it's peak, bone mass begins to decrease at a rate of 0.25–1% per year. Men demonstrate a gradual rate of bone loss that persists throughout the remainder of adult life. Women on the other hand undergo a rapid rate of bone loss in the peri-menopausal and post-menopausal periods [49]. Loss of trabecular bone exceeds that of compact bone. Some investigators have determined that 50% of trabecular bone and 30% of compact bone will eventually be lost [50]. Generally lifetime bone losses for men are 20–30%, while some women may lose 50% or more [48]. In the post-menopausal period, women show a normal age-related annual bone loss of 1–2% in appendicular bone and about 4–8% in the spinal trabecular bone [49, 51, 52]. The factors related to bone loss in the peri-menopausal and post-menopausal periods include age-related factors, estrogen deficiency, calcium deficiency and other factors such as physical activity, smoking, alcohol consumption and medications [53].

Remodeling is crucial in maintaining the integrity of normal bone and altering the bone architecture in response to stress. Trabecular bone is remodeled more rapidly than cortical bone [48]. Trabecular bone has a turnover rate of up to eight times that of compact bone and is highly responsive to metabolic stimuli [54]. This high turnover rate makes it a primary site for detecting early bone loss and for monitoring the response to interventions [50, 55].

Osteoporosis is characterized by abnormal reduction in bone density and hence a decrease in the amount of calcified bone mass per unit volume of skeletal tissue. The basic mechanism behind this condition is decreased bone formation (osteoid formation) even though calcium deposition may be normal. The disease develops when the process of bone resorption and formation (remodeling cycle) is disrupted, leading to an imbalance. The complete remodeling cycle – activation of the basic multicellular units, bone resorption and bone formation – normally takes about 4 months in adults. In patients with osteoporosis this remodeling cycle may require up to 2 years. This can be attributed to the increase in the number of activated basic multicellular units, leading to resorption at more sites, an increased rate of resorption, an increased frequency of activation of basic multicellular units and a delay in bone formation. Osteoporosis also occurs when the number of osteoblasts and osteoclasts in bone is inadequate.

There are numerous causes of osteoporosis [56]; many are metabolic in nature (Table 3.1). Types of osteoporosis not considered metabolic in origin include juvenile osteoporosis, which affects younger individuals and is idiopathic rather than metabolic. The disease may be generalized, involving the major portions of the axial skeleton, or restricted to one region of the appendicular skeleton (Fig. 3.9). Senile osteoporosis, which is the most common type, often produces increased susceptibility to fractures in old age. Since men have a greater peak bone mass than women, men are affected by senile osteoporosis later in life. Post-menopausal osteoporosis is also common, and a deficiency of estrogen leads to decreased bone formation. This is because estrogen is necessary to stimulate the production of new osteoblasts, which otherwise fail to lay down sufficient bone matrix. The prolonged use of steroids, or steroid overproduction (e.g. Cushing's syndrome) may cause osteoporosis since it increases the ability of the body to resorb bone (Table 3.2). Smoking lowers circulating estrogen levels in premenopausal women and accelerates the onset of menopause. Smoking is also a osteoporosis risk factor in men. The disease has also been reported to be prevalent among patients with liver cirrhosis [48, 57 – 62]. In one study, the prevalence of spinal osteoporosis was 20 % in cirrhotic patients compared with 10 % in controls [63]. Regional and transient osteoporosis occurs in portions of the appendicular skeleton when there is disuse, or immobilization, of a limb such as would happen with paralysis, or healing of a fracture in a cast. Osteoporosis usually appears after about 8 weeks of immobilization.

Since the condition results in brittle, or porous, bone, patients suffer more fractures. Compression fractures of the spine, distal radius and femoral neck are more common in the presence of osteoporosis. Repeated and multiple vertebral fractures, often in the thoracic spine, may lead to kyphosis and other spinal deformities [64 – 66]. Fractures of the ribs, sternum, pelvis and feet are also common in osteoporotic patients (Fig. 3.10).

Bone density evaluation can be performed by various densitometry methods which are used for three

Table 3.1. Etiology and classification of osteoporosis [56]

Primary
a. Involutional
   Type I: Postmenopausal
   Type II: Age related (Senile)
b. Idiopathic
   Juvenile
   Adult
 	
Secondary
   1. Prolonged immobilization
   2. Steroid therapy
   3. Diabetes mellitus
   4. Prolonged heparin administration
   5. Sickle-cell disease
   6. Cushing's syndrome
   7. Rheumatoid arthritis
   8. Scurvy
   9. Multiple myeloma
   10. Osteogenesis imperfecta (brittle bone disease).
   11. Disuse or immobilization of a limb (regional osteoporosis)

Table 3.2. Risk factors for primary involutional osteoporosis [48, 57 – 62]

1. Female gender 2. Age, advancing 3. Positive family history 4. Race: Caucasian or Asian 5. Slender body habitus 6. Early or surgical menopause 7. Late menarche 8. Calcium deficiency 9. Alcohol, tobacco, caffeine 10. Medications: steroids, heparin, thyroid hormones, anticonvulsants 11. Sedentary lifestyle 12. Hypogonadism in men 13. Anorexia nervosa 14. Hyperparathyroidism 15. Hyperthyroidism 16. Primary or secondary amenorrhea

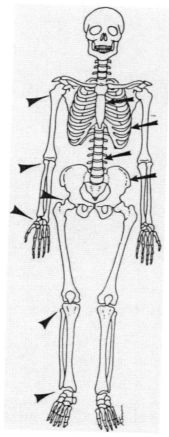

Fig. 3.9. The distribution of abnormalities in generalized versus regional osteoporosis. In generalized osteoporosis (*arrows*, on right-hand side), the spine, the pelvis, the ribs, and the sternum are affected most commonly. In regional osteoporosis (*arrowheads*, on left-hand side), the appendicular skeleton is the predominant site affected, particularly in the peri-articular regions. From Resnick D: Resnick bone and joint imaging. Elsevier, 1996 with permission

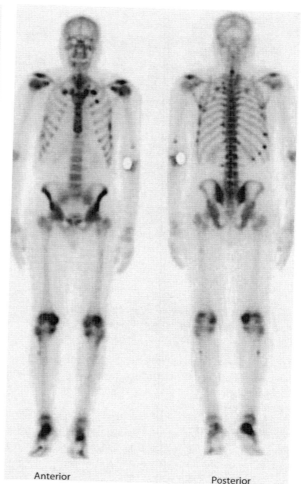

Anterior   Posterior

Fig. 3.10. Multiple insufficiency fractures in a patient with osteoporosis

purposes: (1) assessment of individuals with a high risk for metabolic bone disease and estimate the status of osteoporotic bone loss in perimenopausal women; (2) assessment of fracture risk for the spine, hip and wrist; and (3) evaluation of the effectiveness of treatment, which aims to slow down the rate of calcium and bone loss and avoid complications such as fracture and deformities. These methods measure the radiation absorption by the skeleton to determine bone mass of the peripheral, and total skeleton. Techniques include single and dual-photon absorptiometry and dual-energy X-ray absorptiometry, quantitative computed tomography and radiographic absorptiometry. Although osteoporosis can sometimes be obvious on standard radiographs, quantification of bone density from these radiographs is difficult and inaccurate. Quantitative bone densitometry is now well established in clinical practice. Dual-energy X-ray absorptiometry (DXA), however, is the most widely used technique and is considered currently the gold-standard method for the measurement of bone mineral density. It provides stable calibration, good precision, and short scan times.

A measurement of hip bone mass density (BMD) has been shown to be most reliable in the assessment of the

risk of hip fracture [67, 68]. The spine is considered the optimum site for monitoring the response to therapy [69] because the vertebrae are rich in the metabolically active trabecular bone. The rediation dose to the patient from a DXA scan is very low (1 – 10 μSv) [70]. This is comparable to the average daily natural background radiation dose of 7 μSv. For the interpretation of DXA, T-, and to a lesser extent, Z-scores are used. The T-score relates the individual's density to that of young healthy adults and the Z-score relates the density to that of the same age group. The T-score is calculated by determining the difference between a patient's measured BMD and the mean BMD of healthy young adults, matched for gender and ethnic group, and expressing the difference relative to the young adult population:

$$\text{T-score} = \frac{\text{Measured BMD} - \text{Young adult mean BMD}}{\text{Young adult standard deviation}}$$

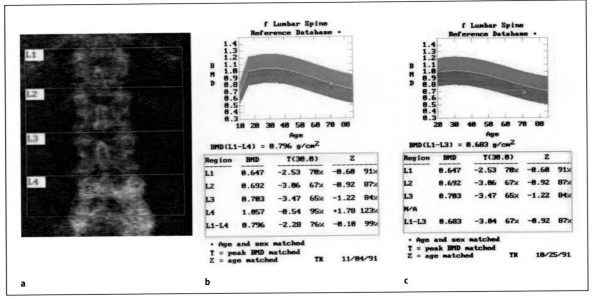

Fig. 3.11a–c. A bone densitometry study of a patient with osteoporosis. Calculation (**b**) was repeated (**c**) after excluding L-4 vertebra since it showed DJD on the scan (**a**). Final T score is < –2.5 SD

A T-score result therefore indicates the difference between the patient's BMD and the ideal peak bone mass of a young adult and it may accordingly have a negative value if decreased.

Based on the T-score values, WHO has defined osteoporosis and osteopenia [71]. An individual with a T-score ≤-2.5 at the spine, hip or forearm is classified as having osteoporosis (Fig. 3.11), a T-score between –2.5 and –1 is classified as osteopenia (Fig. 3.12), while a T-score ≥-1 is regarded as normal (Fig. 3.13). An additional fourth state of 'established osteoporosis' has also been proposed, but in the presence of one or more documented low-trauma, or 'fragility', fractures. According to the WHO definition of osteoporosis, the condition affects around 25–30% of all Caucasian post-menopausal women [72, 73]. This figure approximates to the lifetime risk of fracture for a 50-year-old woman.

Instead of comparing the patient's BMD with the young adult mean, the Z-score compare the bone density of the individual to the mean BMD expected for the patient's peers (age-matched) as expressed in the following formula:

$$Z\text{-score} = \frac{\text{Measured BMD} - \text{Age matched mean BMD}}{\text{Age matched standard deviation}}$$

Although the Z-score is not as widely used as the T-score, it remains a useful concept since it expresses the patient's risk of having an osteoporotic fracture relative to their peers. It is estimated that for every reduction of 1 SD in BMD the likelihood of fracture increases by 1.5–2.5. Accordingly, patients with a Z-score ≤1 are at a substantially increased risk of fracture compared to their peers with a Z-score of 0. Presenting bone density results using T- and Z-scores is advantageous since it avoids the confusion present when using the actual BMD values that differ among between different pieces of equipment [74].

A careful visual examination of the scan image is important in the interpretation of DXA studies before reporting T- and Z-scores to ensure that values are not affected by artifacts. For spinal scans such artifacts include degenerative joint disease (Fig. 3.14), vertebral fractures and metal artifacts, as well as the effects of body habitus such as steatopygia and bands of fat (Fig. 3.15). The affected vertebra(e) should be excluded from analysis. For example, a patient was seen who had a low-normal BMD and a bone mineral density of the L4 vertebra that was lower than the others; image analysis showed a defect in the right part of its body which was proven to be lung cancer metastasis. This again indicates that image analysis of bone densitometry should be evaluated carefully [75].

On the other hand, major sources of error in the case of the proximal femur are a short femoral neck, Paget's disease of the femur or significant osteoarthritis and incorrect rotation or abduction of the leg. The International Committee for Standards in Bone Measurement (ICSBM) have recommended use of a total femur region of interest (ROI), instead of the widely used ROI on the femoral neck site, because of its larger area and therefore improved precision. The total femur ROI cur-

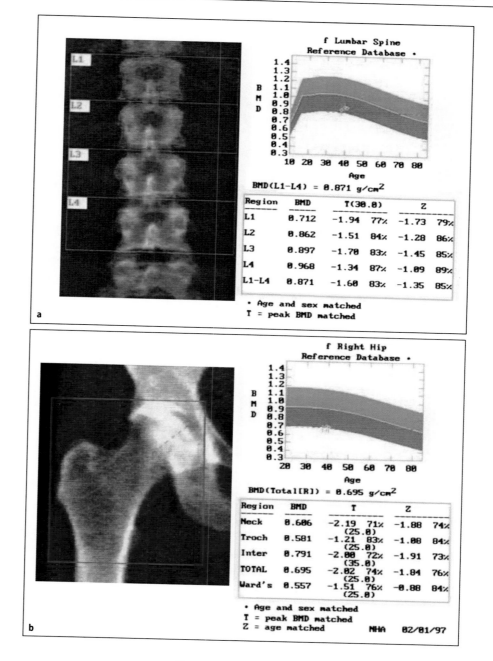

Fig. 3.12a, b. Osteopenia. T scores are between –2.5 and –1 SD

rently is being used increasingly for DXA scan reporting. In fact, using the total femur ROI and the hip BMD reference range of the third US National Health and Nutritional Examination Surveys reference range, significantly fewer patients will be diagnosed as having true osteoporosis than when using the femoral neck ROI and the manufacturer's reference range. Consistency is, however, crucial in clinical practice, particularly when it comes to the follow up of patients with osteoporosis [76–78].

3.4
Osteomalacia and Rickets

Osteomalacia arises from abnormal mineralization of bone, predominantly as a result of vitamin D deficiency, with a decrease in bone density which is secondary to the lack of both calcium and phosphorus. It is worth noting that in osteomalacia, there is a normal amount of osteoid (bone formation) while it is decreased in osteoporosis. In other words, there is inadequate and delayed mineralization of osteoid in spongy and compact

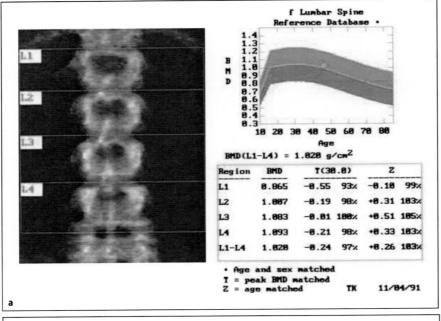

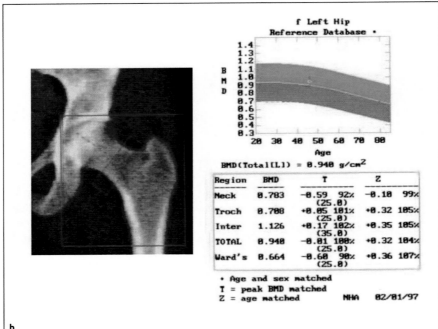

Fig. 3.13a, b. A bone densitometry study with normal T scores of > −1 SD

bone, which have a normal remodeling cycle as opposed to the delayed cycles in osteoporosis. Simply, in osteomalacia the osteoid tissue is normal in amount but soft since it lacks calcium, while in osteoporosis there is a lack of osteoid tissue as a whole. If osteomalacia occurs in growing bones before the closure of the growth plate, it is called infantile osteomalacia or rickets. Growing bones fail to mineralize and become soft with the resultant deformities. Growth plates and meta-physis are disorganized in patients with rickets with a decrease in the length and width of the growth plates.

Clinically, osteomalacia is manifested by progressive generalized bone pain, muscle weakness, hypocalcemia, pseudofractures, and, in the late stages, a waddling gait. Osteomalacia due to vitamin D deficiency is often missed or is not diagnosed promptly in susceptible patients. This is probably because physicians are not sufficiently aware of this rare condition. In a study of 17 patients with osteomalacia due to vitamin D deficiency, only four were suspected by the referring physicians, although a gastrointestinal disorder that can lead to vitamin D deficiency was present in every patient [79].

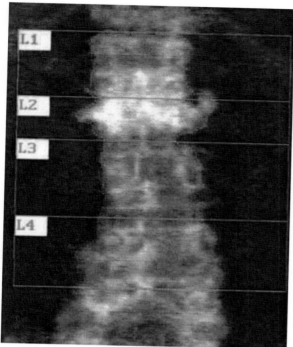

Fig. 3.14. Bone densitometry scan showing severe degenerative joint disease with compression fracture causing falsely increased bone density value which affects the mean value of lumbar spine. When the affected vertebrae are excluded from analysis the mean value reflects better the status of bone density of the spine

Pseudofractures are common in patients with osteomalacia. Among 23 patients studied by Reginato et al. [80] seven showed characteristic pseudofractures, and two showed polyostotic areas of increased uptake on bone scans mimicking metastatic bone disease caused by pseudofractures [80]. Tc-99m (V) DMSA was used in patients with osteomalacia [81]. Eight women aged 17–72 years (six with osteomalacia and two with primary hyperparathyroidism) were studied by bone scans and Tc-99m (V) DMSA scans, and many of the fracture and pseudofracture sites detected on bone scans were also visualized on Tc-99m(V)-DMSA scanning, which was suggested by the authors as having potential as a screening method in patients with metabolic bone disease [81, 82].

3.5
Hyperparathyroidism

Overactivity of the parathyroid gland(s) results in excess secretion of parathyroid hormone (PTH). This promotes bone resorption and consequently leads to hypercalcemia and hypophosphatemia. Primary, secondary and tertiary hyperparathyroidism all share elevated serum calcium and PTH.

Primary hyperparathyroidism is caused by a benign adenoma in approximately 80% of cases. Hyperplasia is essentially the cause in the remainder of cases, and carcinoma is a very rare cause. Secondary hyperparathyroidism results from compensatory hyperplasia in response to hypocalcemia. This may occur, for example, in long-standing renal failure. Reduced renal pro-

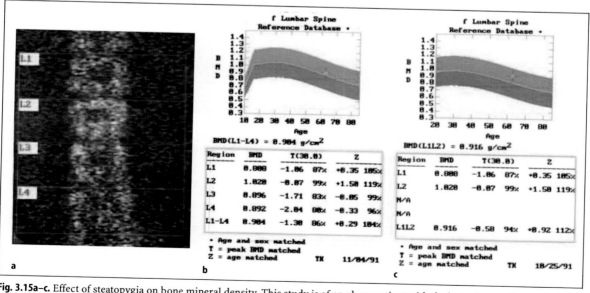

Fig. 3.15a–c. Effect of steatopygia on bone mineral density. This study is of an obese patient with the buttocks causing attenuations artefact on lower lumbar region falsely decreasing the T-value. Exclusion of L-3 and 4 resulted in normal overall T-score of the lumbar vertebra

Table 3.3. Bone scan patterns in advanced metabolic bone disease [147, 148]

Generalized increased uptake with increased contrast between bone and soft tissue
Increased uptake in long bones
Increased uptake in axial skeleton
Increased uptake in periarticular areas
Increased uptake in calvaria
Increased uptake in mandible
Increased uptake in costochondral junctions (beads)
Increased uptake in sternum („tie sternum")
Foci of increased uptake due to fractures, pseudofractures and brown tumor
Faint or absent kidney

duction of 1,25-dihydroxyvitamin D3 (an active metabolite of vitamin D) leads to decreased intestinal absorption of calcium, resulting in hypocalcemia. Failure of the tubules to excrete phosphate results in hyperphosphatemia. The hypocalcemia is compensated by parathyroid hyperplasia and an excessive production of PTH [65, 66]. Tertiary hyperparathyroidism describes a condition of persistent PTH overproduction (even after a low calcium level has been corrected) as a result of autonomous hyperplastic parathyroid tissue.

In all forms of hyperparathyroidism, there is increased bone resorption and an associated increased osteoblastic activity leading to a generalized increased uptake of bone seeking radiopharmaceuticals. This is less prominent in the primary form of the disease than in the other forms of hyperparathyroidism, which show other additional features of metabolic bone disease (Table 3.3).

3.6
Renal Osteodystrophy

Renal osteodystrophy is a metabolic bone condition associated with chronic renal failure. It is a frequent complication of renal insufficiency that has become more prevalent due to the improved survival of renal failure patients. This has lead to increased number of patients with the condition, changed our understanding and defined the forms of the disease [83, 84]. The pathogenesis of renal osteodystrophy is incompletely understood. However, two mechanisms predominate: secondary hyperparathyroidism and abnormal vitamin D metabolism following reduced renal function. Renal insufficiency results in the decreased excretion of phosphate, leading to hyperphosphatemia. This in turn causes a decrease of serum calcium and a consequent secondary hyperparathyroidism. Also, since renal tissue is the site of activation of 25-hydroxy cholecalciferol into the 1, 25-dihydroxy form of vitamin D which is the active form of the vitamin, chronic renal failure causes a decrease of the formation of the active form. This leads to

reduced gastrointestinal absorption of calcium, producing hypocalcemia.

The major skeletal changes of the disease include osteitis fibrosa cystica, rickets, osteomalacia, osteosclerosis and extra-osseous calcification, including tumor calcinosis. Slipped capital femoral epiphysis, avascular necrosis including Legg-Perthes disease in children and brown tumors are other associated pathological features [83–88]. Osteitis fibrosa is characterized by extensive medullary fibrosis and increased osteoclastic resorption linked to PTH hypersecretion. Osteomalacia occurs mainly due to aluminum intoxication, vitamin D insufficiency, hypocalcemia, acidosis and exceptionally due to hypophosphatemia. It should be mentioned that aluminum overload directly inhibits the osteoblast.

The clinical presentation of renal osteodystrophy is influenced by the patient's age at the onset of renal failure, the etiology of the renal disease, the geographical location, dietary intake (protein, phosphate and calcium) and treatment modalities. The reported prevalence of each bone change mentioned varies and does not correlate well with the clinical findings and laboratory data. Currently the disease is believed to occur in three major types: high-turnover disease, low-turnover disease and a mixed disease [65, 89–94]. An additional adynamic, or aplastic, bone disease has also emerged recently; the term has been used synonymously with low-turnover disease, but adynamic/aplastic disease should actually be considered as an extreme variant of the low-turnover type [95, 96]. The prevalence of different forms of the disease has changed significantly over the past decade. The high-turnover form is the most common and presents typically with osteitis fibrosa and is linked to the development of secondary hyperparathyroidism; hence, it is sometimes described as "predominant hyperparathyroid bone disease".

As mentioned above, high turnover can result in other disease processes locally or diffusely (Table 3.4).

Table 3.4. High-turnover disorders

Generalized disorders
Primary hyperparathyroidism
Renal osteodystrophy (certain forms)
Type 1 (post-menopausal) osteoporosis
Localized disorders
Focal osteoporotic syndromes
Disuse atrophy
Complex regional pain syndrome type 1 (reflex sympathetic dystrophy)
Transient osteoporosis (oligodystrophy)
Paget's disease
Stress fractures
Fibrous dysplasia
Myeloproliferative disorders
Wide spread metastases

Local processes include widespread metastases, fibrous dysplasia, Paget's disease and myeloproliferative disorders. The latter include myelofibrosis, leukemia, lymphoma, Waldenström's macroglobulinemia and aplastic anemia. Hyperparathyroidism, hypervitaminosis D, rickets or a combination of these represent diffuse high-turnover states and are seen in renal failure. High-turnover renal osteodystrophy is usually associated with tubular interstitial nephritis as an underlying disease of renal failure, since it is a slowly progressing form of renal pathology compared to glomerular disease, which has a rapidly progressive course with a lesser risk of developing high-turnover disease [91].

The low-turnover type may present with osteomalacia and osteoporosis, which can also occur in the high-turnover disease. The mixed form shows both osteomalacia and osteitis fibrosa. The use of high-dose pulsed intravenous, intraperitoneal and oral calciferol (vitamin D) therapy resulted in significant disease of serum PTH levels and inhibited the growth of osteitis fibrosa. These therapeutic protocols have led also to the increasing prevalence of low-turnover disease and to the development of a dynamic disease variant particularly in the pediatric population [93, 94]

Differentiation of the different forms is usually based on clinical data, laboratory findings and standard radiographs, although it can be difficult.

Radiologically, skeletal deformities, thickening of the cortical bone, thickened irregular trabecular bone, osteonecrosis, extraosseous calcification and brown tumors can all be seen with variable frequency [97]. Brown tumors present as well-defined lytic lesions that may cause expansion seen on standard radiographs since they may involve the cortical bone.

Scintigraphically, diffusely increased uptake with increased skeletal to renal uptake ratio (Fig. 3.16) occurs in the high-turnover form. This uptake may be homogeneous or heterogeneous, with focal findings depending on the predominant pathophysiological process. One or more of the typical findings of metabolic bone disease on bone scan may be seen (Table 3.3). A mixture of these findings are seen in the mixed form, while in the low-turnover form the decreased uptake can be seen if identified. It should be noted that there is

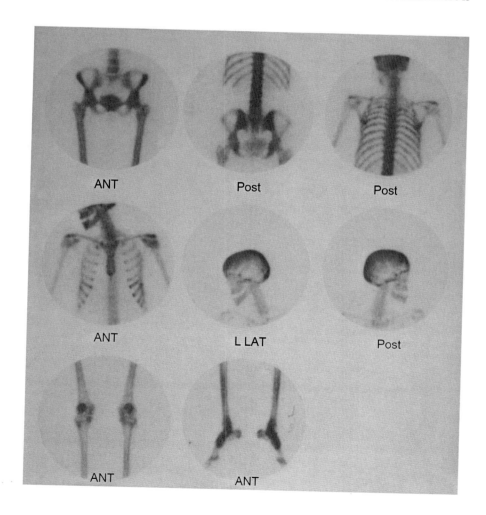

Fig. 3.16. Diffuse increased uptake of metabolic bone disease

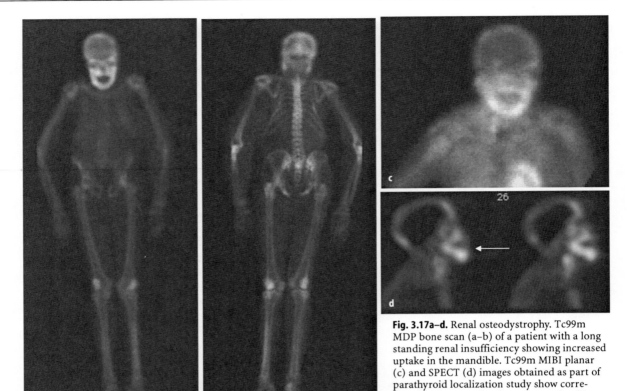

Fig. 3.17a–d. Renal osteodystrophy. Tc99m MDP bone scan (a–b) of a patient with a long standing renal insufficiency showing increased uptake in the mandible. Tc99m MIBI planar (c) and SPECT (d) images obtained as part of parathyroid localization study show corresponding increased radiotracer uptake. (From Reczek J, Elgazzar A [100] with permission)

no consistency in the patterns seen on standard radiographs and bone scans in patients with renal osteodystrophy (Fig. 3.17). Bone scanning can be helpful in differentiating between cases of osteitis fibrosa and osteomalacia [97].

So et al. compared bone scan uptake in patients with renal osteodystrophy with and without diabetes. The authors found that the diabetes group showed significantly lower uptake than the non-diabetic group and indicated that diagnosing renal osteodystrophy in diabetic patients with renal failure by bone scan could be difficult [98].

Recently bone marrow scanning, using Tc-99m antigranulocyte antibody, has been suggested for the detection of bone marrow expansion. This allows an evaluation of the extent of marrow fibrosis in patients with renal osteodystrophy [98]. Pentavalent Tc-99m dimercaptosuccinic acid (DMSA) was shown in one patient to be better than Tc-99m MDP in evaluating the response of osteodystrophy to therapy since it showed markedly decreased uptake with no significant difference before and after therapy [99]. We identified a case of renal osteodystrophy showing intense Tc-99m methoxyisobutylisonitrile (MIBI) uptake in the mandibular region of a scan that had been obtained to localize abnormal parathyroid glands [100]. This suggests that MIBI may

be potentially useful for the evaluation of renal osteodystrophy if the imaging is extended to include the whole skeleton. MRI was also used in patients with renal osteodystrophy and was shown to provide detailed information about the bone marrow [101].

3.7
Complex Regional Pain Syndrome I (Reflex Sympathetic Dystrophy)

A new classification system, collectively called the complex regional pain syndromes, has been devised in order to replace the nomenclature of pain disorders previously termed reflex sympathetic dystrophy and causalgia. A working group of the International Association for the Study of Pain (IASP) has further classified the new terminology into complex regional pain syndrome (CRPS) types I and II [102, 103]. CRPS I (previously reflex sympathetic dystrophy, RSD) is defined as a pain syndrome that usually develops after an initiating noxious event with no identifiable major nerve injury; it is not limited to the distribution of a single peripheral nerve, and the level of pain is out of proportion to the inciting event or expected healing response. It is associated during its course with evidence of edema, changes in skin blood flow, abnormal sudomotor activity in the region of the pain or hyperalgesia. The site is usually the distal aspect of an affected extremity, or has a distal to proximal gradient. CRPS II, on the other hand, replaces the term causalgia and requires identifiable peripheral nerve injury [104, 105].

The pathophysiology of CRPS I (RSD) is not well understood. Investigations of this entity have resulted in confusing and conflicting theories about the etiology and pathophysiology [105]. It is believed that an imbalance between the sympathetic and neuroceptive sensory systems occurs after trauma. Normally, afferent C and A-delta fibers carry information from the skin neuroceptors to the neurons in the dorsal horns of the spinal cord. From this region, information is transferred to the higher central nervous system levels and also directed through sympathetic neurons and their efferent fibers. These sympathetic fibers control the tone of distal arterioles and capillaries. It is postulated that trauma, which could be trivial, minor, or nerve injury, causes an alteration or imbalance of these nociceptive-sympathetic contact sites, resulting in the vasomotor disturbances, pain, and dystrophic changes which form the features of this condition [106]. It also was suggested that the accompanying peripheral edema may be caused by an increased sympathetic stimulus to the lymphatic system [107].

Synovial histopathological changes have been found in patients with CRPS I. The most common findings are proliferation of synovial cells, subsynovial fibrosis, and vascular proliferation. As a result of vasomotor disturbances vasodilatation occurs as a prominent feature, leading to increased blood flow to the synovial and osseous tissues. Vascular changes can be demonstrated on Tc-99m diphosphonate blood pool images, which show increased peri-articular activity. The cell proliferation finding is a result of a synovium reaction which eventually leads to secondary fibrosis. Although inflammatory cellular infiltration is lacking, a recent study has found that lateralization of regional hyperemia, increased micro-vascular permeability and bone metabolism in CRPS I parallel shifts in protein concentrations and blood cell counts. This suggests a subacute inflammatory process, even in patients with no overt signs of inflammation [108]. The adjacent bone undergoes increased turnover locally with some resorption. This explains the presence of radiographic and bone scintigraphic changes typical of RSD, as well as the changes at the level of the synovium.

The disorder has a wide spectrum of clinical presentations. The clinical course of the condition, which is probably under-recognized, consists of three stages: acute, dystrophic and atrophic [109–111]. The first stage is characterized by pain, stiffness, tenderness and swelling of the involved joint. In the second stage, there is still pain, tenderness and wasting of subcutaneous tissues and muscles. Thickened fascia and loss of color with cold skin are also seen. The third stage may last for months or become chronic. This stage is characterized by pronounced wasting of the muscles and subcutaneous tissue. Skin is atrophic and smooth-appearing contractures are frequent. The joints of the upper extremity are most commonly involved; among them, the wrist is the most commonly affected followed by the hand, the shoulder and the elbow [110].

Although the diagnosis of CRPS I (RSD) depends on the clinical evaluation, multiphase bone scanning has an adjunct role in the diagnostic assessment of the disease, the disease staging, predicting the response to therapy, follow-up and in determining the prognosis of the disorder [1–4, 112–115]. MRI has also been reported to be a useful modality by showing bone and soft tissue edema when the disease is clinically active. MRI bone edema was found in some patients to move from one location to another during the follow-up [113].

The scintigraphic patterns and results depend on the duration of the disease, age of the patient population evaluated, the predisposing injury, location of the disease, and the varying scintigraphic scan interpretation criteria used [105, 113]. In the first, or acute stage (20 weeks), all three phases of the bone scan show increased activity. Typically, there is diffuse hyperemia of the affected hand, or foot, and peri-articular increased uptake of the affected region (or the whole extremity) (Figs. 3.18–3.20). This pattern was found reliable for the diagnosis and in differentiating CRPS I from an inactivity atrophy [116]. After 20, and up to 60, weeks during the dystrophic phase, the first two phases normalize while the delayed phase images show increased peri-articular uptake. After 60 weeks (atrophic phase), the flow and blood pool images show a decreased perfusion with normal uptake on delayed images. In CRPS I in children, decreased perfusion and uptake are the most common manifestations (Table 3.5), a pattern that is rarely encountered in adults [117].

Table 3.5. Scintigraphic patterns of CRPS I (RSD)

Pattern on bone scans	Flow	Blood pool	Delayed images
Typical pattern	Increased	Increased	Increased
Atypical patterns			
RSD of children and adolescents	Decreased	Decreased	Increased
Paralysis, immobilization	Decreased	Decreased	Increased
Subacute	Normal	Normal	Increased
Late phase of RSD	Normal, decreased	Normal, decreased	Variable
Persistent use of painful limb	Decreased	Decreased	Decreased

Modified from [149]

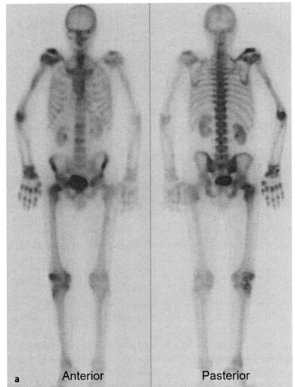

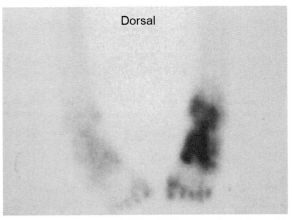

Fig. 3.19. A spot image of Tc99m MDP scan of a patient with CRPS I (RSD) involving left ankle and foot joints regions with increased periarticular uptake in these areas

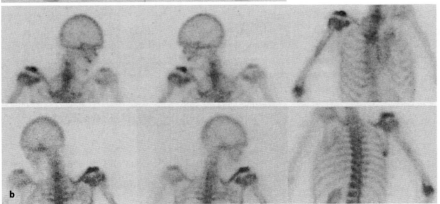

Fig. 3.18a, b. Tc99m MDP whole body (**a**) and spot images (**b**) of a 40-year-old male patient with C RPS-1 (RSD) involving the right upper extremity with periarticular increased uptake in the shoulder, elbow, wrist and hand joints regions. Increased periarticular uptake is also noted in the regions of the right hip and knee indicating possible involvement of the right lower limb as well

Multiphase bone scanning is very sensitive for detecting early CRPS I [118]. The sensitivity ranges between 73 % and 96 %, while the specificity is 86 – 100 %. Since it is a sensitive modality for the disease, it is excellent in excluding CRPS I as it has high negative predictive value [114, 116, 119].

The bone scan assessment of the disease has been found to correspond closely to the clinical course of CRPS I and also in determining the stage of the disease. This is an important determination for therapeutic decisions. Bone scans have proved accurate, and useful, in staging the disease by evaluating the degree of vascular

hyperemia on dynamic flow and early static images and the uptake on delayed static images [119]. Bone edema seen on MRI and scintigraphic radionuclide uptake remained positive for 6 months and were found to fade simultaneously thereafter [113].

When bone scan was serially performed, it was found to be useful in predicting the response to therapy. In patients with good and moderate response to treatment, the mean uptake ratios on bone images at initial scanning were significantly higher than in patients with poor outcomes. This indicates that multiphase bone scan has a prognostic value in CRPS I since

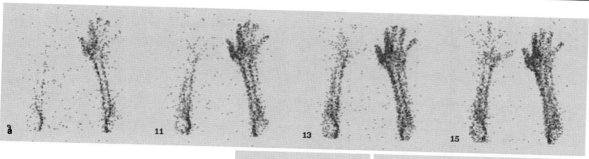

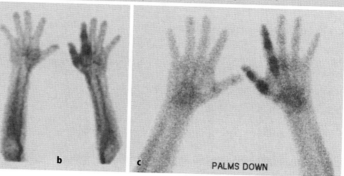

Fig. 3.20a–c. A three phase bone scan of the hands of a 42-year-old male worker complaining of pain in his right hand. There is increased flow (**a**) and blood pool (**b**) activity in the radial aspect of the right hand with increased periarticular delayed uptake around the joints of the thumb and index fingers (**c**) representing CRPS I (RSD) involving only part of the hand

marked uptake of the tracer indicates a better outcome. At post-therapy final scans, the mean uptake ratios of patients with good, moderate and poor response to treatment did not differ significantly [118].

3.8
Hypertrophic Osteoarthropathy

Two types of hypertrophic osteoarthropathy are recognized: primary and secondary. The primary type (also called pachydermoperiostosis) is less common and occurs in adolescence with spontaneous arrest of the process in young adulthood. The secondary form follows a variety of pathological conditions, predominantly intrathoracic. Lung cancer and other intrathoracic malignancies, benign lung pathologies and cyanotic heart disease are common causes. Abdominal malignancies, hepatic and biliary cirrhosis and inflammatory bowel disease are less common causes [120, 121].

The pathological condition is a form of periostitis and may be painful. Additionally clubbing of fingers and toes, sweating and thickening of skin may also be seen. Tubular bones may show periosteal new bone formation. This pathological feature explains the typical scintigraphic pattern of diffusely increased uptake along the cortical margins of long bones giving the appearance of 'parallel tracks'.

The scintigraphic abnormalities are usually confined to the diaphyseal regions, although they may also occur in the epiphyseal bone (Fig. 3.21). The changes

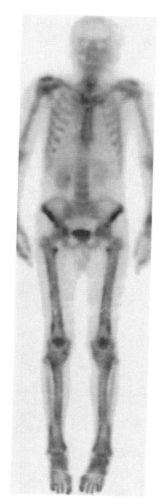

Fig. 3.21. Hypertrophic osteoarthropathy in a patient with lung cancer. Note the diffusely increased uptake in all bones of the lower extremities with a parallel track pattern in the femurs and tibiae

are usually bilateral but can be unilateral in approximately 15% of cases [121]. The tibia and fibula are affected most commonly, followed by the distal femur, radius, ulna, hand, foot and distal humerus. The scapula, patella, maxilla, mandible and clavicle are less commonly affected. The ribs and pelvis are rarely affected. The changes disappear after successful treatment of the lung cancer or other inciting pathology.

3.9
Fibrous Dysplasia

Fibrous dysplasia is a benign bone disorder characterized by the presence of fibrous tissue containing trabeculae of non-lamellar bone (woven bone) which remains essentially unchanged and can be seen in lesions of long duration [122]. The lesions cause thining of the bone cortex and replacement of bone marrow. The condition may present as solitary lesion (monostotic), or with multiple foci (polyostotic). Polyostotic fibrous dysplasia may be associated with cafe-au-lait pigmentation and multiple endocrine hyperfunction, most commonly seen as gonadotropin-independent precocious puberty in girls, Cushing's syndrome, and is called the McCune-Albright syndrome. The etiology of the condition is not entirely clear; however, there is growing evidence of a genetic mechanism. The syn-

drome is believed to be due to a constitutively activating mutation in the gene (*GNAS1*) encoding the subunit of the signal-transducing guanine nucleotide-binding protein (G protein).

Standard radiographs show lucent areas with various amounts of ossification and cyst formation and may show expansion (Fig. 3.22). Fibrous dysplasia, in

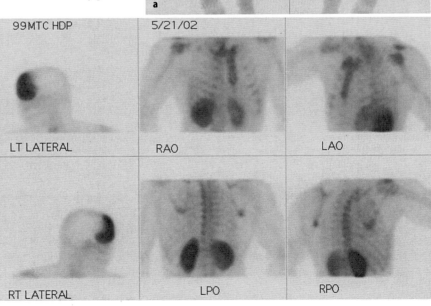

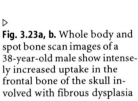

▷
Fig. 3.23a, b. Whole body and spot bone scan images of a 38-year-old male show intensely increased uptake in the frontal bone of the skull involved with fibrous dysplasia

a

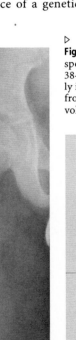

Fig. 3.22. A standard radiograph of a patient with fibrous dysplasia of the proximal right femur. Note the bone expansion

b

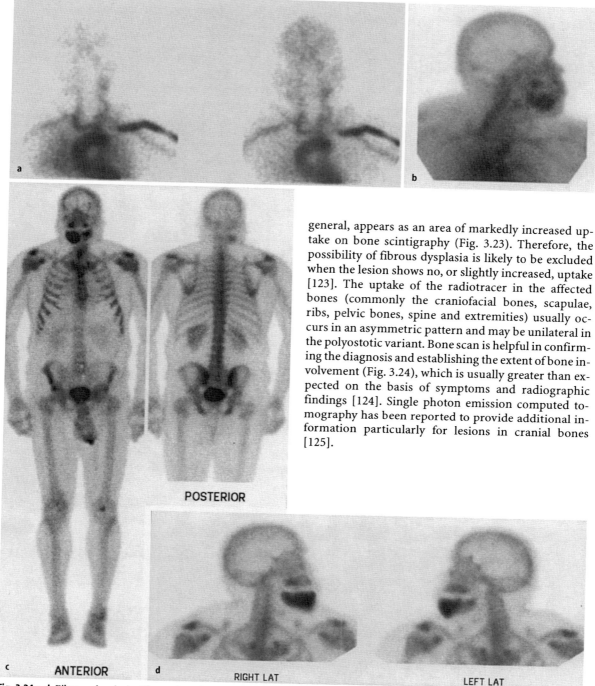

general, appears as an area of markedly increased uptake on bone scintigraphy (Fig. 3.23). Therefore, the possibility of fibrous dysplasia is likely to be excluded when the lesion shows no, or slightly increased, uptake [123]. The uptake of the radiotracer in the affected bones (commonly the craniofacial bones, scapulae, ribs, pelvic bones, spine and extremities) usually occurs in an asymmetric pattern and may be unilateral in the polyostotic variant. Bone scan is helpful in confirming the diagnosis and establishing the extent of bone involvement (Fig. 3.24), which is usually greater than expected on the basis of symptoms and radiographic findings [124]. Single photon emission computed tomography has been reported to provide additional information particularly for lesions in cranial bones [125].

POSTERIOR

ANTERIOR   RIGHT LAT   LEFT LAT

Fig. 3.24a–d. Fibrous dysplasia. Three-phase bone scan of a 61-year-old man with history of pain in the right mandible for years. There is increased flow to the region of the right mandible (**a**) and clearly increased blood pool activity (**b**) to the same region. Whole body delayed scan (**c**) and spot images of the skull (**d**) show intensely increased uptake in the right mandible. Biopsy showed fibrous dysplasia

Images of fibrous dysplasia on computed tomography (CT), or MRI vary depending on the relative proportions of the fibrous and osseous components [126]. Helical CT is the optimal method for the evaluation of the skull lesions [127].

Using MRI, the condition shows a low signal intensity on T1-weighted images while on T2-weighted images it appears as either hyperintense or hypointense [128]. MRI could be particularly useful in the identification of a no-touch lesion, allowing avoidance of an unnecessary bone biopsy [129].

A report on the use of PET on fibrous dysplasia of the craniofacial bone showed signs of the acceleration of bone mineral turnover with an increased uptake on bone scintigraphy without elevated glucose utilization on fluorine-18-FDG PET. Accordingly it has been proposed that the growth of fibrous dysplasia appears to be based on the acceleration of bone mineral turnover without an increase in glucose metabolism [130].

3.10
Other Metabolic and Endocrine Conditions

3.10.1
Hypothyroidism

Hypothyroidism can be associated with certain skeletal manifestations, particularly in children. In adults they are usually mild. In hypothyroidism the rate of bone turnover is decreased and the calcium metabolism becomes abnormal, which may result in a slightly increased bone mass [131]. Ectopic calcifications in the soft tissue may also be seen.

3.10.2
Hyperthyroidism

Hyperthyroidism is associated with accelerated bone maturation in children and increased bone turnover and remodeling in adults. In adults over 50 years, a progressive osteoporosis that is more rapid than the postmenopausal type is seen among patients with hyperthyroidism. Treatment of hyperthyroidism leads to partial recovery of bone mineral content [131].

3.10.3
Fluoride Toxicity

Fluoride accumulates in bone and, when present in abundant amounts, induces modifications of bone remodeling and causes osteoblastic stimulation and trabecular fragility [132]. On scintigraphy this causes diffusely increased uptake of the radionuclide, stress fractures with focal uptake or a pattern of osteomalacia which occurs when impaired renal function is present (even if mild) [133].

3.10.4
Aluminum Toxicity

Excess aluminum leads to blocking of mineralization by the aluminum deposits at the calcification sites. This can occur, for example, in association with renal dialysis using dialysis water containing a high aluminum content, or the use of aluminum-containing antacids, and can also lead to osteomalacia (Fig. 3.25) [134–136]. The scintigraphic pattern of this condition is distinc-

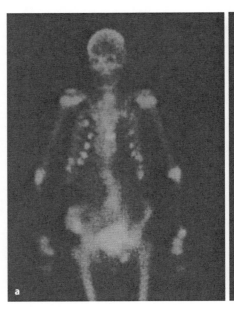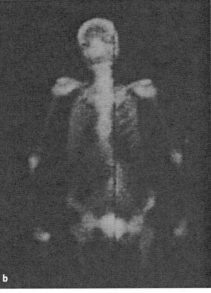

Fig. 3.25a–b. Tc99m MDP bone scan of a patient with antacid induced osteomalacia (**a**) before and (**b**) after 1 year of treatment with calcium phosphate, vitamin D and sodium fluoride. Note the increased uptake in the costochondral junctions. (From [135] with permission)

tive and bone scanning typically shows a lack of tracer uptake by bone and excessive uptake by soft tissue which reverts either to normal or to the pattern of hyperparathyroidism after treatment [136, 137].

3.10.5
Hypervitaminosis A

Hypervitaminosis A causes hyperostosis of the diaphysis of long bones. It is seen scintigraphically as periosteal uptake in the femur, tibia, fibula, ulna and/or sutures of the skull.

3.11
Osteopetrosis

Osteopetrosis is a rare metabolic bone disease characterized by a generalized increase in skeletal mass. It is an inherited disorder characterized by a congenital defect in the development or function of the osteoclasts leading to defective bone resorption. The impaired bone resorption prevents formation of bone marrow cavities, causes delayed or absent tooth eruption and results often in abnormally shaped bones. The infantile malignant form is an autosomal recessive condition and usually results in death in the first years of life. The autosomal dominant type is seen in older children and adults. In recent years the genetic effects of some osteopetrotic mutations have been identified. Colony-timulating factor 1 (CSF-1), the growth factor for cells of the mononuclear phagocytic system, which is also essen-

tial for the development of osteoclasts was found to be deficient in osteopetrotic mice [138]. Standard radiographs show a characteristic pattern of generalized sclerosis of bones. On scintigraphy, there is a diffuse increased uptake that may also be a superscan [139] and can show non-uniform uptake with foci of hyperemia (Fig. 3.26) [140].

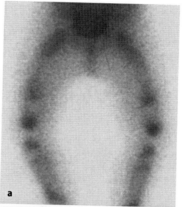

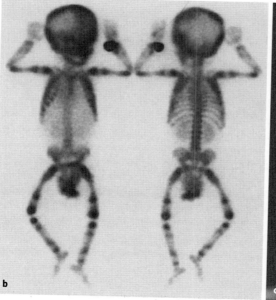

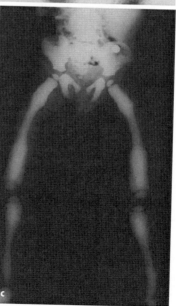

Fig. 3.26a, b. Osteopetrosis showing non-uniform blood pool activity in the lower extremities with foci of hyperemia (**a**). Delayed whole body scan (**b**) shows diffusely increased uptake in the long bones of the lower extremities and humeri. Standard radiograph (**c**) of the lower extremities show diffuse sclerosis in the femurs and tibiae. (From [140] with permission)

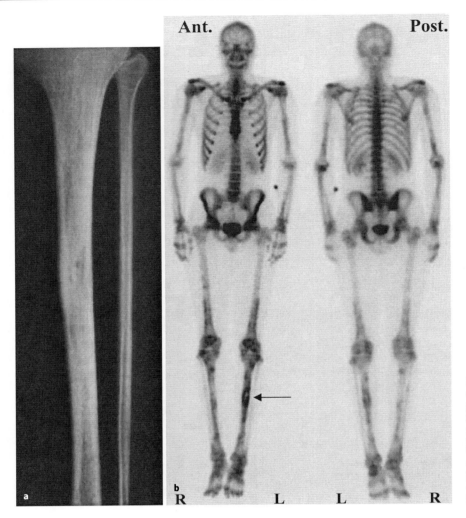

Fig. 3.27a–c. Hardcastle syndrome. A standard radiograph of the left tibia and fibula of a 19-year-old male patient who complained of pain in his left mid tibia. There is marked sclerosis of the tibial shaft. Whole body bone scan (**b**) shows nonuniform increased uptake in both femurs and tibiae.

3.12
Medullary Diaphyseal Sclerosis (Medullary Diaphyseal Stenosis or Hardcastle Syndrome)

This is a hereditary condition believed to be transmitted within families by autosomal dominant inheritance [141]. The condition is characterized by multiple bone infarcts, cortical bone thickening and medullary stenosis along the metaphyseal diaphyseal segments. It can be associated with malignant transformation with development of malignant fibrous histiocytoma [142, 143]. Bone scintigraphy has a pattern of increased uptake along the long bones with an irregular and nonuniform pattern and the malignant lesion can be identified using Tl-201 [144]. (Fig. 3.27) or, potentially, FDG-PET.

3.13
Gorlin's Syndrome

Gorlin's syndrome is an autosomal dominant condition with variable features involving many organs including the skin, teeth, eyes, central nervous system, endocrine system and skeletal system [145, 146]. Nevoid basal cell carcinomas are the most important skin lesions. Mandibular and maxillary keratocysts are the most important odontogenic feature and are of fundamental importance for the diagnosis. Calcification of the falx cerebri and tentorium cerebelli are the most typical CNS features. Skeletal abnormalities include bifid, missing or fused ribs, frontoparietal bossing, dysplastic scapula leading to shoulder deformity (Sprengel's deformity),

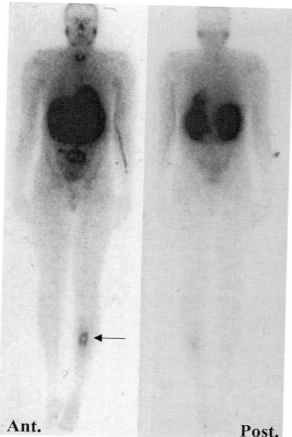

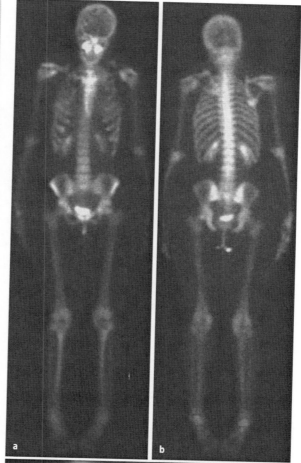

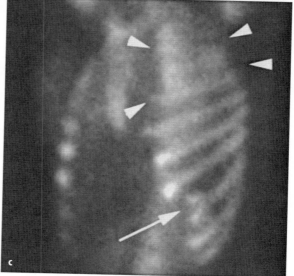

Fig. 3.27 (Cont.) TI-201 image (**c**) obtained for further evaluation of the mid left tibial uptake shows focally increased uptake in the left tibia proven later to be malignant fibrous histocytoma in this patient with Hardcastle syndrome. (From [144] with permission)

spina bifida, polydactyly of the hands and feet, and sclerotic bone lesions of the pelvis and lumbar vertebrae [146]. Awareness of the condition helps its identification on imaging; radiography and scintigraphy can show many of the typical features (Fig. 3.28).

3.14
Progressive diaphyseal dysplasia (Camurati-Engelmann disease)

A rare hereditary disorder characterized by progressive bone formation along the periosteal and endosteal surfaces of long tubular bones with widening of their shafts. Other bones are also involved including the skull. The disease is an autosomal dominant and is usually manifested in childhood but can present later. The most frequent symptoms are pain and muscle weakness. Deafness can also occur due to otosclerosis. On bone scan there is diffusely increased uptake in the

Fig. 3.28a–e. Gorlin's syndrome. Whole body bone scan (**a, b**) of a 31-year-old female known to have Gorlin's syndrome. Note the increased uptake in the maxillary deformed left scapula. Deformed left lower ribs is also seen which is clean on LAO (**c**) showing a bifid rib (*arrow*) and short ribs (*arrow heads*)

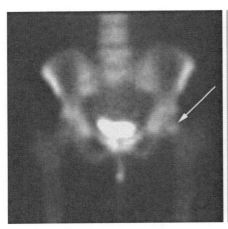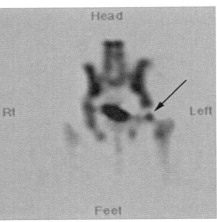

Fig. 3.28 (Cont.) Increased uptake in the left hip focally is seen also in the whole body and is further clarified on spot planar image (**d**) and SPECT coronal section (**e**)

skeleton with relative sparing of the spine, hands and feet. The degree of uptake varies and widening of the long bones may be clearly apparent.

Radiologically there is sclerosis with focal lytic areas that correspond to foci of more intense uptake on bone scan [150–151].

References

1. Paget J (1877) On a form of chronic inflammation of bones. Med Chir Trans 60:37–63
2. Coppes-Zantinga AR, Coppes MJ (2000) Sir James Paget (1814–1889) a great academic Victorian. J Am Coll Surg 191:70–74
3. Hosking DJ (1981) Paget's disease of bone. Br Med J 283:686–688
4. Hamdy RC (1981) Paget's disease of bone: assessment and management. Praeger, London
5. Barker DJP (1984) The epidemiology of Paget's disease of bone. Br Med Bull 40:396–400
6. Coleiro B, Camilleri F, Samuel A, Mallia C (1999) Paget's disease of bone in Malta. A preliminary survey. Adv Exp Med Biol 455:437–450
7. Hsu LF, Rajasoorya C (1998) A case series of Paget's disease of bone: diagnosing a rather uncommon condition in Singapore. Ann Acad Med Singapore 27:289–293
8. Altman RD, Bloch DA, Hochberg MC, Murphy WA (2000) Prevalence of pelvic Paget's disease of bone in the United States. J Bone Miner Res 15:461–465
9. Rothschild BM (2000) Paget's disease of the elderly. Compr Ther 26:251–254
10. Lecuyer N, Grados F, Dargent-Molina P, Deramond H, Meunier PJ, Fardellone P (2000) Prevalence of Paget's disease of bone and spinal hemangioma in French women older than 75 years: data from the EPIDOS study. Joint Bone Spine Rev Rhumat 67:315–318
11. Kurihara N, Reddy SV, Menaa C, Anderson D, Roodman GD (2000) Osteoclasts expressing the measles virus nucleocapsid gene display a Pagetic phenotype. J Clin Invest 105:607–614
12. Perry HM III, Kraezle D, Miller DK (1995) Paget's disease in African Americans. Clin Geriatr 3:69–74
13. Noor M, Shoback D (2000) Paget's disease of bone: diagnosis and treatment update. Curr Rheumatol Rep 2:67–73
14. Burchardt P (1994) Biochemical and scintigraphic assessment of Paget's disease. Semin Arthritis Rheum 23:237–239
15. Ran K (2000) The importance of measles virus in Paget's disease. J Clin Invest 105:555–558
16. Helfrich MH, Hobson RP, Grabowski PS, Zurbriggen A, Cosby SL, Dickson GR, Fraser WD, Ooi CG, Selby PL, Crisp AJ, Wallace RG, Kahn S, Ralston SH (2000) A negative search for a paramyxoviral etiology of Paget's disease of bone: molecular, immunological, and ultrastructural studies in UK patients. J Bone Miner Res 15:2315–2329
17. Mills BG, Singer FR, Weiner LP, et al (1984) Evidence for both respiratory syncytial virus and measles virus antigens in the osteoclasts of patients with Paget's disease of bone. Clin Orthop Relat Res 183:303–311
18. Ooi CG, Walsh CA, Gallagher JA, Fraser WD (2000) Absence of measles virus and canine distemper virus transcripts in long-term bone marrow cultures from patients with Paget's disease of bone. Bone 27:417–421
19. Ankrom M, Shapiro J (1998) Paget's disease of bone (osteitis deformans). Prog Geriatr 46:1025–1033
20. Collier BD, Carrera GF, Johnson RP, Isitman AT, Hellman RS, Knobel J et al (1985) Detection of femoral head avascular necrosis in adults by SPECT. J Nucl Med 26:979–987
21. Renier JC, Audran M (1997) Polyostotic Paget's disease. A search for lesions of different durations and for new lesions. Rev Rhum (Engl Edn) 64:233–242
22. Mills BG, Masuoka LS, Graham CC Jr et al (1988) Gallium-67 citrate localization inosteoclast nuclei of Paget's disease of bone. J Nucl Med 29:1083–1087
23. Lander PH, Hadjipavlou AG (1986) A dynamic classification of Paget's disease. J Bone Joint Surg [Br] 68b:431–438
24. Siris E, Canfield RE (1991) Paget's disease of bone. Trends Endocrinol Metab 2:207–212
25. Hamdy RC, Moore S, LeRoy J (1993) Clinical presentation of Paget's disease of the bone in older patients. South Med J 86:1097–1100
26. Krane SM (1977) Paget's disease of bone. Clin Orthop Rel Res 127:24–36
27. Melton LJ III, Tiegs RD, Atkinson EJ, O'Fallon WM (2000) Fracture risk among patients with Paget's disease: a population-based cohort study. J Bone Miner Res 15:2123–2128
28. Singer FR (1977) Paget's disease of bone. Plenum, New York, pp 103–112
29. Morales-Piga AA, Moya JL, Bachiller FJ, Munoz-Malo MT, Benavides J, Abraira V(2000) Assessment of cardiac function by echocardiography in Paget's disease of bone. Clin Exp Rheumatol 18:31–37

30. Poncelet A (1999)The neurologic complications of Paget's disease. J Bone Miner Res 14 [Suppl 2]:88–91

31. Monsell EM, Cody DD, Bone HG, Divine GW(1999) Hearing loss as a complication of Paget's disease of bone. J Bone Miner Res 14 [Suppl 2]:92–95

32. Price CH, Goldie W (1969) Paget's sarcoma of bone – a study of 80 cases. J Bone Joint Surg 51B:205–244

33. Fogelman I, Carr D (1980) A comparison of bone scanning and radiology in the evaluation of patients with metabolic bone disease. Clin Radiol 31:321–326

34. Vuillemin-Bodaghi V, Parlier-Cuau C, Cywiner-Golenzer C, Quillard A, Kaplan G, Laredo JD (2000) Multifocal osteogenic sarcoma in Paget's disease. Skeletal Radiol 29:349–353

35. Vande Berg BC, Malghem J, Lecouvet FE, Maldague B (2001) Magnetic resonance appearance of uncomplicated Paget's disease of bone. Semin Musculoskeletal Radiol 5:69–77

36. Boutin RD, Spitz DJ, Newman JS, Lenchik L, Steinbach LS (1998) Complications in Paget disease at MR imaging. Radiology 209:641–651

37. Cherian RA, Haddaway MJ, Davies MW, McCall IW, Cassar-Pullicino VN (2000) Effect of Paget's disease of bone on a real lumbar spine bone mineral density measured by DXA, and density of cortical and trabecular bone measured by quantitative CT. Br J Radiol 73:720–726

38. Serafini AN (1976) Paget's disease of bone. Semin Nucl Med 6:47–58

39. King MA, Maxon HR (1984) Paget's disease: the role of nuclear medicine in diagnosis and treatment. In: Silberstein EB (ed) Bone scintigraphy. Futura, Mount Kisco, NY, pp 333–346

40. Elgazzar AH, Yeung HW, Webner PJ (1996) Indium 111 leukocyte and Tc99m sulfur colloid uptake in Paget's disease. J Nucl Med 37:858–861

41. Garnero P, Christgau S, Delmas PD (2001) The bisphosphonate zoledronate decreases type II collagen breakdown in patients with Paget's disease of bone. Bone 28:461–464

42. Pons F, Alvarez L, Peris P, Guanabens N, Vidal-Sicart S, Monegal A, Pavia J, Ballesta AM, Munos-Gomez J, Herranz R (1999) Quantitative evaluation of bone scintigraphy in the assessment of Paget's disease activity. Nucl Med Commun 20:525–258

43. Ettinger B, Genant HK (eds) (1987) Osteoporosis update 1987. Radiology Research and Education Foundation, San Francisco

44. Schwivitz S, Djukic S, Genant HK (1990) The current status of bone densitometry. Appl Radiol; 19:20–25

45. Cooper C, Aihie-Sayer A (1994) Osteoporosis: recent advances in pathogenesis and treatment. Q J Med 87:203–209

46. Kaplan FS (1987) Osteoporosis: pathophysiology and prevention. Clin Symp 39:1–32

47. Matkovic V, De Kanic D (1989) Developing strong bones: the teenage female. In: Kleerehoper M, Krane SM (eds) Clinical disorders of bone and mineral metabolism. Liebert, New York

48. Gillespy T, Gillespy MP (1991) Osteoporosis. Radiol Clin North Am 29:77–84

49. Christiansen C, Riis BJ (1989) Optimizing bone mass in the permenopause. In Kleerehoper M, Krane SM (eds) Clinical disorder of bone and mineral metabolism. Liebert, New York

50. Lang P, Steiger P, Faulkner K et al (1991) Current techniques and recent developments in quantitative bone densitometry. Radiol Clin North Am 29:49–76

51. Snyder W (1975) Report of the task group on reference man. Pergamon, New York

52. Recker RR, Heaney RP (1989) Effects of age, sex and race on bone remodeling. In: Kleerehoper M, Krane SM (eds) Clinical disorders of bone and mineral metabolism. Liebert, New York

53. Genant HK, Cann CE, Ettinger B et al (1982) Quantitave computerized tomography of the vertebral spongiosa: a sensitive method for detecting early bone loss after oophorectomy. Ann Intern Med 97:699–705

54. Heaney RP (1989) Optimizing bone mass in the permenopause: calcium. In: Kleerehoper M, Krane SM (eds) Clinical disorders of bone and mineral metabolism. Liebert, New York

55. Frost HM (1964) Dynamics of bone remodelling. In: Frost HM (ed) Bone biodynamics. Little Brown, Boston, pp 315–334

56. Peck WA, Riggs BL, Bell NH (1987) Physician's resource manual on osteoporosis. National Osteoporosis Foundation,Washington DC

57. Resnick D, Nirvayama G (1988) Diagnosis of bone and joint disorders. Saunders, Philadelphia

58. Riggs BL, Melton JM (1986) Involutional osteoporosis. NEJM 314:1676

59. Weinstein RS, Bell NH (1988) Diminished rates of bone formation in normal black adults. NEJM 319:1698

60. MacMahon B, Trichopoulous D, Cole P et al (1982) Cigarette smoking and urinary estrogens. NEJM 307:1062

61. Seeman E, Melton LJ, O'Fallon WM et al (1983) Risk factors for spinal osteoporosis in men. Am J Med 75:977

62. Slemenda CW, HUI SL, Longcope C et al (1989) Cigarette smoking, obesity and bone mass. J Bone Miner Res 4:737

63. Chen CC, Wang SS, Jeng FS, Lee SD (1996) Metabolic bone disease of liver cirrhosis: is it parallel to the clinical severity of cirrhosis? J Gastroenterol Hepatol 11:417–421

64. Simon SR (1994) Osteoporosis: orthopedic basic science. American Academy of Orthopedic Surgeons, Chicago

65. Fogelman I (1987) The bone scan in metabolic bone disease. In: Fogelman I (ed) Bone scanning in clinical practice. Springer, Berlin Heidelberg New York, pp 73–88

66. Lack CA, Rarber JL, Rubin E (1999) The endocrine system. In: Rubin E, Farber JL (eds) Pathology, 3rd edn. Lippincott-Raven, Philadelphia, pp 1179–1183

67. Marshall D, Johnell O, Wedel H (1996) Meta-analysis of how well measures of bone mineral density predict occurrence of osteoporotic fractures. BMJ 312:1254–1259

68. Cummings SR, Black DM, Nevitt MC et al (1993) Bone density at various sites for prediction of hip fractures. Lancet 341:72–75

69. Eastell R (1998) Treatment of postmenopausal osteoporosis. N Engl J Med 338:736–746

70. Njeh CF, Fuerst T, Hans D, Blake GM, Genant HK (1999) Radiation exposure in bone mineral assessment. Appl Rad Isotope 50:215–236

71. WHO Technical Report Series 843 (1994) Assessment of fracture risk and its application to screening for postmenopausal osteoporosis. World Health Organization, Geneva

72. Kanis JA, Delmas P, Burckhardt P, Cooper C, Torgerson D, on behalf of the European Foundation for Osteoporosis and Bone Disease (1997) Guidelines for diagnosis and treatment for osteoporosis. Osteoporosis Int 7:390–406

73. Ballard PA, Purdie DW, Langton CM, Steel SA, Mussurakis S (1998) Prevalence of osteoporosis and related risk factors in UK women in the seventh decade: osteoporosis case finding by clinical referral criteria or predictive model? Osteoporosis Int 8:535–539

74. Genant HK, Grampp S, Glüer CC et al (1994)Universal standardization for dual x-ray absorptiometrey: patient and phantom cross-calibration results. J Bone Miner Res 9:1503–1514

75. Paspati I, Lyritis GP (2000) Metastatic lung cancer detected by lumbar bone densitometry: a case report. Clin Nucl Med 25:691–693

76. Chen Z, Maricic M, Lund P, Tesser J, Gluck O (1998) How the new Hologic hip reference values affect the densitometric diagnosis of osteoporosis. Osteoporosis Int 8:423–427

77. Hasnon J (1997) Standardization of femur BMD (letter to the editor). J Bone Miner Res 12:1316–1317

78. Looker AC, Wahner HW, Dunn W et al (1998) Updated data on proximal femur bone minerals levels of US adults. Osteoporosis Int 8:468–489

79. Basha B, Rao S, Han Z, Parfitt M (2000) Osteomalacia due to vitamin D depletion: a neglected consequence of intestinal malabsorption. Am J Med 108:296–300

80. Reginato AJ, Falasca GF, Pappu R, McKnight B, Agha A (1999) Musculoskeletal manifestations of osteomalacia: report of 26 cases and literature review. Semin Arthritis Rheum 28:287–304

81. Akbunar AT, Orhan B, Alper E (2000) Bone-scan-like pattern with 99Tcm(V)-DMSA scintigraphy in patients with osteomalacia and primary hyperparathyroidism. Nucl Med Commun 21:181–185

82. Leitha T (1998) Rapid changes in the scintigraphic pattern in Tc-99m DPD whole-body scanning in metabolic bone disease. Clin Nucl Med 23:784–785

83. Olmastroni M, Seracini D, Lavoratti G, Marin E, Masi A, Vichi G (1997) Magnetic resonance imaging of renal osteodystrophy in children. Pediatr Radiol 27:865–868

84. Goen G, Mazzaferro S (1994) Bone metabolism and its assessment in renal failure. Nephron J 67:383–401

85. Rosenberg AE (1991) The pathology of metabolic bone disease. Radiol Clin North Am 29:19–36

86. Dabbagh S (1998) Renal osteodystrophy. Curr Opin Pediatr 10:190–196

87. Cicconetti A, Maffeini C, Piro FR (1999) Differential diagnosis in a case of brown tumor caused by primary hyperparathyroid ism. Minerva Stomatol 48:553–558

88. Loder RT, Hensinger RN (1997) Slipped capital femoral epiphysis associated with renal failure osteodystrophy. J Pediatr Orthop 17:205–211

89. Savaci N, Avunduk MC, Tosum Z, Hosnuter M (2000) Hyperphosphatemic tumoral calcinosis. Plast Reconstr Surg 105:162–165

90. Rosenberg AE, Salusky IB, Ramirez JA, Goodman WG (1994) Disorders of bone and mineral metabolism in chronic renal failure. In: Holliday MA, Barrett TM, Arner ED (eds) Pediatric nephrology. Williams and Wilkins, Baltimore, pp 1287–1304

91. Yalcinkaya F, Ince E, Tumer N, Ensari A, Ozkaya N (2000) Spectrum of renal osteodystrophy in children on continuous ambulatory peritoneal dialysis. Pediatr Int 42:53–57

92. Jorgetti V, Lopez BD, Caorsi H, Ferreira A, Palma A, Menendez P, Douthat W, Olaizola I, Ribeiro S, Jarava C, Moreira E, Cannata J (2000) Different patterns of renal osteodystrophy in IberoAmerica. Am J Med Sci 320:76–80

93. Sanchez CP, Salusky 1B (1996) The renal bone diseases in children treated with dialysis. Adv Renal Replacement Ther 3:14–23

94. Olaizola I, Aznarez A, Jorgetti V, Petroglia A, Caorsi H, Acuna G, Fajardo L, Ambrosoni P, Mazzuchi N (1998) Are there any differences in the parathyroid response in the different types of renal osteodystrophy? Nephrol Dial Transplant 13 [Suppl]:15–18

95. Fukagawa M, Akizawa T, Kurokawa K (2000) Is a plastic osteodytrophy a disease of malnutrition? Curr Opin Nephrol Hypertens 9:363–367

96. Alon US (2001) Preservation of bone mass in pediatric dialysis and transplant patients. Adv Renal Replacement Ther 8:191–205

97. Kim CD, Kim SH, Kim YL, Cho DK, Lee JT (1998) Bone marrow immunoscintigraphy (BMIS) a new and important tool for the assessment of marrow fibrosis in renal osteodystrophy. Adv Perit Dial 14:183–187

98. So Y, Hyun IY, Lee DS, Ahn C, Chung JK, Kim S, Lee MC, Lee JS, Koh CS (1998) Bone scan appearance of renal osteodystrophy in diabetic chronic renal failure patients. Radiat Med 16:417–421

99. Higuchi T, Hirano T, Inone T, Aoki J, Ueki K, Wakamatsu R, Yano S, Naruse T, Endo K (1998) Pentavalent Tc99m dimercapto succinic acid scintigraphy in renal osteodystrophy. J Nucl Med 39:541–543

100. Reczek J, Elgazzar A (2003) Prominent Tc99m MIBI skeletal uptake in renal osteodystrophy: a possible role for whole body scanning. Clin Nucl Med 28:775–777

101. State LJ (2001) Imaging of metabolic bone disease and marrow disorders in children. Radiol Clin North Am 39:749–772

102. Wong GY, Wilson PR (1997) Classification of complex regional pain syndromes. New concepts. Hand Clin 13:319–325

103. Stanton-Hicks M, Janig W, Hassenbusch S, Haddox JD, Boas R, Wilson P (1995) Reflex sympathetic dystrophy: changing concepts and taxonomy. Pain 63:127–133

104. Rowbotham MC (1998) Complex regional pain syndrome type I (reflex sympathetic dystrophy): more than a myth (comment). Neurology 51:4–5

105. Fournier RS. Holder LE (1998) Reflex sympathetic dystrophy: diagnostic controversies. Semin Nucl Med 28:116–123

106. Holder LE, Cole LA, Myerson MS (1992) Reflex sympathetic dystrophy in the foot: clinical and scintigraphic criteria. Radiology 184:531–535

107. Howarth D, Burstal R, Hayes C, Lan L, Lantry G (1999) Autonomic regulation of lymphatic flow in the lower extremity demonstrated on lymphoscintigraphy in patients with reflex sympathetic dystrophy. Clin Nucl Med 24:383–387

108. Leitha T, Korpan M, Staudenherz A, Wunderbaldinger P, Fialka V (1996) Five phase bone scintigraphy supports the pathophysiological concept of a subclinical inflammatory process in reflex sympathetic dystrophy. Quart J Nucl Med 40:188–193

109. Schiepers C, Bormans I, de Roo M (1998) Three-phase bone scan and dynamic vascular scintigraphy in algoneurodystrophy of the upper extremity. Acta Orthop Belg 64:322–327

110. Shehab D, Al-Jarralah K, Al-Awadhi A et al (1999) Reflex sympathetic dystrophy: an under-recognized entity in Kuwait. APLAR J Rheumatol 3:343–347

111. Handa R, Aggarwal P, Wali JP, Pictorial CME (1999) Complex regional pain syndrome, type I. J Assoc Physic India 47:804

112. Zyluk A (1999)The usefulness of quantitative evaluation of three-phase scintigraphy in the diagnosis of post-traumatic reflex sympathetic dystrophy. J Hand Surg (Br) 24:16–21

113. Zufferey P, Boubaker A, Bischof Delaloye A, So AK, Duvoisin B (1999) Prognostic aspects of scintigraphy and MRI during the first 6 months of reflex sympathetic dystrophy of the distal lower limb: a preliminary prospective study of 4 cases. J Radiol 80:373–377

114. Wang YL, Tsau JC, Huang MH, Lee BF, Li CH (1998) sympathetic dystrophy syndrome in stroke patients with hemiplegia-three phase bone scintigraphy and clinical characteristics. Kaohsiung J Med Sci 14:40–47

115. Schiepers C (1997) Clinical value of dynamic bone and vascular scintigraphy in diagnosing reflex sympathetic dystrophy of the upper extremity. Hand Clin 13:423–429

116. Steinert H, Hahn K (1996) The value of 3-phase skeletal scintigraphy for early diagnosis of Sudeck disease. ROFO Fortschr Geb Rontgenstr Bildgeb V 164:318–323

117. Turpin S, Taillefer R, Lambert R, Leveille J (1996) „Cold" reflex sympathetic dystrophy in an adult. Clin Nucl Med 21:94–97

118. Zyluk A, Birkenfeld B (1999) Quantitative evaluation of three-phase bone scintigraphy before and after the treatment of post-traumatic reflex sympathetic dystrophy. Nucl Med Commun 20:327–333

119. Schiepers C (1997) Clinical value of dynamic bone and vascular scintigraphy in diagnosing reflex sympathetic dystrophy of the upper extremity. Hand Clin 13:423–429

120. Howell DS (1985) Hypertrophic osteoarthropathy. In: McCarty DJ (ed) Arthritis and allied conditions, 10th edn. Lea and Febiger, Philadelphia, pp 1195–1201

121. Ali A, Tetalman MR, Fordham EW et al (1980) Distribution of hypertrophic pulmonary osteo-arthropathy. AJR 134:771–780

122. Sissons HA, Malcolm AJ (1997) Fibrous dysplasia of bone: case report with autopsy study 80 years after the original clinical recognition of the bone lesions. Skeletal Radiol 26:177–183

123. Han J, Ryu JS, Shin MJ, Kang GH, Lee HK (2000) Fibrous dysplasia with barely increased uptake on bone scan: a case report. Clin Nucl Med 25:785–788

124. Di Leo C, Ardemagni A, Bestetti A, Tagliabue L, del Sole A, Conte A, Tarolo GL (1999) A rare case of polystotic fibrous dysplasia assessed by bone scintigraphy with Tc-99m methylene diphosphonate (MDP). Nucl Med 38:169–171

125. Kairemo KJ, Verho S, Dunkel L (1999) Imaging of McCune-Albright syndrome using bone single photon emission computed tomography. Eur J Pediatr 158:123–126

126. Tokano H, Sugimoto T, Noguchi Y, Kitamura K (2001) Sequential computed tomography images demonstrating characteristic changes in fibrous dysplasia. J Laryngol Otol 115:757–759

127. Lupescu I, Hermier M, Georgescu SA, Froment JC (2001) Helical CT and diagnostic evaluation of cranio-facial fibrous dysplasia. J Radiol 82:145–149

128. Jee WH, Choi KH, Choe BY, Park JM, Shinn KS (1996) Fibrous dysplasia: MR imaging characteristics with radio-pathologic correlation. Am J Roentgenol 167:1523–1527

129. Karr JC, Black JA, Bernard JM (2001) Magnetic resonance imaging evaluation of monostotic fibrous dysplasia of the tibia. J Am Podiatr Med Assoc 91:306–310

130. Toba M, Hayashida K, Imakita S, Fukuchi K, Kume N, Shimotsu Y, Cho I, Ishida Y, Takamiya M, Kumita S (1998) Increased bone mineral turnover without increased glucose utilization in sclerotic and hyperplastic change in fibrous dysplasia. Ann Nucl Med 12:153–155

131. Chew FS (1991) Radiologic manifestations in musculo-skeletal system of miscellaneous endocrine disorders. Radiol Clin North Am 29:1135–1148

132. Gerster JC, Gharhon SA, Jaeger P, Boivin G, Briancon D, Rostan A, Baud CA, Meunier PJ (1983) Bilateral fractures of the femoral neck in patients with moderate renal failure receiving fluoride for spinal osteoporosis. Br Med J 287:723–725

133. Orcel P, de Vernejoul MC, Prier A, Miravet L, Kuntz D, Kaplan G (1990) Stress fractures of the lower limbs in osteo-porotic patients treated with fluoride. J Bone Miner Res 5 [Suppl 1]:s191–s194

134. Coburn JW, Norris KC, Nebeker HG (1986) Osteomalacia and bone done disease arising from aluminum. Semin Nephrol 21:68–89

135. Kassem M, Eriksen EF, Melsen F, Mosekilde L (1991) Antacid-induced osteomalacia: a case report with a histomorphic analysis. J Intern Med 229:275–279

136. Drueke T, Cournot-Witmer G (1985) Dialysis osteomalacia: clinical aspects and physiopathological mechanisms. Clin Nephrol 24 [Suppl 1]:S26–S29

137. Botella J, Gallego JL, Fernandez-Fenandez J, Sanz-Guajardo D, deMiguel A, Ramos J, Franco P, Enriques R, Sanz-Moreno C (1985) The bone scan in patients with aluminum associated bone disease. Proc Eur Dial Transplant Assoc Eur Renal Assoc 21:403–409

138. Felix R, Hofstetter W, Cecchini MG (1999) Recent developments in the understanding of the pathophysiology of osteopetrosis. Eur J Endocrinol 134:143–156

139. Kim S, Park CH, Kim B (2001) „Superscan" in an autosomal-dominant benign form of osteopetrosis. Clin Nucl Med 26:636–637

140. Ahmed Alkandari F, Abdulla Kazim N, Collier BD, Shah Sayed GN (2003) Osteopetrosis: a potential mimic of oeteomyelitis on three phase bone scintigraphy. Clin Nucl Med 28:54–55

141. Norton KI, Wagreich JM, Granowetter L, Martignetti JA (1996) Diaphyseal medullary stenosis (sclerosis) with bone malignancy (malignant fibrous histiocytoma): Hardcastle syndrome. Pediatric Radiology 26:675–677

142. Arnold WH (1973) Hereditary bone dysplasia with sarcomatous degeneration : study of family. Ann Intern Med 78:902–906

143. Hardcastle P, Nader S, Arnold W (1986) Hereditary bone dysplasia with malignant change. J Bone Joint Dis (Am) 68:1079–1089

144. Kenan S, Abdelwahab IF, Hermann G, Klein MJ (1998) Malignant fibrous histiocytoma associated with a bone infarct in a patient with hereditary bone dysplasia. Skeletal Radiol 27:463–467

145. Gorlin RJ, Goltz RW (1960) Multiple nevoid basal cell epithelioma, jaw cysts and bifid rib syndrome. NEJM 262:908–912

146. Crean SJ, Cunningham SJ (1996) Gorlin's syndrome: main features and recent advances. Br J Hosp Med 56:392–397

147. Ryan PJ (1998) Orthopedic manifestation of sytemic disease. Semin Nucl Med 28:124–131

148. Fogelman I, Citrin DL (1981) Bone scanning in metabolic bone disease: a review. Appl Radiol 10:158–166]

149. Silberstein EB, Elgazzar AH, Fernandez-Uloa M, Nishiyama H (1996) Skeletal scintigraphy in non-neoplastic osseous disorders. In: Henkin RE, Bles MA, Dillehay GL, Halama JR, Karesh SM, Wagner PH, Zimmer AM (eds) Textbook of nuclear medicine. Mosby, New York

150. Vanhoenacker FM, Janssens K, Van Hul W, Gershoni-Baruch R, B De Schepper AM (2003) Camurati-Engelmann disease. Review of radioclinical features. Acta Radiol 44:430–434

151. Inkaoka J, Shuka N, Sato J, Ishikawa Y, Takahashi K, Aburano T, Makita Y (2001) Scintigraphic evaluation of pamidronate and corticosteroid therapy in a patient with progressive diaphyseal dysplasia (Camurati-Engelmann disease). Clinical Nuclear medicine 26:680–682

Diagnosis of Traumatic Disorders

4

Nuclear medicine has a limited but important role in trauma and its complications. It is particularly useful and indicated in radiologically occult acute fractures including those in children who are the victims of physical abuse and in stress fractures. It is also used in the assessment of physeal closure and stimulation after trauma and to predict the outcome of leg length by semi-quantitative analysis. Bone scintigraphy can also detect chronic ligament and acute and chronic meniscal lesions. Certain technical considerations, particularly related to meticulous positioning, use of single-photon emission computed tomography (SPECT) and use of magnification during acquisition, are important to maximize the diagnostic yield of scintigraphic modalities, particularly bone scan in traumatic disorders.

4.1
Introduction

Despite advances in morphological modalities and nuclear medicine conventional, bone scintigraphy remains an important imaging technique in trauma since it is sensitive in detecting stress fractures and in assessing suspected injuries that are difficult to see on plain films. It is non-invasive and easily applied, and being very sensitive, a normal scintigram excludes pathophysiological conditions or mechanical disorders of the bones and joints. Trauma to the musculoskeletal system may affect bone, cartilage, muscles and joints. To each of these structures, trauma may cause immediate damage and late changes. Trauma is a common condition that affects all age groups. Additionally, sports injuries are becoming more frequent because of the increasing recruitment of individuals into fitness programs from the population that live a sedentary lifestyle. This is in addition to the elite athletes engaged in high-level fitness programs. Both groups are prone to injury for different reasons, the former from unaccustomed exercise and the latter from chronic overuse injuries. The childhood and adolescent athlete fall into a separate category due to the unique patterns of injury that affect the growing but immature skeleton. Although scintigraphy does not play a major role in the diagnosis and management of most fractures, it is valuable in certain situations such as occult fractures of the ribs and small bones of the hands and feet, fractures of physically abused children, and delayed union or nonunion of fractures and in assessing the healing of fractures and bone grafts. Bone scintigraphy, however, is often used to detect stress fractures and can also play a role in the follow-up of these injuries.

4.2
Pathophysiology

4.2.1
Acute Fractures

Fracture is defined as a break in the continuity of a bone. Classification of fractures is not an easy issue since many of the classifications in current use mainly focused on particular anatomical locations, such as the acetabulum or the talar bone. Classifying fractures is an abbreviated way of describing the configuration of the fracture which can be used by clinical orthopedics to guide treatment, predict prognosis and possible complications [1]. For the purpose of simplification and for the purpose of this text, fractures generally can be classified according to several features (Table 4.1). Based on the extent of the break, fractures are classified as complete or incomplete. A complete fracture breaks the bone all the way through, while with incomplete fracture the bone is broken but stays as one piece. Fractures are also classified into open (previously called compound) if the skin is broken and closed [previously called simple] when the skin at the site of fracture is not broken [2]. The pattern of a fracture depends on the mechanism of injury. A compressive load produces compaction or oblique fracture. A bend-

ing load has a tendency to produce flat transverse fractures; however, a bending load on one side only is associated with compression on the other side, which may affect the pattern of the fracture. A torsional force tends to produce spiral fractures.

Other classifications are based on the number of bone pieces and the direction of the fracture line and other factors (Table 4.1). Pathological fractures occur at the sites of pre-existing abnormalities that weaken bone. A minimal force that usually would not cause a fracture of a normal bone may produce a pathological fracture. Transchondral fractures (osteochondritis dissicans) represents fragmentation and separation of portions of cartilage, or cartilage and bone. This type is most prevalent in adolescents and occurs typically in the head of the femur, ankle, kneecap, elbow and wrist.

Bone contusion (bone bruise) is a term describing microfractures of the trabecular bone and edema or hemorrhage within the bone marrow. It normally resolves spontaneously within 8–12 weeks.

4.2.2
Stress Fractures

Stress fractures occur due to repeated stress; each episode is less forceful than that needed to cause acute fractures of the bony cortex. If this occurs in normal bones, the resulting fractures are called fatigue fractures while if they occur in abnormal bones (e.g. osteoporosis), they are termed insufficiency fractures. These

Table 4.1. Classifications of fractures

Based on extent of break:
Complete: bone is broken all the way through
Incomplete: bone is still one piece
Based on skin condition:
Open: broken skin
Closed: intact skin
Based on resulting number of bone fragments:
Comminuted: multiple bone fragment
Non-comminuted: only two fragments
Based on direction of fracture line:
Linear: line is parallel to the long axis of bone.
Oblique: line is at oblique angle to the shaft of the bone
Spiral: line encircles the bone
Transverse: line is perpendicular to the long axis of bone
Based on cause of fracture:
Excessive force on normal non-violated bone: classic acute fracture
Pathological fracture: break at the site of pre existing pathology
Stress fractures: (localized or generalized)
Fatigue fractures: Abnormal stresses applied to normal bones
Insufficiency fractures: Usual stresses to abnormal bones

Table 4.2. Location of common stress fractures and associated physical activity

Location	Activity or event
Sesamoids of metatarsal bones	Prolonged standing
Metatarsal shaft	Marching; stamping on ground; prolonged standing; ballet dancing
Navicular	Stamping on ground; marching; long-distance running
Calcaneus	Jumping; prolonged standing; parachuting
Tibia	Running
Fibula	Running
Patella	Hurdling
Femur shaft	Ballet; long-distance running; marching; gymnastics
Lumbar vertebra (pars interarticularis)	Ballet; gymnastics; tennis; diving; lifting heavy objects
Ribs	Carrying heavy pack; golf; coughing

Data adapted from [79], [106] and [113]

fractures commonly occur in the vertebrae, pelvis and ribs due to trivial, commonly unnoticed, trauma since the bones are fragile. Fatigue fractures are common in athletes, military recruits and dancers (Table 4.2). Stress fractures are not, as previously thought, due to repeated traumatic microfractures; they are a focal area of increased bone turnover secondary to the repeated stress. The process starts with resorption cavities before being coupled by an osteoblastic response to replace the absorbed bone [3]. The process of rarefaction is faster than the osteoblastic process and will progress if the individual continues the stressful activity and trauma resulting in complete fracture through the zone of rarefaction. With repeated loading bone develops loss of its stiffness and strength. If scintigraphy is performed in the acute phase of less than 4 weeks, the flow and blood pool images show increased activity (Fig. 4.1). Later, only delayed uptake will be seen while flow and blood pool activity gradually normalize. This is different from the pattern of shin splints, which are another consequence of stress and may present in the same patient population as fatigue fractures. Shin splints typically show normal flow and blood pool images with an elongated linear increased uptake on de-

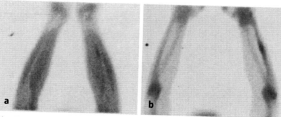

Fig. 4.1a, b. An early-stage stress fracture of a 28 year old male athlete. Blood pool (**a**) shows focally increased hyperemia in the left arm with corresponding intense uptake in the left ulna on delayed image (**b**)

layed images. This is most commonly found in the tibiae and may coexist with fatigue fractures in the same patient. Most stress fractures affect the lower extremity; however, injuries to the upper extremities account for more than 25 % of all sports-related injuries, but receive disproportionately less attention than lower extremity injuries [4].

4.2.3
Spondylolysis

Spondylolysis is a condition in which there is a loss of continuity of bone of the neural arch of the vertebra. This is believed to be due to trauma or more probably stress. The gap, or loss of continuity, most commonly occurs at the junction of the lamina when the vertebra is viewed from above, or between the superior and inferior articular processes (pars interarticularis or facetal joints) when viewed from the side (Fig. 4.2a). This condition, which most commonly affects the fourth and fifth lumbar vertebra, may or may not be symptomatic and usually does not result in any neurological deficit, but is a common cause of low back pain, particularly in

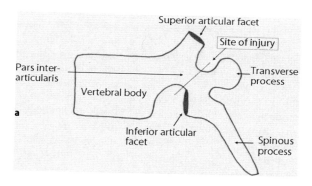

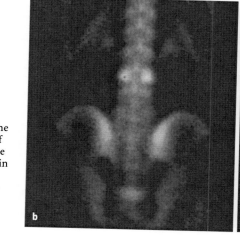

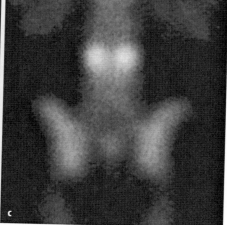

Fig. 4.2. a A diagram illustrating the site of injury causing spondylolysis as seen from lateral view of the vertebra. **b** A spot image of the pelvis and lumbar spine showing increased uptake in L-3 vertebra affected by spondylolysis. Representative coronal section of SPECT study (**c**) show the abnormalities

children and young adults. The diagnosis is usually made using standard radiographs, and scintigraphy is reserved for the detection of radiologically occult cases and for assessing the metabolic activity of the condition. Typically, focally increased uptake is seen in the region of pars interarticularis (Fig. 4.2b–c). SPECT is much more sensitive than planar imaging in detecting this abnormality. The treatment of this condition is usually conservative and the use of back support usually corrects the problem.

4.2.4
Spondylolisthesis

Spondylolisthesis is the forward movement of one vertebra on another (Fig. 4.3), usually as a result of fracture of the neural arch. It is again most commonly seen in the fifth lumbar vertebra in which case there is a forward shift of L5 on the sacrum. It is less commonly seen at L4. In addition to the acquisition using parallel-hole high-resolution collimators, pinhole collimators and/or SPECT again are needed since they are more sensitive.

4.2.5
Fracture Healing

Fracture union is defined as sufficient growth of bone across the fracture line. The healing process of a fracture is outlined as follows:

1. There is formation of a hematoma following a fracture event: When a fracture disrupts the periosteum and blood vessels in the cortex, marrow and the adjacent soft tissue, bleeding occurs and a hematoma forms between the bony fracture ends, beneath the periosteum and within the medullary cavity.
2. Invasion of granulation tissue occurs into the hematoma: Necrosis of the bone tissue adjacent to the fracture takes place immediately. This necrotic tissue, along with the effect of the traumatic injury, in-

duces an inflammatory response with features of acute non-specific inflammation, including vasodilatation, extravasation of plasma and leukocytes and infiltration with leukocytes. Within 48 h, blood flow to the entire bone increases with organization of the hematoma around the broken ends of bone into a fibrous network.

3. A procallus is formed along the outer surface of the shaft and over the broken ends of bone by the bone forming cells in the periosteum, endosteum and marrow.
4. The callus starts to form with synthesis of collagen and matrix by osteoblasts. Mineralization with calcium deposition follows to complete the formation of calluses (woven bone).
5. Remodeling: Any unnecessary callus is resorbed as the process of healing continues, trabeculae are formed, and the remodeling leads to alignment of the cortical bony margins and marrow cavity. Bone accordingly heals by forming new tissue rather than scar tissue.
6. Modeling: reshaping of cortex.

Several factors affect this fracture healing process (Table 4.3), and if disturbances happen, delayed, non- or mal-union can result. *Delayed union* indicates that union does not occur at the expected time. This is difficult to determine objectively and varies with the site of fracture, although it is usually 3–4 months after the fracture. *Non-union* indicates the failure of the bone ends to grow together. Instead of new bone, dense fibrous tissue fills the gap between the broken ends and uncommonly it may be filled by fibrocartilaginous tissue. Necrotic tissue is not seen unless infection is present in the area of non-union. Delayed union and non-union are commonly seen in the tibia, fibula and scaphoid bones. Less common sites are humerus, radius, ulna, and clavicle [5]. Occasionally, the gap between the bone ends contains a space filled with fluid. In this case, the term 'false joint', or *pseudoarthrosis*, is applied and persistent uptake of Tc-99m MDP continues to be seen

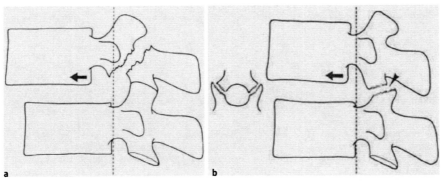

Fig. 4.3.a Spondylolisthesis with spondylolysis. Bilateral defects through the pars interarticularis allow anterior displacement of the vertebral body onto its neighbor. The alignment of the apophyseal joints is normal. **b** Spondylolisthesis without spondylolysis (Degenerative anterior spondylolisthesis). Apophyseal joint osteoarthritis (*arrowhead*) allows the inferior articular processes to move anteriorly, producing forward subluxation of the superior vertebra onto the inferior vertebra. The *inset* demonstrates the manner in which the abnormal apophyseal joints may allow anterior subluxation. (From Resnick [107], with permission)

Table 4.3. Factors affecting fracture healing

1. Patient age: Non-union is rare in children unless there is other condition present as neurofibromatosis, infection, or extensive soft tissue damage

2. Weight bearing: stimulates healing of fractures

3. Fixation: Stimulates union but does not accelerate repair itself

4. Nerve damage: Is associated with rapid union with unknown mechanism

5. Damage of intramedullary canal and nailing: this may lead to delayed repair or to extensive reactive osteogenic activity

6. Blood supply: interrupted blood supply may cause delayed healing

7. Infection: May lead to delayed healing

8. Excessive use of steroids can cause delayed healing

9. Extent of fracture: severely displaced fractures, open fractures, loss of fragments and extensive soft tissue damage cause delayed healing

Table 4.4. Features of the major types of fracture non-union

Feature	Hypertrophic non-union	Atrophic non-union
Blood supply to ends of fragments	Rich	Poor
Potential to heal under stable and correct environment	Yes	Unable to heal
Amount of new bone formation	Good amount	Small amount
Method of ossification of new bone formation	Endochondral and intramembranous	Endochondral
Apoptotic cell death	Increased[a]	Increased
Management	Typically no need for open debridement	Open decortication and cancellous bone graft

[a] Thought previously to be decreased

after the usual period of healing or post-operative changes. The fracture is considered non-united after 6 months, although certain fractures, such as a central fracture of the femoral neck, are considered non-united after only 3 months. Non-union is classified predominantly according to the radiological appearance into hypervascular (hypertrophic) and avascular (atrophic) and is based on the capability to produce a biological reaction. Standard radiographs show that hypertrophic non-union is rich in callus and have a rich blood supply in the ends of the fragments. These have the potential to heal under the correct stable environment [6]. Atrophic non-union, on the other hand, is considered to be relatively avascular at the ends of the fragments, acellular and inert, and consequently it lacks the ability to heal under the correct stable environment [6]. This type is typically seen in tibial fractures treated by plate and screws. Both types contain fibrous tissue, hyaline cartilage, fibrocartilage and areas of bone formation. However, the amount and type of bone formation may differ between the two types. As expected, the hypertrophic type contains more areas of new bone which ossifies by both endochondral and intramembranous ossification (Table 4.4). Atrophic non-union, on the other hand, has only few areas of bone formation which form predominantly by endochondral ossification [6]. Radiographs reflect most of these changes but do not show the biological changes which were studied by Reed and associates [6], who found that hypertrophic non-union shows increased apoptosis, or programmed cell death (PCD), in both types (Table 4.4). *Mal-union* describes the healing of a bone in a non-anatomic orientation.

4.2.6
Trauma to Bone-adjacent Structures

Skeletal muscle damage: Muscle damage of variable degrees is commonly associated with fractures. The incidence of sepsis and other fracture-related complications, and, importantly, fracture healing, are significantly influenced by the severity of muscle and soft tissue damage. The classical criteria of skeletal muscle damage, such as color, consistency, bleeding and contractility, are subjective. Research in animals and humans has shown the feasibility of more accurate objective ways to assess skeletal muscle damage using radionuclide imaging techniques [6]. Injury to skeletal muscle and soft tissue may result in the formation of regional ectopic calcification or heterotopic calcification in the soft tissue.

Tendon and ligament injuries: Tears to tendons are called *sprains*, while ligament tears are called *strains*. These injuries usually do not cause abnormal uptake on bone scintigraphy. On the other hand, complete separation of tendons or ligaments, with or without a portion of bone and/or cartilage, from their attachments are called *avulsions* and cause abnormal uptake on bone scans.

4.3
Scintigraphic Diagnosis of Acute Fractures
4.3.1
Role of Scintigraphy in Acute Fracture

Although standard radiography is the modality of choice for the diagnosis of acute fractures, along with computed tomography (CT) and magnetic resonance imaging (MRI) as complementary modalities in certain cases, bone scintigraphy still has a well-defined role in acute fracture diagnosis and follow-up. In certain locations of the skeleton, it is particularly valuable and can provide information that other modalities cannot supply, such as fractures of the ribs, sternum, pelvis, vertebrae and the small bones of the hands and feet. Differentiation between an old and a recent vertebral fracture, hands/wrists and feet/ankles is another important application. This was found to be also useful in detecting occult, or excluding active, bone damage after a traffic or industrial accident [7–10]. In many of these cases initial radiographs are normal or non-diagnostic. In patients with osteopenia this occurs mainly when radiographs are obtained before the appearance of a fracture line or new bone formation, since their detection is difficult, and when the fracture involves areas of the skeleton that are not easily seen with plain films, such as the pelvis and feet [11].

4.3.2
Scintigraphic Appearance of Acute Fractures

Most fractures are visualized scintigraphically within hours after the trauma event [12, 13]; the optimal timing of imaging a fracture is unclear, however, since in a small minority of older patients the fractures may take several days to be visualized. It is, however, recommended that scintigraphy should be used at any time when there is uncertainty concerning the existence of a fracture [14]. Using this approach, Holder et al. [14] reported sensitivity of 95% and specificity of 97% for fractures if scintigraphy is performed within 48 h and 100% sensitivity if it is performed within 72 h or longer after injury. A few case reports have reported that scintigraphy may only show the fracture as late as 12 days after the injury [15, 16]. It has to be realized, however, that in addition to the patient's age, the bone metabolic activity and mineral content and the imaging technique are all factors that can significantly affect the timing of visualization of a fracture as well as the ability to detect it. Meticulous technique is crucial in achieving an accurate diagnosis, which can be achieved in the majority of cases by following certain technical principles [17]. The study of the patient should be tailored to the history and examination to maximize the scintigraphic diagnostic yield. Knowledge of the date and mechanism of injury, associated diseases and interventions is crucial. Efforts should be made to position the region of suspected fracture with a minimum degree of overlap with other bony structures. Zoomed images in multiple projections with proper utilization of SPECT can increase the diagnostic yield of both bone and soft tissue pathology (Table 4.5). The val-

Table 4.5. Guide to positioning for scintigraphic diagnosis of fracture and traumatic injuries

Location	Position
Wrist	Zoom or pinhole in ulnar deviation
	Zoom lateral view of wrist
Elbow	Zoom anterior, posterior and skyline views
Shoulder	Zoom blood pools and delayed anterior and posterior views; pinhole anterior view; neutral versus abducted
Cervical spine	Zoom SPECT; pinhole
Thoracic spine	Zoom views in prone position with a pillow beneath, collimator against skin; SPECT
Lumbar spine	Zoom planar in flexed position, collimator against skin, SPECT with oblique reconstruction
Pelvis	Subpubic and lateral views
Hips	Pinhole or zoom views in abduction/external rotation, SPECT
Knees	SPECT; pinhole
Ankle	Pinhole or zoom lateral and medial views; SPECT
Foot	Pinhole or zoom views in anterior oblique, lateral, medial and plantar

Modified from [17], with permission

Table 4.6. Bone scan findings in different forms of trauma in correlation with standard radiographs

Pathology	Flow phase	Blood pool phase	Delayed phase	Radiograph
Contusion	Increased	Increased	Increased	Negative
Shin splints	Normal	Normal	Increased	Negative
Stress fracture	Increased	Increased	Increased	Negative for 2–4 weeks
Acute fracture	Increased	Increased	Increased	Usually abnormal
Old fracture	Normal	Normal	Increased	Usually abnormal
Avulsion fracture	Increased	Increased	Increased	Commonly equivocal
Transchondral fracture	Increased	Increased	Increased	Usually abnormal
Battered child	+/–	+/–	Increased	Commonly negative
Growth plate injury				
Early phase	Increased	Increased	Non-uniform uptake	Usually negative
Late phase	Decreased	Decreased	Non-uniform uptake	Difficult to detect
Lisfranc	Increased	Increased	Increased	Difficult to detect
Enthesopathies				
Active	Increased	Increased	Increased	Negative
Inactive	Normal	Normal	Fainter increased uptake	Negative

Table 4.7. Scintigraphic appearance of acute fractures on multi-phase bone scintigraphy

Phase of fracture	Duration	Scintigraphic appearance
First (acute) phase	3–4 weeks	Increased flow and blood pool activity at site of fracture; diffuse area of increased activity around fracture site on delayed images
Second (sub-acute) phase	8–12 weeks	Increased flow and blood pool activity at fracture site which may become more localized; well-defined intense uptake at fracture site on delayed images
Third (healing) phase	Variable	Gradual diminution of flow, blood pool activity and delayed uptake intensity

ue of the bone scan in the early diagnosis and management of fractures can be also increased by the accurate registration with radiographs, or at a minimum level careful correlation with the radiographs (Table 4.6) and a skeleton model (at the time of interpretation) [17–19].

The scintigraphic appearance of fractures depends on the time elapsed after injury (Table 4.7) [13, 20]. The scan can appear abnormal a few hours after the injury. Early on, fractures show focally increased flow and blood pool activity with a correspondingly increased activity on delayed images (Fig. 4.4). Later, flow and blood pool activity decreases progressively till they normalize. This may take up to 6 months (as determined experimentally and by following human fractures at different times after the trauma) [13, 21], while delayed uptake remains positive for a longer time. This has been reported to be as long as 40 years, depending on the age and healing status of the patient [13].

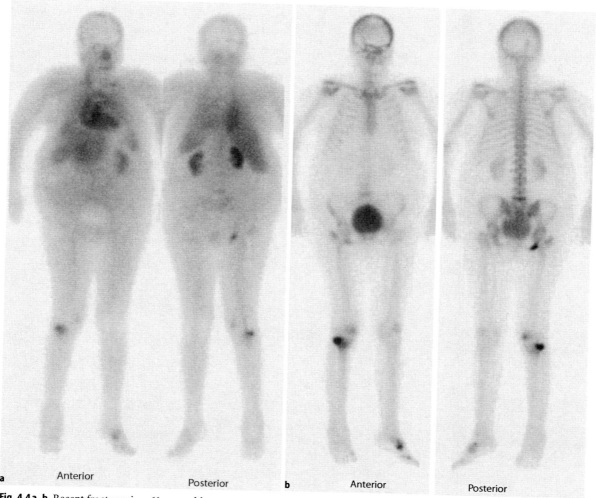

a   Anterior   Posterior   b   Anterior   Posterior

Fig. 4.4a, b. Recent fractures in a 61-year-old woman (with a history of recent car accident). Tc99m MDP bone scan obtained 10 days later shows abnormal uptake at the sites of fractures in L-5, right ischium, right proximal tibia and left foot on both blood pool imaging (**a**) and delayed images (**b**)

4.3.3
Scintigraphic Imaging of Specific Fractures
4.3.3.1
Rib and Sternal Fractures

Rib and sternal fractures can be difficult to detect using standard radiographs and scintigraphy can be of help in many cases. Erhan et al. [22], compared radiography to bone scintigraphy in the same patients and found that scintigraphy was more sensitive in both rib and sternal fractures during the early period of thoracic trauma. Standard radiography should, however, as in other bone diseases, be the initial imaging modality used, since it saves time and can show hemothorax, or pneumothorax, as well as the osseous abnormality being investigated [22]. Scintigraphically, rib fractures may be solitary and appear as a focus of increased uptake (Fig. 4.5), and in

such cases it is difficult to differentiate the fracture by pattern alone from other conditions such as tumors. Fractures may also present as multiple and are typically oriented vertically (Fig. 4.6), a pattern that is very suggestive of rib fractures. Occasionally, spiral rib fractures can appear as an elongated area of increased uptake and in such situations it is again difficult to separate the entity from a malignancy scintigraphically. Sternal fractures are particularly difficult to be detected by radiographs and bone scintigraphy has a crucial role in their diagnosis (Fig. 4.7).

4.3.3.2
Scaphoid Bone Fractures

Occult fractures of the scaphoid bone occur frequently after carpal injuries and may lead to non-union. The diagnosis of scaphoid fracture is often difficult because of the low sensitivity of radiographs. Multiphase bone scintigraphy is considered to be the modality of choice for patients with normal radiographs. Pinhole imaging is particularly useful in showing the focal uptake and localizing it (Fig. 4.8). Bayer et al. [23] studied 40 patients, approximately 2 weeks after trauma, who had negative radiographs but clinically suspected scaphoid fracture, using a rapid version of bone scintigraphy

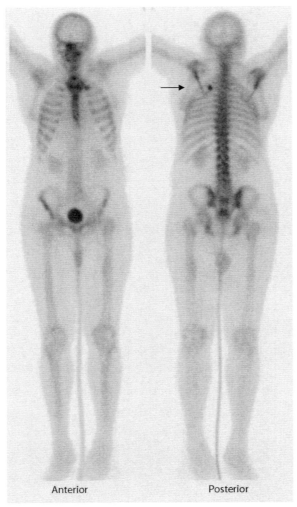

Anterior   Posterior

Fig. 4.5. Whole-body bone scan of a 39-year-old woman with a history of a fall showing a single focus of increased uptake in the left posterior third rib illustrating an example of a single rib fracture (*arrow*)

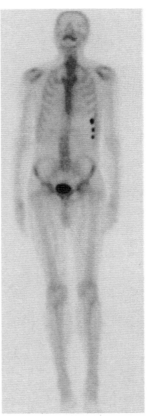

Anterior

Fig. 4.6. Typical pattern of vertically oriented multiple rib fractures, which should not be confused with the typical pattern of metastases

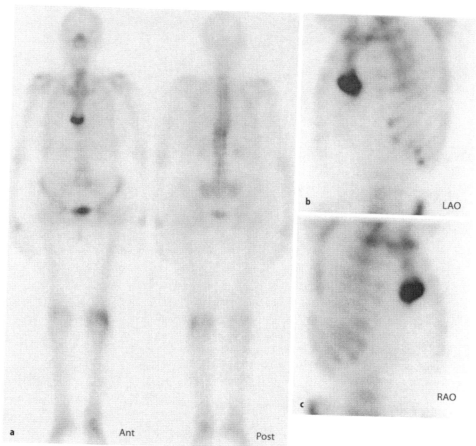

Fig. 4.7a–c. Fracture of the sternum seen on whole body Tc99m MDP bone scan (**a**) and anterior oblique chest views (**b, c**)

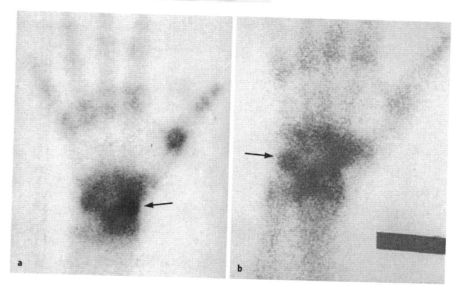

Fig. 4.8a–c. Fractures of the small bones of the hand for which a bone scan is useful. **a** Scaphoid (carpal navicular) fracture as seen using a high resolution bone image. **b** High-resolution image showing right triquetrum fracture.

(with images taken 15 min after radiotracer injection); 8 fractures of the scaphoid bone and 13 of other carpal bones were detected scintigraphically but not on radiographs [23]. In another prospective study of 50 patients with suspected scaphoid fractures, all the patients who had fractures demonstrated using standard radiography (either at the initial visit, or at 2 weeks) had positive bone scans (sensitivity 100%). Four of six patients who

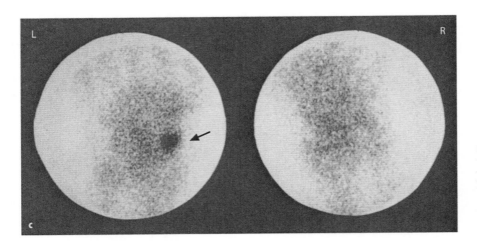

Fig. 4.8 (contin.) c Fracture of the left scaphoid (carpal navicular) bone as seen on pinhole imaging, which has the additional advantage of magnification and better localization of abnormalities

had a positive scan but negative first and second radiographs had persistent tenderness on clinical examination which required extended immobilization in a plaster cast. The overall positive predictive value of scintigraphy was 93%. All patients with a negative scan were clinically and radiologically negative at 2 weeks (negative predictive value 100%). Evidence of multifocal injury was present in 12 scans, but only in one radiograph [24].

Initial experience with MRI suggests that it can be a sensitive modality for the diagnosis of scaphoid fractures and may prove more specific than scintigraphy. Additionally, significant ligamentous injury and carpal instability seen by MRI are not evident on scintigraphy [25, 26].

4.3.3.3
Lisfranc Fracture

Lisfranc injury includes fracture and fracture-dislocation of the tarsometatarsal (Lisfranc) joints that is difficult to diagnose since it is not easy to visualize on radiographs [27]. In a study of 59 patients with Lisfranc injury, Vuori and Aro [27] reported only 39% sensitivity for radiographs. Bone scintigraphy is more sensitive and shows increased flow, blood pool and delayed activity focally or in a transverse fashion (Fig. 4.9).

4.3.3.4
Pediatric Fractures and Traumatic Injuries

Growth Plate Injuries
Injury to the physis, or growth plate, in children may lead to the arrest of growth and/or angular deformities of the limbs. On scintigraphy, normal growth plates appear as thin, well-demarcated lines. The physis is recognized as the site of endochondral ossification and is responsible for a bone's growth in length. Although the

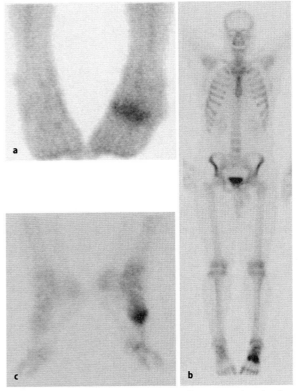

Fig. 4.9a–c. Lisfranc fracture pattern on bone scan showing increased blood pool (**a**) and delayed uptake (**b, c**) at the site of left tarso-metatarsal joints

band of increased uptake seen on scintigraphic bone images is referred to as the growth plate, it actually does not correspond to the lucent band present on a bone radiograph that is also referred to as the growth plate. The radionuclide growth plate corresponds to the dense band of bone in the metaphysis adjacent to the radiographic growth plate and is described in radiographic anatomy as the zone of provisional calcification. The normal scintigraphic appearance of the growth plate varies with age. In infants and young children the physis has a thick and oval-shaped appearance. With

maturation it becomes linear, and in adolescence it shows progressively decreasing activity. Growth plates in different regions of the skeleton close at different times. Skeletal maturation occurs earlier in females than in males [28]. Using quantitative data from nor-

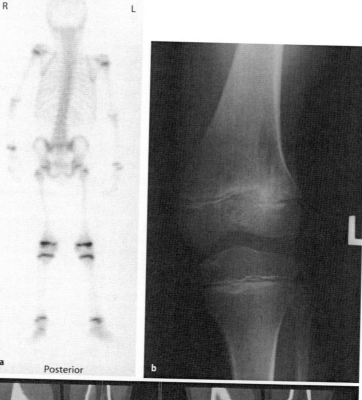

Fig. 4.10a–c. Growth plate injury. Whole body anterior (**a**) and posterior bone scan of a 4-year-old boy with pain in his left knee. The scan shows increased uptake in the lateral aspect of the left distal femoral growth plate. Standard radiograph (**c**) and MRI images of the same patient illustrating the same injury

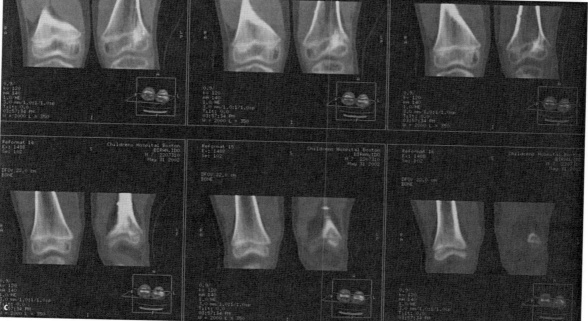

mal children, greater activity is present in the medial half of the distal femoral growth plate than the lateral half, while in the proximal tibial growth plate (Fig. 4.10) the lateral half shows more activity than the medial [28]. Stress factors and mechanical loading influence the scintigraphic uptake at the growth plate. For example, when an extremity is placed at rest, as with prolonged immobilization, activity in the growth plate decreases in comparison with the contralateral weight-bearing extremity. This can occur also in ambulatory patients with a gait disturbance which results in differential weight bearing. On the other hand, increased growth plate uptake can occur on generalized or regional basis. Systemic and metabolic diseases may result in a generalized increase in growth plate uptake throughout the skeleton. Trauma, infection, and other conditions that relates to increased metabolic bone activity may result in uniform increased activity in the plate, or segmental abnormal uptake. Fractures and slipped capital femoral epiphysis result in uniformly increased plate activity at the involved location. Segmental increase, and decrease, in a growth plate is of particular importance, since it is associated with the development of angular deformities. When an incident such as trauma and infection directly involves the growth plate, or occurs near the growth plate, segmental abnormal uptake will be seen and deformity may follow. Also a fracture in the metaphysis of a long bone can, provoke angular deformity by stimulating an adjacent growth plate. Harcke [28] described the increased growth plate activity with metabolic bone disease and documented a return to normal after successful treatment. Such injuries particularly fractures, may cause permanent closure of segments of growth plates [29]. Partial arrest of the growth plate occurs when an osseous or cartilaginous bridge forms across the plate. If this occurs laterally, the relatively accelerated activity of the medial growth plate will result in a valgus deformity while if the barrier is located on the medial side and normal physis continues to grow laterally, it will cause a varus deformity [30]. These angular deformities can also occur secondary to contiguous chronic hyperemia of a metaphysis, or epiphysis, (such as after a fracture to these locations which stimulates the activity of the adjacent part of the physis) resulting in unequal growth with a subsequent deformity [31]. CT and MRI are accurate in identifying segmental closure [32]. The physiological status of the growth plate is difficult to evaluate using morphological imaging. Scintigraphic imaging complements anatomical studies by reflecting the physiological status of the growth plate and has the advantage of being quantitative. It can also detect the abnormalities earlier than morphological modalities and can help particularly in detecting segmental growth plate arrests that are difficult to determine using these modalities [33–36]. A key to the comparison of growth plate uptake is having both plates symmetrically positioned on the same large view. On scintigraphy, differences in activity and configuration of the growth plates can be identified particularly on early blood pool images which show the differences better than delayed images [37]. Both sides must be symmetrically positioned within the field of view. Segmental closure can be better identified using a pinhole view [28, 37]. In addition to asymmetric and segmental differences in uptake, a blurred growth plate appearance can also be seen with adjacent epiphyseal and or metaphyseal injuries [37]. These findings are not permanent, as shown by Etchebehere et al. [38], who studied 18 children with uncomplicated femoral fractures using multiphase bone scintigraphy at three different times (2–5 months, 6–12 months and 18–24 months). Visual analysis of the blood flow, equilibrium and delayed images showed increased activity in the distal femoral growth plates during the first and second time intervals, but not during the third [38]. Scintigraphy is considered to be the only imaging modality capable of assessing the magnitude of physeal stimulus caused by femoral fractures and to predict a favorable, or unfavorable, outcome of leg length by semi-quantitative analysis. SPECT imaging can detect, and locate, the decreased metabolism associated with post-traumatic closure of the physeal plate which predicts growth arrest and deformities [11, 28, 33].

Surgical closure of a growth plate (epiphysiodesis) is performed in children who develop progressive leg length deformity. Scintigraphy can be used to determine the success of the procedure. At 4 months the blood pool and delayed images should demonstrate a decreased uptake in the surgically treated physis. An unsuccessful procedure shows persistent uptake at an above-normal level. Assessment earlier than 4 months may show normal or increased uptake that is due to the healing process. By 4 months a growth plate that is closing can be identified. Complete closure after epiphysiodesis appears to take approximately 8 months (28).

Toddler's Fracture

Although this has been considered typically a non-displaced spiral fracture of the mid-tibia in preschool children, the term is also applied to fractures of other bones in this age group, including the fibula, calcaneus, talus, metatarsals and cuboid. Scintigraphy has a great value in identifying these fractures, which are commonly occult radiographically [39–41]. The toddler fracture of the cuboid bone is relatively common and may be due to forced plantar hyperflexion of the foot and shows a radiological abnormality close to the articular surface of the cuboid with the calcaneus [42]. A focus of increased uptake is seen at the site of the fracture which can be seen and localized better by pinhole imaging.

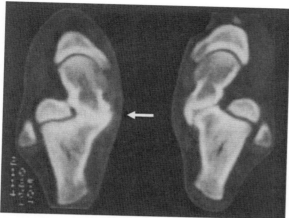

Fig. 4.11. Tarsal coalition (*arrow*) as seen in an illustrative cut of C.T. scan of the feet. Compare to the normal contra-lateral side

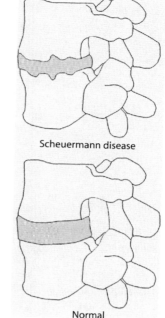

Fig. 4.12. A diagram illustrating the erosions of the end plates and narrowing of the intervertebral space associated with Scheuermann disease (upper diagram). A normal intervertebral space and adjacent end plates (lower diagram) is shown for comparison

Tarsal Coalition

This condition is due to fusion of the talus and calcaneus or the navicular and calcaneus bones. It occurs due to failure of normal segmentation of the ossification centers during embryogenesis but does not become symptomatic before the second decade of life. Radiographic modalities are the primary diagnostic tools (Fig. 4.11); however, when they are equivocal, bone scintigraphy with pinhole imaging can be of significant value by showing focal uptake in the subtalar region indicating coalition. This activity is due to the abnormal motion of the fused bones inducing a stress reaction at the adjacent bone because of the abnormal motion created by the fused bones [37, 43, 44].

Increased radionuclide accumulation in a hypertrophic spur, the talar beak, is a frequent finding in patients with symptomatic subtalar coalition. It results from the abnormal joint mechanics which produce repetitive trauma on the talar periosteum. Bone scintigraphy therefore is useful in identifying talocalcaneal coalition as the cause of foot pain.

Battered Child Syndrome

Bone scintigraphy is useful in identifying abused children. It is more sensitive than radiographs, with up to 50% additional sensitivity by showing foci of increased uptake at different sites, particularly those known to be common for radiographically occult fractures, such as the ribs and pelvis [45, 46].

Scheuermann's Disease

Although this condition is not clearly due to trauma and the etiology has not been defined, it is included here since it occurs in the active age of 13–17 years and trauma is a suspected underlying cause. It is a destruc-

tive form of osteochondrosis featuring erosions of the endplates of two adjacent vertebrae with a decrease in the height of the intervertebral space (Fig. 4.12) and anterior wedging of thoracic vertebrae by 5 deg or more, as seen on lateral standard radiographs, and may lead to kyphosis. Scheuermann's disease also occurs less commonly in the lumbar spine. On scintigraphy, there is no, or only mild, increase of uptake by the vertebrae, a feature that may help separate this condition from others such as tumors and infections which show a significant degree of abnormal uptake [47, 48].

Osteochondritis Dissecans (Transchondral Fractures)

This condition affects young adults and children, with males affected three times more frequently than females. The proposed causes include trauma, ischemia, and a genetic predisposition The theory of ischemia is not widely accepted since the common site of the condition, namely the lower end of the femur, is rich in vascular supply. Although the exact cause remains unsettled, the trauma theory is more widely accepted as prior trauma has been reported in up to 60% of patients [11, 49–51]. The condition results from separation of a segment of cartilage and the subchondral bone from the articular surface whether completely or partially. It most commonly affects the medial femoral condyle, followed by the lateral femoral condyle, the lateral tibial condyle and the patellofemoral compartment. Osteochondritis dissecans also occurs in the bones around the elbow, commonly among baseball players, as reported by Takahara et al. and others [51, 52]. The condition is also common among individuals who have played baseball actively since childhood [51, 52], and repetitive throwing is considered to be one of the main etiological factors of this disease [52–54]. During the acceleration phase of throwing, the elbow joint may be stressed into a valgus position [55] and the capitellum may be subjected to compression and shear forces [56–58].

Minzuta et al. [59] described the clinical presentation of six athletically active children, aged 6–12 years, with symptomatic osteochondritis dissecans of the lateral femoral condyle developed after total resection of the discoid lateral meniscus. The condition presented as a recurrent pain in the treated knee which started 36–65 months after surgery. All patients had been continuously engaged in sports activity after surgery before the recurrence of pain. On arthroscopy, softening was found in two knees, a separated fragment in two knees, and a completely loose fragment in two further knees. The authors suggested that repeated impaction in sports activities on the immature osteochondral structures under altered mechanical force transmission after total resection of the discoid meniscus might be a predisposing factor in the development of osteochondritis dissecans of the lateral femoral condyle [59].

Multiphase bone scanning is used when other modalities are equivocal and there is a need to determine the stability of the joint and prognosis. Standard radiographs and MRI are usually adequate to make the diagnosis, and MRI provides a good assessment of the separated segment. The pattern of abnormalities on scintigraphy depends on the time elapsed and the severity of injury. Accordingly, a scintigraphic classification (Table 4.8) has been proposed which can be of value in determining the prognosis and management [60, 61]. Paletta et al. [62] more recently found a very high prognostic value for scintigraphy among patients with open physes. The authors reviewed the records of 12 patients,

aged 9–16 years, with osteochondritis dissecans of the knee, including bone scan results, clinical course, healing time, and final outcome, to determine the prognostic value of scintigraphy. Patients were divided into those with open physes (distal femoral and proximal tibial) and those with closed physes. Four of the six patients with open physes had increased activity on the bone scan and all achieved healing with non-surgical treatment. The remaining two patients had decreased activity on bone scan and non-surgical treatment failed, necessitating surgery. On the other hand, all the six patients with closed physes had increased activity on the bone scan, but only two had healing of the osteochondral lesions without surgery. Accordingly, the authors found that quantitative bone scanning had a 100% predictive value for the prognosis in this group of osteochondritis dissecans patients with open physes, but for those with closed physes the predictive value was lower [62].

Slipped Capital Femoral Epiphysis

This term describes displacement of the femoral head from the femoral neck at the site of the growth plate during growth. The condition affects adolescent boys more often than girls and is more frequent among patients of African descent [63]. The condition can be unilateral or bilateral and is usually diagnosed with standard radiographs. Scintigraphy is used when it is difficult to make a diagnosis using radiography, such as in cases of bilateral displacement or when the clinical situation is complicated by osteonecrosis, which occurs in approximately 15% of cases [37].

On bone images, there is increased uptake at the site of the growth plate and the adjacent femoral metaphysis, a finding that probably reflects the increased metabolic activity at the site of the plate disruption [37]. Additionally, significant displacement is due to the abnormal posteromedial relationship of the femoral head to the femoral neck. When osteonecrosis is present, other scintigraphic findings include increased peri-articular uptake, illustrating an associated reactive synovitis, and photon deficiency of the femoral head. Scintigraphy can also be useful in assessing whether the treatment is adequate. This is determined by demonstrating fusion of the growth plate.

Table 4.8. Scintigraphic classification of osteochondritis dissecans of the femoral condyle

Stage	Scintigraphic pattern	Clinical significance
0	Normal multiphase scan	
I	Normal multiphase scan with abnormal radiographs	Stable lesion, asymptomatic
II	Focally increased activity on delayed images	Stable lesion, pain starts
	Focally increased blood pool and delayed uptake at site of lesion	Unstable lesion
III	Focally increased activity on all phases in and around lesion	Unstable lesion
IV	Same as in stage III with increased uptake in juxtaarticular tibial Plateau	Unstable lesion

4.4
Scintigraphic Diagnosis of Stress Fractures

4.4.1
Role of Scintigraphy in Stress Fractures

Contrary to the case of acute fracture diagnosis, scintigraphy has a major role in the diagnosis of stress fractures, whether due to fatigue or insufficiency, since

Table 4.9. Diagnosis of stress fractures: accuracy of bone scanning compared with standard radiographs

Author	Year	Number of patients	Sensitivity		Specificity	
			Bone scan	Radiographs	Bone scan	Radiographs
Geslin	1976 [109]	200	100%	0%	100%	–
Wilcox	1977 [110]	34	100%	85%	100%	100%
Prather	1977 [111]	42	100%	29%	76%	100%
Roub	1979 [112]	42	100%	41%	–	–
Rupani	1985 [108]	238	100%	41%	100%	100%
Zwas	1987 [69]	310	100%	18%	–	–
Holder	1998 [65]	16	100%	–	100%	–

standard radiographs take additional time to show the fractures (Table 4.9). Additionally scintigraphy can differentiate more reliably between recent and old fractures [64]. Holder et al. [65] studied 16 patients with stress-related bone injuries and normal standard radiographs with MRI and two-phase bone scanning. The average sensitivity, specificity, and positive and negative predictive values for the presence of stress-related injuries of MRI were 66%, 90%, 96%, and 45%, respectively, while for scintigraphy, all abnormal and normal findings were correctly identified. Those authors recommend bone scintigraphy as the initial imaging modality of choice for patients with clinically suspected stress-related injuries and a low probability of other active bone diseases such as infection or neoplasm [65].

4.4.2
Scintigraphic Appearance of Stress Fractures

If scintigraphy is performed in the acute phase within 4 weeks, the flow and blood pool images show increased activity. The delayed uptake typically involves less than one fifth of the bone in this phase. Later, only a delayed uptake will be seen. In general, three patterns of uptake on delayed images can be recognized in fractures: a focal band of uptake, diffuse uptake, or peripheral linear uptake parallel to the periosteum [66]. Complete, or partial, scintigraphic resolution occurs within 4–6 months in the presence of normal healing [66]. Fractures may be single, or multiple (Fig. 4.13), particularly in athletes and patients with osteoporosis. Multiple fractures, particularly in osteoporotic patients, may simulate metastatic disease (Fig. 4.14) [67]. Scintigraphically, stress fractures can be staged into five stages based

on the amount of bone involvement (Fig. 4.15): stage I involves less than 20%, as mentioned earlier; stage II involves 20–40%; stage 3, 40–60%; stage 4, 60–80%; and in stage V 80–100% of the bone is involved (complete fractures). Localization of stress fractures is important and should be included in the report since the prognosis can be different. The less frequently encountered anterior tibial stress fractures are more prone to

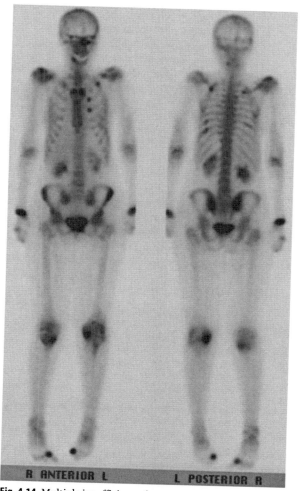

Fig. 4.14. Multiple insufficiency fractures seen on a whole body bone scan of a 67-year-old woman after a fall

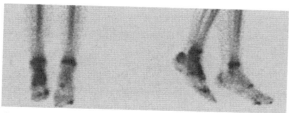

Fig. 4.13. Spot image of the feet of a 23-year-old dancer demonstrating multiple fatigue fractures of feet

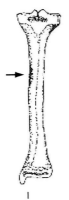
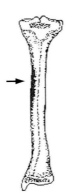
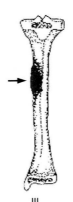
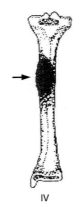

I

Small ill defined
cortical area of
mildly increased
activity

II

Larger well defined
elongated cortical area
of moderately
increased activity

III

Wide-fusiform
cortico-medullary
area of highly
increased activity

IV

Extensive
transcortical area of
intensely increased
activity

Fig. 4.15. A diagram illustrating 4 stages of stress fracture. Stage V represents complete fracture. (Diagram from Zwas [66] with permission)

complications such as non-union and avascular necrosis. It is important to note that sometimes anterior fractures show decreased rather that the typical increased uptake focally. Fractures of the femoral neck have the potential for avascular necrosis and displacement. These fractures may show focal uptake along the medial femoral neck but less commonly show a transverse band of increased uptake extending across the femoral neck.

Shin splint which results from extreme tension on the muscles, or muscle groups, inserting onto the tibia and to a lesser extent the femur. This leads to periosteal elevation with reactive bone formation. It is most commonly found in the tibia and may coexist with fatigue fractures. It is characterized by exercise-induced pain and tenderness typically along the posterior medial and anterior lateral aspects of the tibia and anterior medial aspect of the femur. Differentiating shin splints from stress fractures is crucial since the management is different. Radiographs are normal. Scintigraphically, the flow and blood pool are typically normal, although slightly increased activity may occasionally be seen. Using delayed images, there is longitudinal increased uptake along the diaphysis which can be faint and most commonly involve the posteromedial and antero-lateral aspects of the tibial cortex(affecting usually one third of the bone length) and the anteromedial border of the femur, affecting usually the upper or mid-portions of the bone (Fig. 4.16). Both posterior and anterior tibial changes may present in the same individual. The locations of abnormalities suggest that the entity is related to the soleus muscle in the case of tibial splints and the adductor muscle group in the case of the femoral splints [68–70]. Shin splints also occur in the upper extremity bones.

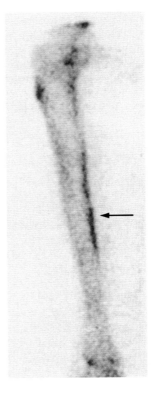

Fig. 4.16. A linear pattern of increased uptake seen at the posterior border of a tibia illustrating typical bone scintigraphic pattern of skin splint

4.4.3
Scintigraphic Diagnosis of Specific Stress Fractures
4.4.3.1
Stress Fractures of the Feet

Stress fractures of the feet and ankle, fatigue or insufficiency are frequently radiographically occult in their acute and sub-acute phases. The sensitivity of radiography is low and was 18% in one series [66].

Common sites of these fractures in this region include the distal fibula, metatarsals, calcaneus, talus, sesamoid and navicular bones [71]. Scintigraphy is useful in detecting such fractures [72].

4.4.3.2
Stress Fractures of the Ribs

Stress fractures of the ribs are common and may be due to repetitive mechanical movement of the upper extremities as seen in golf and rowing sports or in older patients after coughing, hard straining or other trivial trauma.

In a collaborative review study at three institutions, Lord et al. [73] documented 19 cases of stress fractures of the ribs in golfers (the 4th to 6th ribs were the most commonly injured). All fractures occurred along the posterolateral aspect of the ribs, and nine patients had fractures in more than one rib. Plain radiographs were helpful diagnostically. However, bone scintigraphy was necessary to reach a diagnosis in three cases. Stress fractures of the ribs in golfers may be more common than previously realized and it is believed that fatigue of the serratus anterior is the mechanism of injury [74].

A case of multiple cough-induced stress fractures and arthropathy has been documented using Tc-99 bone scanning in a high-altitude climber. It has been proposed to add the term 'high-altitude cough syndrome' to the medical terminology to identify this discrete medical problem of exposure to very high altitude [75].

Single a multiple foci of increased uptake are seen on bone scan with corresponding blood pool activity in recent fractures.

4.4.3.3
Stress Fractures of the Tibia

Tibia is the most common location of stress fractures. These fractures cause severe pain focally and if neglected may cause complete fracture which commonly is complicated by non union. They occur most frequently in the anterior proximal third in children and at the junction of the middle and distal thirds in adults.

Fifty-two patients with a history and physical examination suggestive of tibial stress fracture underwent a tuning fork test (TFT) followed by a bone scan in order to compare the performance of the TFT with nuclear scintigraphy for the identification of tibial stress fractures. The TFT was performed by applying a 128-Hz tuning fork to the anterior surface of the bared tibia. If the patient reported a marked exacerbation, or reproduction, of the shin pain in a localized area of the tibia, the TFT was considered positive. The sensitivity and specificity of the tuning fork test were 75 and 67%, re-

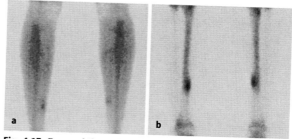

Fig. 4.17. Recent bilateral tibial stress fractures in an athletic young man. Note the typical focally increased uptake at the site of fractures on both blood pool (**a**) and delayed (**b**) images

spectively. The TFT is not sensitive enough to rule out a stress fracture on the basis of a negative test [76] and cannot replace bone scan (Fig. 4.17).

4.4.3.4
Stress Fractures of the Femur

Stress fractures of the femur may involve the femoral neck, intertrochanteric region and/or the shaft of the bone. The fractures may be fatigue fractures, which mainly occur in athletes, or insufficiency fractures occuring, particularly in older individuals. In either situation, these fractures may lead to significant morbidity, particularly if not treated promptly. Fatigue fractures of the femoral neck may be compressive, typically at the inferior border due to a compressive effect created when the supero-inferior and infero-superior forces meet, or tensile at the superior margin due to injury in adduction [14, 77, 78]. On multiphase bone scanning, which is indicated when radiographs are normal, the fractures present with increased flow, blood pool activity and varying degrees of increased delayed uptake [14, 78, 79]. Fernandez et al. [79] indicated that the fractures of the neck may show only subtle degree of uptake and may be missed unless the images are analyzed carefully along with careful looking at the pelvis and other bones for associated abnormalities. In our experience, SPECT is important in detecting abnormalities of the femoral neck and can provide important information.

4.4.3.5
Pelvic Fractures

Pelvic insufficiency fractures are a complication of osteoporosis. This may be due to post-menopausal status, high-dose corticosteroids, or local irradiation. The fractures usually occur in the sacroiliac joint and in the pubis and can mimic bone metastases on bone scans. Knowledge of the nature of the trauma and osteoporosis is essential in order to rule out metastatic disease and thus avoid inappropriate treatment. Although ra-

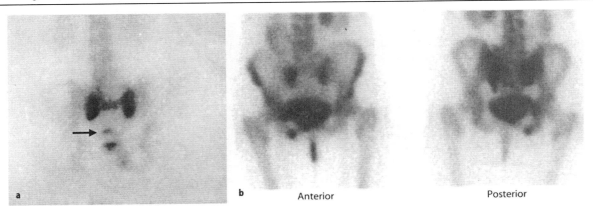

Fig. 4.18. a An example of sacral fractures showing the H pattern with two vertical fractures and connecting horizontal fracture. Smaller horizontal sacral fracture is also noted (*arrow*). **b** Bilateral vertical fractures

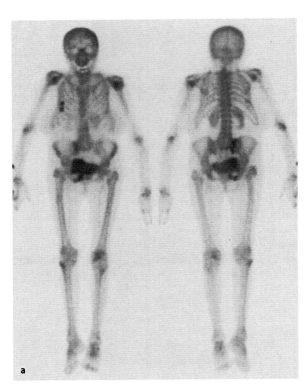

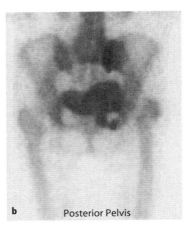

Fig. 4.19a, b. Unilateral vertical uptake with a fainter horizontal uptake at the site of a right sacral fracture representing another pattern of sacral fractures. Note additional fractures of the left rib cage and pelvic bones

dionuclide bone scanning is useful in the early detection of pelvic insufficiency fractures, CT can provide a definitive diagnosis in many patients [80]. Insufficiency fracture of the sacrum as a cause of lower back pain is not uncommon, especially in post-menopausal women with risk factors. Insufficiency fracture of the sacrum is often radiographically occult. Bone scintigraphy is the method of choice for the diagnosis. The typical scintigraphic pattern is H-shaped uptake (Fig. 4.18), which presents in approximately 20% of cases. The most common pattern, however, is unilateral vertical uptake, which is present in approximately 32%

of cases (Fig. 4.19), followed by horizontal uptake in 27% (Fig. 4.20), half H-shaped uptake in 14% and bilateral vertical uptake in the sacral wings (Fig. 4.21) in 7% of cases [81, 82]. Bone scintigraphy is not only an adequate procedure for the detection of often radiographically occult sacral fractures, but also for revealing the often concomitant fractures, since further fractures are identified in 85% of cases, with the main locations in the pubic bone, spine and ribs [81]. Bilateral fracture of the sacrum has also been associated with pregnancy, and it is not clear whether it represents an insufficiency fracture due to transient osteoporosis of the sacrum associated with pregnancy, or a fatigue fracture due to unaccustomed stress related to rapid and excessive weight gain in the last trimester of pregnancy (Fig. 4.22) [83].

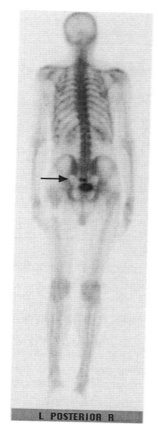

Fig. 4.20. A horizontal uptake in the mid-sacrum (*arrow*) illustrating another pattern of sacral fractures

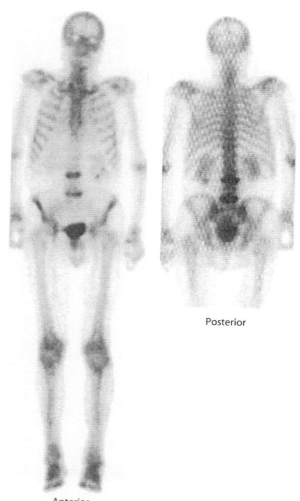

Posterior

Anterior

Fig. 4.22. Compression fractures at the lumbar spine showing typical scintigraphic pattern

4.4.3.6
Vertebral Fractures

Vertebral stress fractures are mostly due to insufficiency. Vertebral insufficiency fractures are known to show a marked female predominance and a concave deformity of the affected vertebra. They show a wide range of

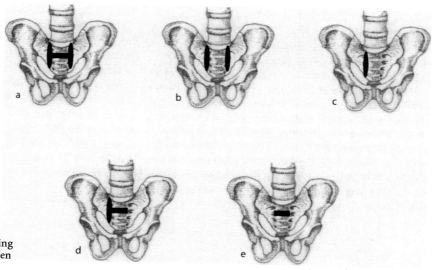

Fig. 4.21a–e. A diagram illustrating patterns of sacral fractures as seen on scintigraphy

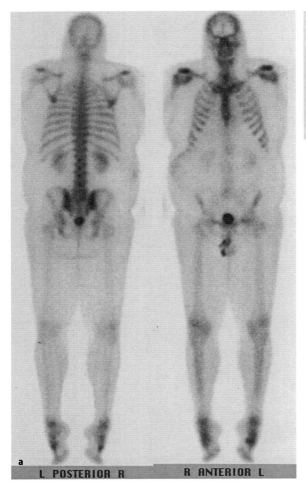

a   L POSTERIOR R   R ANTERIOR L

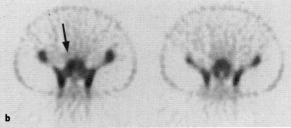

b

Fig. 4.23. a A whole body bone scan of a patient complaining of low back pain. The scan shows no definite abnormalities.
b Representative transaxial cuts of the SPECT study shows focally increased uptake in the right side of L-5 vertebra, illustrating the value of SPECT to identify and localize spine abnormalities

4.5
Scintigraphic Evaluation of Fracture and Bone Graft Healing

4.5.1
Evaluation of Fracture Healing

Approximately 60% of fractures heal scintigraphically within 1 year and 90% by 2 years [87]. However, healing also depends on the location of the fracture. Vertebral fractures, for example, take longer to normalize, with only 59% returning to normal by 1 year after the fracture compared to 79% for rib fractures [13].

A scintigraphic study of the healing process of closed tibial shaft fractures was carried out in 40 patients treated non-operatively, comprising 32 men and 8 women; the average age was 30.6 years. Scintigraphic scans were obtained at 6, 12 and 24 weeks after the fracture, and an activity index was calculated taking the mean of three consecutive uptake counts for both the fractured leg and the normal opposite leg, used for comparison. The results showed that the activity index in general decreased progressively from the first to the third evaluation during healing [88].

Multiphase bone imaging is essential for differentiating hypervascular from avascular (atrophic) non-unions (Fig. 4.24) and for monitoring delayed union [11]. As the name implies, in hypervascular non-union, there is increased flow and blood pool activity along with varying degrees of delayed uptake. On the other hand, in avascular non-unions which require surgical intervention (since nothing will be added by waiting), there is no increased flow, or blood pool activity, and the activity at the site of fracture is decreased on delayed images.

fracture distribution and the vertebral height and low consistency between the vertebral deformity seen on the lateral radiograph and positive abnormality on bone scanning. These findings emphasize the difficulty of radiographic diagnosis of vertebral fractures [84]. Scintigraphy, including SPECT, is a sensitive modality for the diagnosis of vertebral fractures and is useful in determining the age of fractures [85].

Fatigue fractures of the vertebrae mainly occur in active young adults and children. Thirty-three athletes complaining of back pain of more than 1 month's duration and with normal radiography of the lower spine were all studied using scintigraphy. From this group 24 were studied with SPECT, which detected 28% more lesions than planar imaging [86]. SPECT has an additional value in localizing the abnormalities of vertebra; this can also aid in the etiologic classification of the abnormality based on the location (Fig. 4.23).

4.5.2
Evaluation of Bone Graft Viability

Multiphase bone scanning is an excellent modality for monitoring graft viability non-invasively and offers a

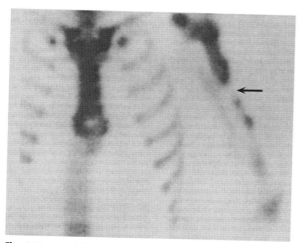

Fig. 4.24. Atrophic non-union. A comminuted fracture of the right humerus due to a gunshot is bridged by a long fibular strut graft placed medially 8 months prior to the bone scan. There is absence of uptake (*arrow*) corresponding to the non union fracture site. Linear uptake in the medial aspect is at the viable fibular graft. (From [113] with permission)

simple method for the assessment of the graft's physiological status. Autologous graft revascularization shows an increased uptake on all phases of the scan and eventually becomes uniform to adjacent bone as it is incorporated. Allografting initially shows a photon deficient area and gradually shows filling by uptake on serial scans. As initially shown in experimental studies by Stevenson et al. [89], the revascularization of a conventional graft commences at the host-graft junctions with subsequent extension from these sites throughout the graft until finally there is complete integration. Velasco et al. [90] for example, utilizing split rib grafts in ten patients, observed this pattern in nine patients in whom there was consolidation of the graft but observed no uptake in the remaining graft, which failed. With micro-vascularized bone grafts, three-phase scintigraphy is particularly useful because it permits assessment of both the integrity of the blood supply to the bone graft and the viability of the bone demonstrated by functioning osteocytes. Breggren et al. [91] emphasized the importance of the timing of such studies. If they are performed more than 1 week postoperatively, there may be a false-positive bone image due to the onset of creeping substitution whereby new bone is formed on the surface of the graft. However, Itoh et al. [92], favored serial three-phase imaging, since it not only permitted assessment of the vascular potency at an early stage but also allowed continuing observation of any complications. They also drew attention to a patient with an iliac bone graft in whom, following the demonstration of negative findings in all phases of scintigraphy, hyperbaric therapy was undertaken with subsequent serial bone images showing an improve-

ment in the vascularity and in the bone uptake in the grafted bone.

The utility of planar bone scintigraphy was evaluated for discerning bony union after spinal-fusion surgery, especially in cases of clinically and radiologically suggested pseudarthrosis. Between 1991 and 1996, Bohnsack et al. [93] performed bone scintigraphy on 42 patients (21 women, 21 men; mean age: 42 years) after spinal fusion surgery and just before their admission to the hospital for material removal. The fusions comprised 29 lumbosacral, 6 thoracolumbar, 3 lumbar, 2 thoracolumbosacral, 1 thoracic, and 1 cervical. The mean fusion spanned four segments, and the mean time between spinal fusion and material removal was 27 months. Based on scintigraphy, pseudarthrosis was suspected in five patients, and the condition was confirmed in four patients during operation, two diagnosed and two undiagnosed. The accuracy of the method was 88%; sensitivity, 50%, specificity, 93%; the positive predictive value was 40%; and the negative predictive value was 95%. The authors concluded that the sensitivity and positive predictive value of bone scintigraphy are low for possible instability after spinal fusion and that the method is not sufficient to reliably diagnose pseudarthrosis after spondylodesis [93].

4.5.3
Evaluation of Metallic Implants for Removal

The decision to remove metallic implants from patients with fractures with bridging plates, or interlocking nails, is based on subjective criteria. Recently multiphase bone scanning was found to be a useful guide in timing the removal of the implants. Mild uptake indicates consolidation and implants can be removed, while intense uptake indicates an unconsolidated fracture and implants should not yet be removed [94].

4.6
Scintigraphic Diagnosis of Injuries to Bone-adjacent Structures
4.6.1
Avulsion Injury

Apophyseal growth cartilage is the weakest point in the musculotendinous unit until they become ossified and is hence particularly prone to being avulsed due to the sudden forceful or repetitive muscular traction. Figure 4.25 illustrates the major apophyses sites focusing on the pelvic and proximal femoral apophyses and the muscles that attach to them. Common locations of such injuries, at the site of insertion of certain muscles (e.g. the powerful hamstring muscles attaching to the ischium and the brachioradialis muscle to the distal radius), are the ischium, greater and lesser trochanters, anterior

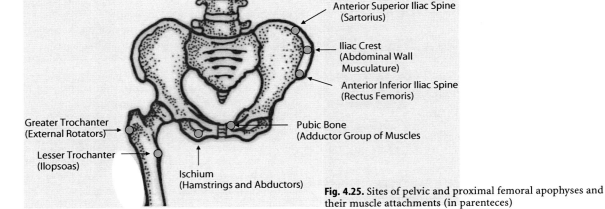

Fig. 4.25. Sites of pelvic and proximal femoral apophyses and their muscle attachments (in parenteces)

superior and anterior inferior iliac spine, iliac crest and distal radius [95–97]. Avulsion injuries present with acute pain and are common in adolescents. Early diagnosis is important in order to reduce the continuing displacement of the fragment which occurs particularly in avulsions of the ischium, a common injury caused by the power of the hamstring muscles. The condition needs at least 6 weeks of reduced activity for healing. Some avulsions can be readily identified by standard radiography, where displacement of the apophysis from its normal position is seen. CT and/or MRI are able to define the separation better; however, in other cases, particularly locations such as iliac crest and anterior inferior iliac spine, the displacement may be difficult to detect radiographically. In such cases scintigraphy is helpful and may be the first investigative technique to point to the diagnosis [95]. The scintigraphic findings depend on the displacement and the time of the study since the injury. The fragment may be clearly seen in its displaced site but, as healing proceeds, a localized increase in uptake, often intense, may be seen along with focally increased uptake on blood pool images (Fig. 4.26) and may also be possibly shown on flow study analysis [4, 79, 96]. Bone scintigraphy has the capability of detecting early avulsion before the onset of edema or changes in the bone marrow that are detected by MRI. If this capability is combined with precise anatomical localization of lesions, it enriches the diagnostic value of this modality in sports medicine [17].

4.6.2
Skeletal Muscle Injury

Since muscle injury cause release of muscle protein myosin from the injured cells, In-111-labeled antimyosin antibodies can be used to detect and assess the extent of skeletal muscle damage [6, 98] which is an important parameter affecting fracture healing.

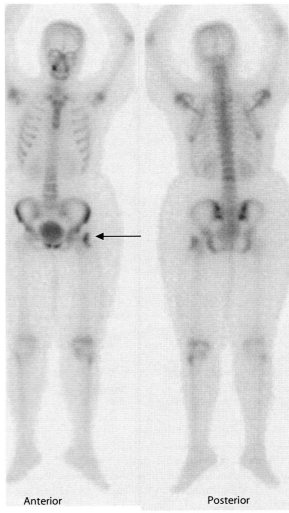

Anterior   Posterior

Fig. 4.26. Avulsion injury in the region of the left greater trochanter in a patient with history of recent trauma

4.6.3
Post-traumatic Soft Tissue Calcification

Heterotopic bone formation may be associated with trauma (but not exclusively). Bone scanning has a valuable role in its diagnosis, and more importantly follow-up, in order to determine the maturity and appropriate time for surgical intervention [99]. Early in the immature phase there is increased flow, blood pool activity and delayed uptake. The flow and blood pool activity decrease gradually until they stabilize, indicating normalization (see Chap. 8 for more details).

4.6.4
Meniscal and Ligament Tears

MRI is known to be the modality of choice for the diagnosis of these tears. However, it may not be possible to perform MRI due to a contraindication or lack of availability. In addition, it is associated with a false-negative rate of approximately 20%. Planar imaging has limited value, and SPECT and/or pinhole imaging help in the diagnosis. For acute tears it has a sensitivity of 88%, negative predictive value of 91% and positive predictive value of 83% [11]. Pinhole imaging can significantly facilitate the localization of the abnormal uptake.

4.6.5
Enthesopathies (see also Chap. 7)

The sites of insertion of tendons, ligaments and articular capsule to bone are called entheses. These sites are metabolically active and can act in manner similar to the periosteum at their sites. Trauma, degeneration and or inflammation of these sites can result in regional periosteal reaction with osteoblastic bone activity. Plantar fasciitis and Achilles tendinitis, which typically show increased flow and blood pool activity with varying degrees of focally increased activity on delayed images on scintigraphy, are major examples. Enthesopathies are commonly seen as sporting injuries and are associated with conditions as spondyloarthropathies [100].

4.6.6
Impingement Syndromes

This is a group of painful conditions caused by friction of joint tissue. They are classified into bone impingement, soft tissue impingement and entrapment neuropathy. Although occurring less frequently than meniscal and ligamental injuries, impingement syndromes must be taken into consideration when looking for skeletal disorders. Diagnostic imaging, particularly MRI, is very useful as it allows a proper and correct diagnosis procedure for any single condition. Scintigraphy is a complementary modality; however, physicians interpreting bone scans should be aware of the entity and its findings for proper diagnosis of skeletal conditions. The disorders can be seen in the joint regions of the upper and lower extremities, including the shoulders, elbows, knees, ankles and hands and feet [101–103].

Rotator cuff impingement syndrome is an example of an upper extremity disorder. Carpal tunnel syndrome is the most common peripheral entrapment neuropathy of the upper limb; it is caused by compression of the median nerve at the wrist. Tarsal tunnel syndrome is the most important ankle entrapment neuropathy causing burning pain and paresthesias in the toes and sole of the foot [104]. The ankle impingement syndrome is a frequent condition in both athletes and the normal population. Examples of this syndrome include anterior tibiotalar impingement, found frequently in dancers following repeated extension of the ankle joint (dorsiflexion). Posterior impingement syndrome of the ankle results from repeated plantar flexion, often among ballet dancers and gymnasts. Consequently, the os trigonum, an accessory ossicle that occasionally forms a synostosis with the posterior aspect of the talus, can become compressed between the calcaneus and the posterior lip of the tibia, eventually creating a fracture [105].

Knee impingement syndromes are very frequently reported in both professional and amateur sportsmen. The sites of symptom onset is divided into the medial, lateral, anterior and posterior portions. Patellofemoral disorders are the most frequent anterior knee syndromes and are associated with incorrect torsional movements of the lower limbs or local dysplasia. Among posterior impingement syndromes, the most frequent abnormalities involve the insertional tract of the mid-calf muscle, associated with a bursa reaction and insertional popliteus hypertrophy. The most frequent abnormality in medial syndromes involve the parapatellar synovial fold whose symptoms can be often mistaken for a meniscal injury. In lateral syndromes, involvement of the distal insertional tract of the broad fascia tensor tendon with bursa reaction is the most frequent [106]. Scintigraphically, focal area of increased uptake at the site of injury is characteristic and pinhole views can again help significantly in localization of the abnormality.

References

1. Martin JS, Marsh JL (1997) Current classification of fractures. Radiol Clin North Am 35:491–506
2. Mourad A (1998) Alterations of musculoskeletal function. In: McCance KL, Huether SE (eds) Pathophysiology, 3rd edn. Mosby, Philadelphia, pp 1435–1485
3. McCarthy EF (1997) Histopathologic correlates of a positive bone scan. Seminars in Nuclear Medicine 27:309–320

4. Patel M (1998) Upper extremity radionuclide bone imaging: shoulder, arm, elbow, and forearm. Semin Nucl Med 28:3–13

5. Shigeru E (1997) Complications of skeletal trauma. Radiol Clin North Am 35:767–781

6. Malki A, Owunwanne A, Elgazzar A, Abdel-Dayem AH (1999) Assessment of skeletal muscle damage in experimental animal using in-111 antimyosin. J Surg Invest 1:99–105

7. Reed A, Joyner C, Brawnlow H, Simpson H (2001) Radiological classification of human non-unions does not reflect biological activity. Proceeding of the 47th annual meeting, Orthopedic Research Society, San Francisco

8. Hain SF, O'Doherty MJ, Smith MA (2002) Functional imaging and the orthopedic surgeon. J Bone Joint Surg (Br) 84B:315–321

9. Maguire WB (2000) Pelvic fractures diagnosed by bone scintigraphy in patients with normal radiographs after a fall. Med J Austr 172:302–303

10. Versijpt J, Dierckx RA, de Bondt P, Dierckx I, Lambrecht L, de Sadeleer C (1999) The contribution of bone scintigraphy in occupational health or medical insurance claims: a retrospective study. Eur J Nucl Med 26:804–811

11. Etchebehere EC, Etchebehere M, Gamba R, Belangero W, Camargo EE (1998) Orthopedic pathology of the lower extremities: scintigraphic evaluation in the thigh, knee, and leg. Semin Nucl Med 28:41–61

12. Rosenthall L, Hill RO, Chuang S (1978) Observation on the use of Tc99m phosphate imaging in peripheral bone trauma. Radiology 119:637–741

13. Matin P (1979) The appearance of bone scan following fractures including intermediate and long term studies. J Nucl Med 20:1227–1231

14. Holder LE, Schwarz C, Wernicke PG et al (1990) Radionuclide bone imaging in early detection of fractures of the proximal femur (hip): multifactorial analysis. Radiology 152:509–515

15. Spitz J, Lauer I, Tittel K (1993) Scintimetric evaluation of remodeling after bone fractures in man. J Nucl Med 34:1403–1409

16. Skarzynski JJ, Skiklas JJ, Spencer RP (1985) Delayed appearance of positive bone scan following fracture. Clin Nucl Med 10:663–667

17. Van der Wall H, Storey G, Frater C, Murray IPC (2001) Importance of positioning and technical factors in anatomic localisation of sporting injuries in scintigraphic imaging. Semin Nucl Med 26:17–27

18. Mohamed A, Ryan P, Lewis M, Jarosz JM, Fogelman I, Spencer JD, Clarke SE (1997) Registration bone scan in the evaluation of wrist pain. J Hand Surg (Br) 22:161–166

19. Roolker W, Tiel-van Buul MM, Broekhuizen AH, Eikelenboom AK, van Royen EA (1997) Improved wrist fracture localization with digital overlay of bone scintigrams and radiographs. J Nucl Med 38:1600–1603

20. Wahler HM (1978) Radionuclide diagnosis of fracture healing. J Nucl Med 19:1356–1358

21. Elsaid M, Hamouda A, Newman D, Woodcock J, Elgazzar A (2000) When do flow and blood pool activity at fracture sites on bone scintigraphy normalize? An experimental study. J Nucl Med 41:327P

22. Erhan Y, Solak I, Kocabas S, Sozbilen M, Kumanlioglu K, Moral AR (2001) The evaluation of diagnostic accordance between plain radiography and bone scintigraphy for the assessment of sternum and rib fractures in the early period of blunt trauma. Turk J Trauma Emerg Surg 7:242–245

23. Bayer LR, Widding A, Diemer H (2000) Fifteen minutes bone scintigraphy in patients with clinically suspected scaphoid fracture and normal x-rays. Injury 31:243–248

24. Vrettos BC, Adams BK, Knottenbelt JD, Lee A (1996) Is there a place for radionuclide bone scintigraphy in the management of radiograph-negative scaphoid trauma? South Afr Med J 86:540–542

25. Fowler C, Sullivan B, Williams LA, McCarthy G, Savage R, Palmer A (1998) A comparison of bone scintigraphy and MRI in the early diagnosis of the occult scaphoid waist fracture. Skeletal Radiol 27:683–687

26. Thorpe AP, Murray AD, Smith FW, Ferguson J (1996) Clinically suspected scaphoid fracture: a comparison of magnetic resonance imaging and bone scintigraphy. Br J Radiol 69:109–113

27. Vuori JP, Aro HT (1993) Lisfranc joint injuries: trauma mechanisms and associated injuries. J Trauma 36:40–45

28. Harcke HT, Mandell GA (1993) Scintigraphic evaluation of the growth plate. Semin Nucl Med 23:266–273

29. Wioland M, Bonnerot V (1993) Diagnosis of partial and total physeal arrest by single photon emission computed tomography. J Nucl Med 34:1410–1415

30. Peterson HA (1984) Partial growth plate arrest and its treatment. J Pediatr Orthop 4:246–258

31. DeCampo JF, Boldt DW (1986) Computed tomography in partial growth plate arrest: Initial experience. Skeletal Radiol 183:119–123

32. Jaramillo D, Hoffer EA, Shapiro F et al (1990) MR imaging of fracture of the growth plate. AJR 155:1261–265

33. Sharkey CA, Harcke HT, Mandell GA et al (1986) SPECT techniques in the evaluation of growth plate abnormalities about the knee. J Nucl Med Tech 14:13

34. Harcke HT, Zapf SE, Mandell GA et al (1987) Angular deformity of the lower extremity: evaluation with quantitative bone scintigraphy. Radiology 164:437–440

35. Gates GF, Dore EK (1975) Detection of craniosynostosis by bone scanning. Radiology 115:665–671

36. Harcke HT (1978) Bone imaging in infants and children: a review. J Nucl Med 19:324–329

37. Mandell GA (1998) Nuclear medicine in pediatric orthopedics. Semin Nuclear Med 28:95–115

38. Etchebehere EC, Caron M, Pereira JA, Lima MC, Santos AO, Ramos CD, Barros FB, Sanches A, Santos-Jesus R, Belangero W, Camargo EE (2001) Activation of the growth plates on three-phase bone scintigraphy: the explanation for the overgrowth of fractured femurs. Eur J Nucl Med 28:72–80

39. Anglaro EE, Gelfand MJ, Paltiel HJ (1992) Bone scintigraphy in preschool children with lower extremity pain of unknown origin. J Nucl Med 33:351–354

40. Newman L (1990) Acute plastic bowing fractures of both the tibia and fibula in a child. Injury; 21:122–123

41. Aronson J, Karvin K, Siebert J et al (1992) Efficiency of the bone scan for occult limping toddlers. J Pediatr Orthop 12:38–44

42. Blumberg K, Patterson RJ (1991) The toddler's cuboid fracture. Radiology 179:93–94

43. Deutsch AL, Resnick D, Campbell G (1982) Computed tomography and bone scintigraphy: in evaluation of tarsal coalition. Radiology 144:137–140

44. Sarno RC, Carter BL, Semine MC (1984) Computed tomography in tarsal coalition. J Comput Assist Tomogr 8:1155–1160

45. Sty JR, Starshak RJ (1983) The role of bone scintigraphy in the evaluation of the suspected abused child. Radiology 146:369–375

46. Smith FW, Gilday DL, Ash JM et al (1980) Unsuspected costovertebral fractures demonstrated by bone scanning in the child abuse syndrome. Pediatr Radiol 10:103–106

47. Lowe TG (1990) Scheuermann disease. J Bone Joint Surg (Am) 72:940–945

48. Cleveland RH, Delong GR (1981) The relationship of juvenile lumbar disc disease and Scheuermann's disease. Pediatr Radiol 10:161–164

49. Bohndorf K (1996) Injuries at the articulating surfaces of bone (chondral, osteochondral, subchondral fractures and osteochondrosis dissecans). Eur J Radiol 22:22–29

50. Kumar R, Dilip S, Padhy AK, Malhotra R, Malhotra A, Machineni S, Sharma R (1998) Three-phase bone imaging in the early diagnosis of osteochondritis dissecans of the patella. Clin Nucl Med 23:540–541

51. Takahara, M; Shundo Mo, Kondo M, Suzuki K, Nambu T, Ogino T (1998) Early detection of osteochondritis dissecans of the capitellum in young baseball players: report of three cases. J Bone Joint Surg 80-A:892–897

52. Adams JE (1965) Injury to the throwing arm. A study of traumatic changes in the elbow joints of boy baseball players. Calif Med J 102:127–132

53. Barbes DA, Tullos HS (1978) An analysis of 100 symptomatic baseball players. Am J Sports Med 6:62–67

54. Brown R, Blazina ME, Kerlan RK, Carter VS, Jobe FW, Carlson GJ (1974) Osteochondritis of the capitellum. J Sports Med 2:27–46

55. Hang YS, Lippert FG III, Spolek GA, Frankel VH, Harrington RM (1979) Biomechanical study of the pitching elbow. Int Orthop 3:217–222

56. Andrews JR (1985) Bony injuries about the elbow in the throwing athlete. In: American Academy of Orthopaedic Surgeons: Instructional course lectures, vol 34. Mosby, St Louis, pp 323–331

57. Jobe FW, Nuber G (1986) Throwing injuries of the elbow. Clin Sports Med 5:621–636

58. Masatoshi T, Motoyuki S, Makoto K, Katsunori S, Toshikazu N, Toshihiko O (1998) Early detection of osteochondritis dissecans of the capitellum in young baseball players: report of three cases. J Bone Joint Surg 80-A:892–897

59. Mizuta H, Nakamura E, Otsuka Y, Kudo S, Takagi K (2001) Osteochondritis dissecans of the lateral femoral condyle following total resection of the discoid lateral meniscus. Arthroscopy 17:608–612

60. Cahill BR, Berg BC (1983) Technetium-99m phosphate compound joint scintigraphy in the management of juvenile osteochondrotis dissicans of the femoral condyle. Am J Sports Med 11:329–335

61. Mesgarzadeh M, Sapega AA, Bonakdarpour A et al (1987) Osteochondrotis dissicans: analysis of mechanical stability with radiography, scintigraphy and MR inaging. Osteochondrotis dissicans: analysis of mechanical stability with radiography, scintigraphy and MR imaging. Radiology 165:775–780

62. Paletta GA Jr, Bednarz PA, Stanitski CL, Sandman GA, Stanitski DF, Kottamasu S (1998) The prognostic value of quantitative bone scan in knee osteochondritis dissecans. A preliminary experience. Am J Sports Med 26:7–14

63. Andersen PE, Schantz K, Ballerslev J et al (1988) Bilateral femoral head dysplasia and osteochondrosis. Multiple epiphyseal dysplasia and osteochodritis. Multiple epiphyseal dysplasia tarda, spondyloepiphyseal dysplasia tarda and bilateral leg perthes siaease. Acta Radiol 29:705–709

64. Miyakoshi N, Sato K, Murai H, Tamura Y (2000) Insufficiency fractures of the distal tibiae. J Orthop Sci 5:71–74

65. Holder J, Steinert H, Zanetti M, Frolicher U, Rogala J, Stumpe K, von Schulthess GK (1998) Radiographically negative stress related bone injury. MR imaging versus two-phase bone scintigraphy. Acta Radiol 39:416–420

66. Zwas ST, Elkanovitch R, Frank G (1987) Interpretation and classification of bone scintigraphic findings in stress fractures. J Nucl Med 28:452–457

67. Baron E, Sheinfeld M, Migdal EA, Hardoff R (1996) Multiple pathologic fractures mimicking bone metastases in a patient with Cushing's syndrome. Clin Nucl Med 21:506–508

68. Charkes ND, Siddhivarn N, Schneck CD (1987) Bone scan-

ning in the adductor insertion avulsion syndrome („thigh splints"). J Nucl Med 28:1835–1838

69. Spencer RP, Levinson ED, Baldwin RD et al (1979) Diverse bone scan abnormalities in „shin splints". J Nucl Med 20:1271

70. Holder LE, Michael RH (1984) The specific scintigraphic pattern of „shin splints in the lower leg". Concise communication. J Nucl Med 25:865–869

71. Geslien GE, Thrall JH, Espinosa JL et al (1976) Early detection of stress fractures using Tc99m polyphosphate. Radiology 121:683–687

72. Sopov V, Liberson A, Groshar D (2000) Bone scintigraphic findings of os trigonum: a prospective study of 100 soldiers on active duty. Foot Ankle Int 21:822–824

73. Lord MJ, Ha KI, Song KS (1996) Stress fractures of the ribs in golfers. Am J Sports Med 24:118–122

74. Jamard B, Constantin A, Cantagrel A, Mazieres B, Laroche M (1999) Multiple rib fractures caused by coughing in a young woman without bone loss. Rev Rhum (Engl Edn) 66:237–238

75. Litch JA, Tuggy M (1998) Cough induced stress fracture and arthropathy of the ribs at extreme altitude. Int J Sports Med 19:220–222

76. Lesho EP (1997) Can tuning forks replace bone scans for identification of tibial stress fractures? Milit Med 162:802–803

77. Erne P, Burkhardt A (1980) Femoral neck fatigue fracture. Arch Orthop Trauma Surg 97:213–220

78. Elkhoury GY, Wehbe MA, Bonfigalio M et al (1980) Stress fractures of the femoral neck: a scintigraphic sign for early diagnosis. Skeletal Radiol 6:271–273

79. Fernandez Ulloa M, Klostermeier T, Lancaster K (1998) Orthopedic nuclear medicine: the pelvis and hip. Semin Nucl Med 28:25–40

80. Moreno A, Clemente J, Crespo C, Martinez A, Navarro M, Fernandez L, Minguell J, Vazquez G, Andreu FJ (1999) Pelvic insufficiency fractures in patients with pelvic irradiation. Int J Radiat Oncol Biol Phys 44:61–66

81. Hatzl-Griesenhofer M, Pichler R, Huber H, Maschek W (2001) The insufficiency fracture of the sacrum. An often unrecognized cause of low back pain: results of bone scanning in a major hospital. Nuklearmedizin 40:221–227

82. Peh WC (2001) Clinics in diagnostic imaging: insufficiency fractures of the pelvis. Singapore Med J 42:183–186

83. Schmid L, Pfirrmann C, Hess T, Schlumpf U (1999) Bilateral fracture of the sacrum associated with pregnancy: a case report. Osteoporosis Int 10:91–93

84. Kawaguchi S, Yamashita T, Koshio H, Kirita T, Minaki Y, Yokogushi K (2001) Insufficiency fracture of the spine: a prospective analysis based on radiographic and scintigraphic diagnosis. J Bone Miner Metab 19:312–316

85. Hendler A, Hershkop M (1998) When to use bone scintigraphy. It can reveal things other studies cannot. Postgrad Med 104:59–66

86. Garces GL, Gonzalez-Montoro I, Rasines JL, Santonja F (1999) Early diagnosis of stress fracture of the lumbar spine in athletes. Int Orthop 23:213–215

87. Pavlov H (1990) Imaging of the foot and ankle. Radiol Clin North Am 28:991–1017

88. Barros JW, Barbieri CH, Fernandes CD (2000) Scintigraphic evaluation of tibial shaft fracture healing. Injury 31:51–54

89. Setvenson JS, Bright RW, Dunson GL, Nelson FR (1974) Technetium-99m phosphate bone imaging: a method of assessing bone graft healing. Radiology 110:391–396

90. Velasco JG, Vega A, Leisorek A, Callejas F (1976) The early detection of free bone graft viability with 99mTc: a preliminary report. Br J Plast Surg 29:344–346

91. Breggren A, Weiland AJ, Ostrup LT (1982) Bone scintigraphy in evaluating the viability of composite bone grafts revascularised by microvascular anastomoses, conventional autogenous bone grafts and free nonvascularized periosteal grafts. J Bone Joint Surg 64A:799–809

92. Itoh K, Minami A, Sakuma T, Furudate M (1989) The use of three-phase bone imaging in vascularised fibular and iliac bone grafts. Clin Nucl Med 14:494–500

93. Bohnsack M, Gosse F, Ruhmann O, Wenger K (1999) The value of scintigraphy in the diagnosis of pseudarthrosis after spinal fusion surgery. J Spin Disord 12:482–484

94. Etchebehere EC, Pereira Neto CA, Zippi GN, Angelini JA, Lima MC, Santo AO, Ramos CD et al (1998) Three phase bone scintigraphy to guide the removal of metallic implants in fracture: preliminary study. Rev Bras Orthop 35:67–72

95. Connoly LA (2001) Scintigraphic manifestations of sports injuries. Proceedings of the 48th Annual Meeting of the Society of Nuclear Medicine, pp 180–185

96. Metzmaker JN, Pappas AM (1985) Avulsion fractures of the pelvis. Am J Sports Med 13:349–358

97. Stevens MA, El Khoury GY, Kathol MH, Brandser EA, Chow S (1994) Imaging features of avulsion injuries. Radiographics 19:655–672

98. Malki A, Elgazzar A, Ashqar T, Owunwanne B, Abdel-Dayem AH (1992) New technique for assessing muscle damage after trauma. J R Coll Surg Edinb 37:131–133

99. Shihab D, Elgazzar AH, Collier D (2002) Heterotopic ossification. J Nucl 43:346–353

100. Benjamin M, Kumai T, Mitz S, Boszczyk BM, Boszczyk AA, Ralphs JR (2002) The skeletal attachment of tendons – tendon "entheses". Comp Biochem Physiol A Mol Integ Physiol 133:931–945

101. Kleiger B (1982) Anterior tibiotalar impingement syndromes in dancers. Foot Ankle 3:69–73

102. Woertler K, Lindner N, Gosheger G, Brinkschmidt C, Heindel W (2000) Osteochondroma: MR imaging of tumor-related complications. Eur Radiol 10:832–340

103. Stabler A, Heuck A, Reiser M (1997) Imaging of the hand: degeneration, impingement and overuse. Eur J Radiol 25:118–128

104. Billi A, Catalucci A, Barile A, Masciocchi C (1998) Joint impingement syndrome: clinical features. Eur J Radiol 27 [Suppl 1]:S39–S41

105. Masciocchi C, Catalucci A, Barile A (1998) Ankle impingement syndromes. Eur J Radiol 27 [Suppl 1]:S70–S73

106. Faletti C, DeStefano N, Giudice G, Larciprete M (1998) Knee impingement syndromes. Eur J Radiol 27 [Suppl 1]:S60–S69

107. Resnick D (1989) Bone and joint imaging. Saunders, Philadelphia

108. Rupani HD, Holder LE, Espinola DA et al (1985) Three phase radionuclide bone imaging in sports medicine. Radiology 156:187–196

109. Geslin GE, Thrall JH, Espinosa JL et al (1976) Early detection of stress fractures using Tc-99m-polyphosphate. Radiology 121:683–687

110. Wilcox JR Jr, Moniot AL, Green JP (1977) Bone scanning in the evaluation of exercise related stress injuries. Radiology 123:699–703

111. Prather JL, Nusynowitz ML, Snowdy HA et al (1977) Scintigraphic findings in stress fractures. J Bone Joint Surg 59:869–874

112. Roub LW, Gumerman LW, Hanley EN Jr et al (1979) Bone stress: a radionuclide imaging prospective. Radiology 132:431–438

113. Silberstein EB, Elgazzar AH, Fernandez-Uloa M, Nishiyama H (1996) Skeletal scintigraphy in non-neoplastic osseous disorders. In: Henkin RE, Bles MA, Billehay GL, Halama JR, Karosh SM, Wagner PH, Zimmer AM (eds) Textbook of Nuclear Medicine. Mosby, New York pp 1141–1147

Diagnosis of Circulatory Disorders

Osteonecrosis is a common condition that is believed to develop after an ischemic event in bone and bone marrow and is likely due to intravascular coagulopathy. It may be secondary to many other known causes, such as trauma, sickle-cell disease and steroid intake. It may also be primary, or idiopathic, with no apparent cause such as Legg-Calvé-Perthes disease in the pediatric age group, spontaneous osteonecrosis of the femoral head and knee in adults. Bone scintigraphy is more sensitive than standard radiographs. MRI is an excellent complementary modality. Generally, early on, bone scanning shows decreased activity with a subsequent progressive increase in uptake, which starts at the periphery. SPECT is more sensitive than planar imaging, and pinhole imaging is particularly useful in children and small bones. Osteonecrosis may affect one bone or can be multifocal. The osteochondroses are a group of conditions mostly affecting children and adolescents that are characterized by the alteration of endochondral ossification; some forms feature osteonecrosis, such as Freiberg's disease (affecting the second metatarsal head), Kohler's disease (affecting the navicular bone and occasionally the patella) and Osgood-Schlatter disease (affecting the tibial tuberosity).

5.1 Introduction

Bone infarction, or osteonecrosis, is a relatively common condition that most typically occurs in the metaphyseal region of the long bones, often around the knee. The terms aseptic and avascular necrosis (AVN) are generally applied to areas of epiphyseal or subarticular involvement, as is commonly seen in the femoral head. The terms bone infarct or osteonecrosis are used for the metaphyseal and diaphyseal regions. Since there is a synonymous use of these terms, they are used interchangeably. A variety of conditions predispose to bone infarction, including exposure to compressed air, such as occurs in caisson workers and divers; Gaucher's disease; chronic pancreatitis; gout; pregnancy; exposure to radiation; and collagen or vascular disorders. Osteonecrosis also occurs with no recognizable cause.

The classification of vascular bone disorders is difficult to unify, as is the case with other categories of bone diseases. When osteonecrosis occurs in the growing skeleton it is included in the group of disorders collectively called osteochondroses. These involve the epiphyses or apophyses of the growing bones. The process is due to osteonecrosis in some cases and to trauma or stress in others. In addition to avascular necrosis, the osteochondroses often demonstrate similar pathological features, such as transchondral fractures, reactive synovitis, degeneration and cyst formation. This group is discussed elsewhere in the book and only the diseases that feature necrosis are discussed here.

5.2
Pathophysiology

Osteonecrosis is thought to develop after an ischemic event in bone and bone marrow [1]. Although the cause of ischemia remains unknown, Jones claimed that intravascular coagulopathy is an intermediary event initiated by several seemingly unrelated risk factors, including alcoholism, hypercortisolism, hyperlipidemia, and allograft organ rejection (hypersensitivity reactions) [2]. Intravascular coagulopathy occurs in the capillary-sinusoidal beds, arteries, or veins. The resulting vascular compromise leads to imbalances between the demand and supply of oxygen to osseous tissues and consequently avascular necrosis of the bone or osteonecrosis. There are many causes for osteonecrosis (Table 5.1). In some cases the underlying cause cannot be determined, and in this situation the condition is called primary, idiopathic or spontaneous osteonecrosis. This commonly affects the femoral head, distal femur, tibial plateau, carpal bones and humoral heads. Following the interruption of blood supply, blood-forming and mesenchymal cells of the marrow as well as primitive osteoblasts are involved first and die 6–12 h after the cessation of blood flow. Bone cells including osteocytes and mature osteoblasts die 12–48 h later, followed by the fat cells, which are most resistant to ischemia and die 2–5 days after the interruption of blood flow (Fig. 5.1). This sequence of events may explain why bone marrow scintigraphic changes, with decreased uptake, appear earlier than bone scan abnormalities [3, 4]. Ischemia does not directly affect the cartilage. The articular cartilage receives most of its nutrition by direct absorption from the synovial fluid. Cartilage, however, cannot resist persistent elevation of intracapsular pressure for more than 5 days, after which time degeneration begins.

Table 5.1. Causes of osteonecrosis

1. Trauma (fracture or dislocation)
2. Hemoglobinopathies (sickle cell anemia)
3. Exogenous or endogenous hypercortisolism (corticosteroid medication, Cushing's syndrome)
4. Renal transplantation
5. Alcoholism
6. Pancreatitis
7. Dysbaric (Caisson disease)
8. Small vessel disease (collagen vascular disorders)
9. Gaucher's disease
10. Hyperuricemia
11. Irradiation
12. Synovitis with elevation of intraarticular pressure (infection, hemophilia)
13. Idiopathic (spontaneous osteonecrosis)

When the reparative process is initiated it is carried out by neovascularization through the collateral circulation advancing from the periphery of the area of necrosis, or by recanalization of the occluded vessels. This newly formed granulation tissue provides all the elements necessary for the formation of bone matrix and new bone deposition by young osteoblasts. This repair process may, however, be altered. Bone collapse may occur, resulting from structural weakening and external stress. Bone collapse and cartilage damage can result in significant deformity [4, 5].

5.3
General Scintigraphic Features and Staging

The different scintigraphic patterns of femoral head avascular necrosis correlate with the sequence of pathological events. During the first 48 h (stage I), the mor-

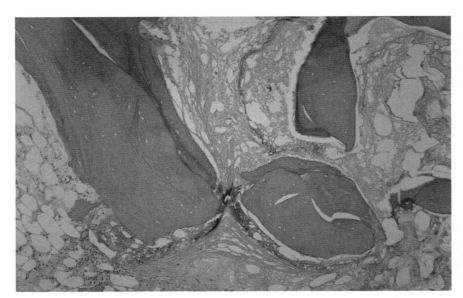

Fig. 5.1. A photomicrograph of a necrotic bone. Note the paucity of cells in marrow spaces

phology of bone is preserved and the radiographs are normal. Osteoblastic uptake on bone scanning varies from absent to almost normal which reflects the greater relative resistance of mature osteoblast to ischemia. Subsequently a cold area of necrosis develops. This avascular pattern will be seen immediately if interruption of the blood supply is abrupt and severe.

The next stage (stage II) begins with the reparative process. In this stage, hyperemia is frequent and there is diffuse demineralization of the area surrounding the necrotic tissue. This stage is characterized scintigraphically by progressively increased technetium diphosphonate uptake starting at the boundaries between the site of necrosis and the normal tissue and beginning after 1–3 weeks. This increased uptake will eventually advance around a central photopenic area and lasts for a few months.

As the reparative process is completed, uptake returns to normal. However, in cases with bone collapse (stage III), increased uptake may persist indefinitely. Stage IV is characterized by collapse of the articular cartilage with degenerative changes on both sides of the joint with a resultant increased peri-articular uptake. Single-photon emission computed tomography (SPECT) should be used in the diagnosis of femoral head avascular necrosis, particularly when the reparative process is thought to have started. SPECT may detect a center of decreased uptake a finding that increases the accuracy of bone scanning for the diagnosis of the condition. It should be noted, however, that no uniform method of evaluating and staging osteonecrosis is yet available, and depending on the site of the disease, three to five stages may be used by different investigators [6–20].

The patterns of abnormalities seen on bone scintigraphy vary according to the site of osteonecrosis. Specifically, the pattern in the knee region is different from the pattern in the femoral head. Since the knee is richly supplied by blood, we see hot, or increased, uptake as the usual pattern. In the femoral head, on the other hand, one sees a decreased uptake and later a 'cold in hot' pattern or only a hot pattern. The 'cold in hot pattern' is very specific since most patients will not show the classic cold pattern by the time they have the scintigraphy. SPECT is useful in resolving the cold center in an apparently hot lesion on planar images (Fig. 5.2). In patients with osteonecrosis of the femoral head, the blood supply is absent from the avascular segment and the area appears cold, whereas the reparative area with new vascular formation around the necrotic lesion appears hot on bone scanning. On the other hand, in the distal femur and the proximal tibia (knee region), the anteroposterior bone volume is larger and the blood supply from vascular anastomosis is richer than in the femoral head. Thus, bone uptake on the anteroposterior or posteroanterior plane tends to increase. Therefore, all lesions are thought to demonstrate focally increased bone uptake. The patterns of increased bone uptake look partially similar to the patterns in osteoarthritis of the knee [21–22].

Bone scans and magnetic resonance imaging (MRI) are the most valuable imaging modalities in the diagnosis, and follow-up, of avascular necrosis. In a 10-year retrospective study, MacLeod and Houston found that the overall accuracy of multiphase bone scintigraphy using functional imaging in the diagnosis of osteonecrosis in 327 patients was 97%, with a sensitivity of 98% and a specificity of 96% [23].

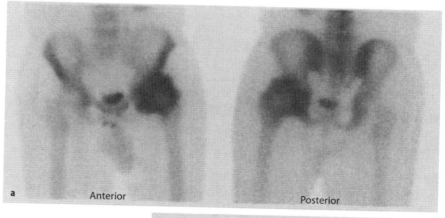

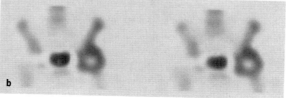

Fig. 5.2a, b. Planar (**a**) and SPECT (**b**) imaging of osteonecrosis of the left femoral head illustrating the additional diagnostic value of the technique in resolving the specific scintigraphic pattern of the condition

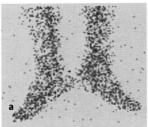
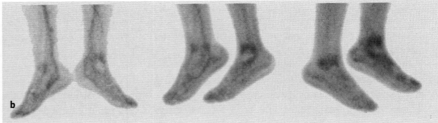
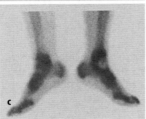

Fig. 5.3a–c. Post-traumatic osteonecrosis. Osteonecrosis of the talus bone in a 34-year-old male with history of foot trauma 2 months earlier. Flow images (**a**) show an ill-defined area of decreased flow in the region of the left talus, better seen on blood pool images (**b**), which also show a rim of increased blood pool activity. On delayed images (**c**) there is a photon-deficient area in the left talus surrounded by a rim of increased activity, indicating healing

5.4
Distinctive Forms of Osteonecrosis

5.4.1
Post-traumatic Osteonecrosis

Following a fracture, bone death of variable extent on either side of a fracture line is relatively common. Necrosis of a relatively large segment of bone following fracture or dislocation is, however, generally restricted to sites that possess a vulnerable blood supply with few arterial anastomoses. The femoral head, the body of the talus (Fig. 5.3), scaphoid bone and the humeral head are such sites [5]. Other locations include the carpal hamate and lunate and the tarsal navicular bone. These bones are characterized by an intra-articular location and limited attachment of soft tissue in addition to the peculiarities of their blood supply [4].

5.4.2
Osteonecrosis of the Femoral Head in Children
(Legg-Calvé-Perthes Disease)

This condition represents osteonecrosis of the femoral head in pediatric populations and predominates in boys aged 4–7 years old. The blood supply to the adult femoral heads is via the circumflex femoral branches of the profunda femoris artery (Fig. 5.4). This adult pattern of femoral head vascularity usually becomes established with closure of the growth plate at approximately 18 years of age. Before this, in infancy and childhood variable vascular patterns are noted (Fig. 5.5). The changing pattern of femoral head vascular supply with age may explain the prevalence of Legg-Calvé-Perthes disease in individuals between the age of 4 and 7 years and the high frequency of necrosis following femoral neck injury in children. Fractures of the femoral neck (occurring more often as intracapsular than ex-

tracapsular fractures) are the most common cause. Other causes include dislocation of the hip and slipped capital femoral epiphysis. Table 5.2 summarizes the stages of the disease. Bone scintigraphy is a sensitive, as well as specific, modality for the diagnosis of this condition typically showing a cold area with, or without, a rim of increased uptake. In our own experience pinhole imaging (Fig. 5.6) has proved to be a valuable tool in the evaluation of this condition and is preferred to SPECT in this age group. The sensitivity and predictive value

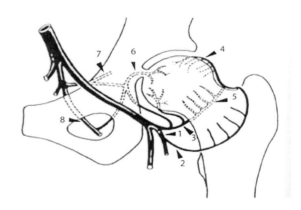

Fig. 5.4. Femoral head vascularity in adults. The major blood supply is derived from the profunda femoris artery (*1*) from which arise the lateral (*2*) and the medial (*3*) circumflex arteries (the medial and lateral circumflex arteries may arise from the femoral artery rather than the profunda femoris artery in some individuals). As these latter vessels pass anterior and posterior to the femur to anastomose at the level of the trochanters they send of small branches beneath the capsule of the hip joint. These branches, including the superior retinacular (lateral epiphyseal) arteries (*4*) and the inferior retinacular (inferior metaphyseal) arteries (*5*), raise the synovial membrane into folds or retinacula. A second supply of blood is derived from the vessels of the ligamentum teres. Here, the foveal (medial epiphyseal) arteries (*6*) can be noted. Additional regional vessels are the inferior gluteal artery (*7*) and the obturator artery (*8*). (From Resnick and Niwayama (eds), Diagnosis of Bone and Joint Disorders, (2nd edn) Saunders, Philadelphia, with permission)

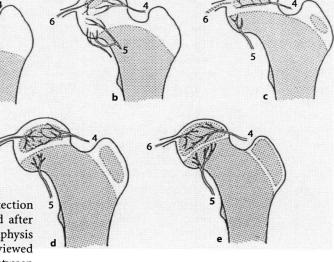

Fig. 5.5. Femoral head vascularity in infancy and childhood. Blood supply to neonates (**a**), infant and child between 4 months and 4 years of age (**b**), child between 4 and 7 years of age (**c**), preadolescent between 7 and 12 years of age (**d**), and adolescent between 12 and the time of closure of the growth plate (**e**). Illustrated are the superior retinacular (*4*), inferior retinacular (*5*), and foveal (*6*) arteries. (From Resnick and Niwayama (eds), Diagnosis of Bone and Joint Disorders, (2nd edn) Saunders, Philadelphia, with permission)

of early post-operative bone scanning for the detection of early avascular necrosis of the femoral head after surgical treatment of slipped capital femoral epiphysis were evaluated by Fragniere et al. The authors reviewed records of 49 patients (64 hips) operated on between 1980 and 1997 with a mean follow-up of 3 years. Sixty-one out of 64 hips went through an early postoperative bone scan. The three hips that developed AVN showed a significant decrease in radionuclide uptake. There were neither false-positive nor false-negative cases in this series [24]. The authors concluded that bone scintigraphy has excellent sensitivity and predictive value for detection of AVN after surgical treatment of slipped capital femoral epiphysis.

The value of scintigraphy in predicting the course of the disease was illustrated by Tsao, who studied 44 consecutive patients treated for Legg-Calvé-Perthes disease. The patients underwent serial technetium-99m diphosphonate bone scintigraphy and were followed up for an average period of 4.4 years. The bone scintigraphy classification characterizes cases into two pathways: the A pathway is characterized by early lateral column formation, which is not seen in the B pathway. Pathway A had 20 hips. The average age at presentation

Table 5.2. Stages of Legg-Calvé-Perthes disease

First stage (incipient): few weeks	Edema Hyperemia Joint fluid in many cases Widening of joint space Bulging of joint capsule
Second stage (necrotic): several months to 1 year	Death of femoral head (usually starts in interior half and may extend to other parts) Softening of the metaphyseal bone at the junction of the femoral neck and capital epiphyseal plate Cysts may be present
Third stage (regenerative)	Procallus formation replacing dead head Collapse and flattening of the femoral head Femoral neck may become short and wide
Fourth stage (residual)	Remodeling occurs Newly formed bone becomes organized into a line of spongy bone Restoration of femoral head to normal shape, more likely if only anterior portion is involved

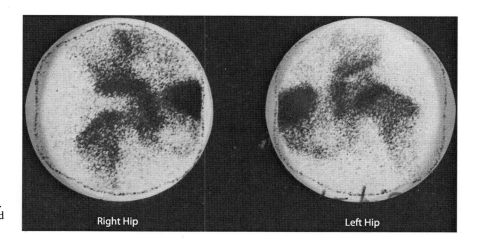

Right Hip   **Left Hip**

Fig. 5.6. Bone scan pinhole image showing the typical pattern of Legg-Calvé-Perthes disease of the right hip. Typically a cold area is noted involving the femoral head

was 6.1 years. At last follow-up, this group had an average Mose classification of 1.2 and Catterall score of 2.4, without any patient having head-at-risk signs or requiring operative treatment. Pathway B had 20 hips. The average age at presentation was 5.8 years. At last follow-up, this group had an average Mose classification of 5.2, a Catterall score of 3.5, and 18 patients had head-at-risk signs, with 11 requiring operative treatment. Bone-scintigraphy classification preceded the radiographic head-at-risk signs by an average of 3 months, allowing earlier treatment and correlated with subsequent femoral head involvement [25]. MRI is also very useful in predicting the course of the disease particularly later in the course of the disease during the fragmentation stage [26]. In patients with Legg-Calvé-Perthes disease, progressive degenerative changes may develop in subsequent years.

5.4.3
Osteonecrosis of the Femoral Head in Adults

Femoral head is a common site of osteonecrosis in adults as is the case in pediatric population. It is a common disease entity with approximately 20,000 new cases reported each year in the USA [27, 28]. The condition commonly occurs secondary to trauma, renal transplantation, systemic lupus erythematosus and others. As many as 30% of individuals with conditions such as systemic lupus erythematosus or sickle cell anemia will develop osteonecrosis of the femoral head. Additionally, osteonecrosis is the underlying diagnosis in as many as 10% of the 500,000 total hip arthroplasties performed in the United States. When the cause or an underlying condition cannot be identified, the condition is classified as spontaneous or primary osteonecrosis of the femoral head; this is usually seen in older patients. Scintigraphy is valuable in the early diagnosis, follow-up and in determining the prognosis in both primary and secondary forms. SPECT was found more sensitive than MRI for the detection of femoral head osteonecrosis in renal transplant recipients. The diagnostic sensitivity of the two modalities was compared in the early detection of femoral head osteonecrosis in 24 patients after renal transplantation, with 32 femoral heads confirmed as having secondary osteonecrosis. The patients underwent both bone SPECT and MRI within 1 month of each other because of hip pain but had normal findings on plain radiography. SPECT was considered positive for osteonecrosis when a cold defect was detected in the femoral head, and the defect was further classified according to the presence of an adjacent increased uptake: type 1 = a cold defect with no adjacent increased uptake; type 2 = a cold defect with adjacent increased uptake. MRI was considered positive for osteonecrosis when a focal region with low signal intensity on T1-weighted images was seen in the

femoral head. SPECT detected osteonecrosis in all 32 femoral heads, resulting in a sensitivity of 100%, whereas MRI detected osteonecrosis in 21 femoral heads, with a sensitivity of 66%. SPECT showed the type 1 pattern in 13 and type 2 in 19 cases. Ten of the 13 femoral heads with the type 1 pattern were false-negative on MRI, whereas only 1 of 19 with the type 2 pattern was normal on MRI. There were six femoral heads with normal MRI findings and abnormal SPECT findings (type 1 pattern) in three patients, for whom hip pain decreased and radiographic findings were normal during follow-up. Follow-up bone SPECT showed a decreasing area of cold defect in four femoral heads [29]. Bone scintigraphy with SPECT is particularly necessary for the diagnosis of osteonecrosis in patients with hip pain and normal radiographs.

Blood pool imaging, or the early static phase of the multiphase bone scan, was also found to be useful in establishing early the hemodynamic changes in patients with osteonecrosis of the femoral head and in estimating early the hemodynamic changes. Three-phase bone scintigraphy was performed on 19 renal allograft recipients between 3 and 9 weeks after they underwent renal transplantation by Kubota et al. [30]. Regions of interest were assigned bilaterally in the femoral heads, diaphyses, and soft tissue. The head-to-diaphysis ratio in each phase was then calculated. Osteonecrosis occurred in eight femoral heads of four patients; three had no abnormal MRI findings at the time of bone scintigraphy. On blood pool imaging and delayed bone scan phases, the head-to-diaphysis ratio was significantly lower than that in the non-osteonecrosis patients [30].

5.4.3.1
Spontaneous Osteonecrosis of the Femoral Head in Adults

Although no specific cause is recognized for this condition, abnormality of the fat metabolism, leading to fatty marrow infiltration or vascular embolization, is the most popular hypothesis [31]. Primary osteonecrosis of the femoral head affects men more frequently then women and is usually seen between the fourth and the seventh decade of life. Unilateral and bilateral involvement may be seen. The reported incidence of bilateral disease has varied from 35–70%, influenced mainly by the method of examination and the duration of follow-up. Despite the high frequency of bilateral involvement, the condition is usually first manifested as unilateral. The pathological findings are virtually identical to those in other varieties of osteonecrosis. SPECT is more sensitive (85%) than planar imaging (55%) in demonstrating photopenia in the femoral heads [32].

The sensitivity for the diagnosis of osteonecrosis of the femoral head for bone scintigraphy equipped with a pinhole collimator and with a high resolution parallel collimator was compared by Maillefert et al. in 16 patients. A total of seven patients were found with bilateral osteonecrosis, while nine had unilateral osteonecrosis of the femoral head. Pinhole scintigraphy documented a photopenic defect in 78% of the necrotic hips, while imaging with a high-resolution parallel collimator documented a defect in 48%. There was no false-positive diagnosis of osteonecrosis of the femoral head using either technique [33]. However SPECT is preferred for diagnosis of femoral head osteonecrosis in adult patients.

Staudenherz documented the value of bone scintigraphy in differentiating osteonecrosis and the bone marrow edema syndrome [34]. Forty-eight symptomatic adult patients (with a final diagnosis of osteonecrosis, bone marrow edema syndrome, other hip pathologies and one normal hip) were examined with dynamic bone scintigraphy visually and qualitatively. A cold spot in the femoral head in both the blood pool and the delayed bone phases was seen only in 24% of osteonecrotic hips. Only 36% of patients with bone marrow edema syndrome of the hips showed diffuse tracer accumulation in the femoral head, neck and the intertrochanteric region in the blood pool phases. The presence of this uptake increased the accuracy of differentiating osteonecrosis and bone marrow edema syndrome. The authors found that osteonecrosis could be differentiated from bone marrow edema syndrome with an accuracy of 86% if the signs of the femoral head and inter-trochanteric uptake were taken into consideration.

Scintigraphy also has a prognostic implication. Large cold areas are associated with a higher rate of collapse. Hasegawa reported that all four patients with large cold areas on scintigraphy had bone collapse within 1 year after osteotomy surgery for osteonecrosis despite good recovery of the weight-bearing surfaces immediately after operation on standard radiographs [35] Another study found similar results in pediatric patients who had surgery for slipped capital femoral epiphysis [24].

5.4.4
Spontaneous Osteonecrosis of the Knee

Although osteonecrosis around the knee is observed in association with steroid therapy, sickle-cell anemia, other hemoglobinopathies and renal transplantation, it may also occur as a spontaneous or idiopathic pathology. The first description of idiopathic osteonecrosis of the medial femoral condyle as a pathologic entity was by Ahlback and colleagues in 1968 [36]. The blood supply in the knee joint is derived from a rich anastomosis of the five major constant arteries- namely, the superior medial and lateral, the middle, and the inferior medial and lateral genicular arteries [37]. Spontaneous osteo-

necrosis can affect any part of the knee [38–43]. It occurs most characteristically in the medial femoral condyle but can also affect the medial portion of the tibial plateau; the lateral femoral condyle or lateral portion of the tibial plateau; the distal femoral metaphysis; and the proximal tibial metaphysis. It rarely affects the patella alone or in combination with the medial femoral condyle [38].

The condition affects predominantly women above 60 years and is characterized by the abrupt onset of knee pain, localized tenderness, stiffness, effusion and restricted motion. Unilateral involvement is more common than bilateral. The pathogenesis of this condition is not clear. Vascular insufficiency associated with age is a proposed etiology. The finding of micro-fractures in the sub-chondral bone with secondary disruption of the local blood supply has also been emphasized. A predominant role of meniscus injury in the pathogenesis of spontaneous osteonecrosis has also been proposed. Radiographs are usually normal at the time of presentation, and weeks or months may pass before changes are seen. Scintigraphy is a more sensitive modality and is helpful in early detection. Scintigraphy may reflect the likely pathogenesis of micro-fractures and vascular disruption. In up to 6 months after the onset, there is increased blood flow, blood pool activity and uptake on delayed images. From 6 months to approximately 2 years, the blood flow and blood pool activity decrease,while delayed uptake may persist. The bone scan tends to return to normal after 2 years, except in patients who develop joint collapse and secondary osteoarthritis [32]. Osteochondritis dissecans, which affects young patients and does not classically involve the weight-bearing surface of the femoral condyle, should not be confused with spontaneous osteonecrosis (see Chap. 4). Osteoarthritis, which commonly affects the knee, can also be confused with the condition but is usually limited to the joint sub-chondral bone, whereas osteonecrosis tends also to involve the adjacent shaft [40].

The disease follows a four-stage course, which consists of a progression from no radiographic findings (stage I); to a slight flattening of the medial femoral condyle (stage II); followed by the appearance of a radiolucent lesion (stage III); and finally, articular cartilage collapse(stage IV). Although stages I and II are potentially reversible, stages III and IV are associated with irreversible destruction of the sub-chondral bone and articular cartilage. Overall, all four stages have somewhat similar signs and symptoms (pain, tenderness, effusion, and synovitis). However, radiographic findings and radionuclide bone scans, computed tomography (CT), and MRI findings, vary considerably according to the clinical stage of the disease. In general, stages I and II are considered early stages in the natural history and potentially are reversible or show no progression.

5.4.4.1
Stage I

Stage I is the earliest stage and also is referred to as the incipient stage. Often the patient has intense symptoms that last for a relatively short period (6–8 weeks), after which they may subside. These patients then may become asymptomatic. Standard radiographs are typically normal. Although MRI has not been accepted widely as a reliable diagnostic method for detecting stage I osteonecrosis, it has been shown that patients with normal T2-weighted images tend to show no progression and even may present with spontaneous resolution of the disease. In contrast, abnormalities in T2-weighted images have been related to further progression of the disease (Fig. 5.7) [44, 45].

Bone scanning, however, is a reliable tool for the diagnosis of stage I idiopathic osteonecrosis of the knee. Bone scans are always positive in these cases and show an increased uptake of the radionuclide at the site of the lesion. This is indicative of sub-chondral bone necrosis. Even though bone scan is not a specific imaging modality for the diagnosis of idiopathic osteonecrosis of the knee, when considered in association with the clinical

signs and symptoms of the patient, it clearly can help the clinician to establish a diagnosis.

Patients with stage I osteonecrosis of the knee usually do not require surgery and can be treated conservatively. In the minority patients with stage I osteonecrosis of the knee who have only limited destruction of the subchondral bone, the knee may remain stable or even show spontaneous resolution. However, the majority of these patients progress to stage II.

5.4.4.2
Stage II

Two to four months after the onset of the disease, a characteristic slight flattening of the medial femoral condyle can be observed. This can be detected mainly in anteroposterior or tangential radiographs of the knee. Flattening of the medial femoral condyle is indicative of stage II. The radiographic findings in this stage may still be somewhat obscure, but abnormal MRI findings are commonly suggestive of osteonecrosis. In addition, radionuclide scintigraphy can be of major assistance in establishing the diagnosis, because radionuclide uptake is as much as 5–15 times greater in the af-

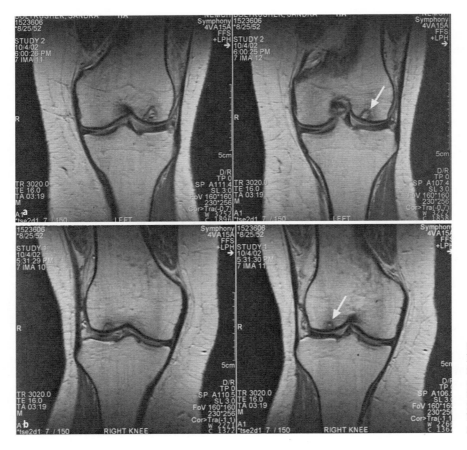

Fig. 5.7a, b. MR images of bilateral osteonecrosis of the femoral condyles. Small low signal intensity lesion is seen in the subarticular end of the femur bilaterally surrounded by a rim of hypo-intense signal (*arrows*)

fected knee. CT scanning, even though it is not diagnostic, can provide more details regarding the appearance of the osteonecrotic lesion, because it permits good resolution and makes it possible to measure the size of the lesion.

5.4.4.3
Stage III

Three to six months after the onset of the disease, a radiolucent lesion can be observed in plain radiographs. This is the so-called crescent or rim sign, and is indicative of segmental necrosis of the sub-chondral bone with articular cartilage destruction. Bone scans, CT and MRI are not essential to make the diagnosis, because plain radiographs usually provide a clear and characteristic picture when positive.

5.4.4.4
Stage IV

Nine months to 1 year after the disease onset, and sometimes even earlier, typical radiographic findings of this stage are usually present. These include additional sub-chondral bone and articular cartilage destruction that may extend over the entire transverse diameter of the medial femoral condyle, leading to complete articular collapse.

Bone scintigraphy has an important diagnostic role especially in stages I and II, where radiographic changes are often obscure (Fig. 5.7) while in stage III and IV radiographs usually suffice.

Stages I and II idiopathic osteonecrosis of the knee are treated conservatively with aspirin, anti-inflammatory drugs, and partial weight-bearing, and in most cases show spontaneous recovery, while patients with stage III or IV usually need surgery. Overall, the prognosis of the disease is severe because approximately 80% of the patients deteriorate to the extent that they need surgical reconstruction, whereas less than 20% have either spontaneous resolution or no additional deterioration of the lesion.

There are significant differences between idiopathic and secondary osteonecrosis (Table 5.3), especially regarding the clinical presentation and the location, extent and MRI appearance of the lesions. These differences are probably due to a difference in the pathogenic mechanism. Secondary osteonecrosis generally occurs in younger patients (Fig. 5.8) and typically has an insid-

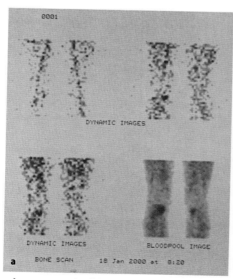

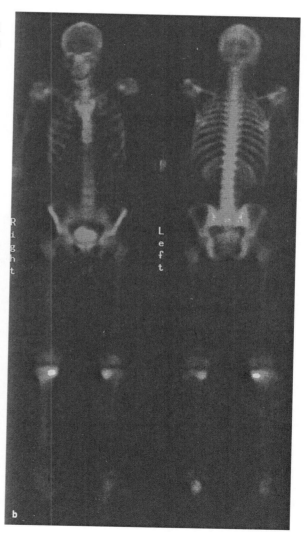

Fig. 5.8. Bilateral osteonecrosis of the knee illustrating the typical pattern on bone scintigraphy. Note the focal increased flow and blood pool (**a**) with corresponding focally increased uptake on delayed image (**b**)

Table 5.3. Comparison of forms of osteonecrosis of the knee

Characteristic	Primary	Secondary
Patient's age	Typically elderly	Young
Onset	Sudden	Insidious
Pain	Severe	Mild
Size of lesions	Small	Large
Distribution of lesions	Unilateral	Commonly bilateral

ious onset with mild or vague pain, the lateral compartment of the knee are often involved, and the lesions seen are usually larger than spontaneous ; in the great majority of cases they involve the femoral condyles and/or tibial plateaus. Bilateral distribution and multifocal involvement are often seen in this form. Additionally, MRI is able to demonstrate different patterns of abnormalities between the idiopathic and secondary types [46]. A retrospective review of 37 consecutive patients with osteonecrosis of the knee confirmed by bone scintigraphy and/or MRI was reported by Narvaez et al. [46] and focused on the comparison of idiopathic and secondary types of osteonecrosis. Idiopathic osteonecrosis of the knee was typically a disease of the elderly, characterized by severe knee pain of sudden onset, unilateral involvement, and restriction of the lesions generally to one femoral condyle or tibial plateau, with predilection for the medial compartment of the joint [46].

5.4.5
Multifocal or Multiple Osteonecrosis

Non-traumatic osteonecrosis of the femoral head is often accompanied by other sites of osteonecrosis. Multifocal osteonecrosis [47, 48] or multiple osteonecrosis is defined as a disease affecting two or more separate anatomical sites. LaPorte et al. reported that when multifocal osteonecrosis was defined as a disease affecting three or more separate anatomical sites, it could be found in 32/1056 (3%) patients with osteonecrosis [47]. All 32 of those patients had osteonecrosis of the femoral head and knee. The authors also reported that osteonecrosis was seen in the shoulder (28 patients) and ankle (8 patients) [47]. In a multi-center study, using the same definition of multi-focal osteonecrosis [48], 101 patients with femoral head disease additionally had osteonecrosis of the knee (96%), shoulder (80%), and/ or ankle (44%). On the other hand, Shimizu et al. reported that multiple osteonecrosis which affected two or more separate anatomical sites was observed by MRI screening in 167 of 250 patients (67%) with steroid-related osteonecrosis of the femoral head and that the most common site beside the femoral head was the lateral femoral condyle (49%), followed by the distal femoral metaphysis (37%), the medial femoral condyle (32%), and the humeral head (24%) [49]. Accordingly, among patients with multifocal osteonecrosis, the knee is a major affected site, second only to the femoral head. A total of 214 knee joints in 107 patients with osteonecrosis of the femoral head were studied by Sakai [43] using bone scintigraphy compared with MRI. Associated osteonecrosis of the knee was classified into five sites: the femoral condyles, distal femoral metaphysis, tibial plateau, proximal tibial metaphysis, and patella. Based on the diagnosis by MRI, osteonecrosis of the femoral condyles was the most common (40%), followed by osteonecrosis of the distal femoral metaphysis (15%), proximal tibial metaphysis (10%), patella (3%), and tibial plateau (0.9%). The sensitivity and specificity of bone scintigraphy for femoral condyle lesions was 63% and 71% respectively, and sensitivity was 89% for the large, or medium, sized lesions (as judged by MRI). The sensitivity for other locations mentioned was poor but these lesions have a low likelihood of collapse. Accordingly, the authors concluded that bone scintigraphy is useful for screening since it is highly sensitive for disease of the femoral condyles which bears a high risk of collapse of the knee [50]. The limitation of this study is the use of MRI as a gold standard.

Overall, technetium bone scintigraphy is valuable for screening for multi-focal osteonecrosis in patients with osteonecrosis of the femoral head [51, 52]. Bone scintigraphy has several advantages which make it suitable for this task: many joints can be visualized at one time on total body images to determine whether multiple osteonecrosis exists, and it can be used for patients with cardiac pacemakers, intracranial clips, and claustrophobia, who cannot undergo MRI.

5.4.6
Sickle-Cell Disease Osteonecrosis

Sickle-cell disease is a relatively common hereditary hematological disorder. The disease is caused by the replacement of glutamic acid of β-chains with valine. The disease has numerous consequences; one of the most common is injury to bone. Osteonecrosis and osteomyelitis are the most common complications [53]. The bone manifestations occur similarly in other hemoglobinopathies and most commonly affect the femora, tibiae and humeri [54, 55]. Since-sickle cell osteonecrosis most commonly involves the femoral and humeral heads, although it can affect any bone of the skeleton, it is possible that the increased length of the nutrient arteries supplying the marrow in the long bones makes them more susceptible to occlusion. Necrosis of the femoral head is one of the significant skeletal disorders in sickle-cell disease patients. Neonates who have sickle-cell disease do not often develop osteonecrosis because of the high fetal hemoglobin level. Although the pathogenesis of the vascular occlusion leading to an infarct is not entirely clear, vaso-occlusion of the marrow is considered to be one of the main culprits in sickle-cell crises. Since hemoglobin S is sensitive to hypoxemia, erythrocytes become viscous and sickle abruptly when exposed to hypoxia. This may compromise the micro-vascular flow and cause necrosis, the most common skeletal complication of sickle-cell disease [56]. The signs of acute infarction can include warmth, tenderness, erythema, and swelling over the site of vaso-occlusion [55]. However, these clinical signs are non-specific and may also be seen in acute osteomyelitis, which may occur as a primary event or may be superimposed on infarcts; necrotic bone is a fertile site for

such secondary infections [54, 55]. Thus, recognition of bone marrow infarction often relies on the use of imaging modalities. MRI has not been found to have the specificity or sensitivity of radionuclide studies [57].

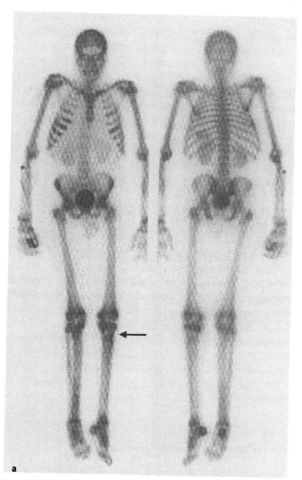

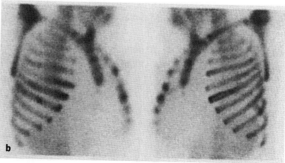

Fig. 5.10a, b. Sickle cell disease infarcts with recent pain in the left knee corresponding to a relatively acute infarct of the proximal left tibia (arrow). Other infarcts are healing, including those in the long bones of the upper and lower extremities, skull and ribs, as seen on the whole-body bone scan (**a**). There is a history of chest pain representing acute chest syndrome associated with the multiple rib infarcts, as clearly demonstrated by anterior oblique views (**b**) (From Sisayan R, Elgazzar A [58] with permission)

Fig. 5.9. Sickle cell disease infarcts: whole body scan show multiple foci of increased uptake in the humeric, femora and ribs representing healing infarcts. An area of decreased uptake is noted in the medial aspect of the left distal femur representing a more acute infarct (*arrow*)

The scintigraphic diagnosis may be straightforward using Tc-99m MDP scan (Fig. 5.9), which shows photon-deficient areas early on. SPECT and pinhole images are very valuable, particularly in resolving a photon-deficient area in the middle of the increased uptake at the reparative process. During this phase it can be difficult to differentiate osteonecrosis from osteomyelitis, and adding gallium-67 or bone marrow scanning may be essential (see Chap. 2). Acute chest syndrome in sickle cell patients is characterized by chest pain that can mimic several pulmonary disorders, including pulmonary embolism and pneumonia [58]. This condition is believed to be a sequela of osteonecrosis of the ribs (Fig. 5.10) and is usually associated with pulmonary infiltrates on chest radiography. Whole-body imaging cannot be overemphasized and should include the ribs in addition to the area of interest if different.

5.4.7
Dysbaric Osteonecrosis

This type of osteonecrosis occurs in patients subjected to a high-pressure environment such as deep-sea divers. The exact cause of ischemia is debated. Immobilization of gas bubbles blocking the vascular channels is considered to be the major factor by many investigators. This occurs due to the liberation of gas bubbles (mainly nitrogen) into the blood and tissue of an individual who was exposed to a hyperbaric environment and has then undergone decompression too rapidly [59]. The shoulders, hips, knees and ankles are commonly involved in this type of osteonecrosis.

5.4.8
Osteochondroses Featuring Osteonecrosis

The osteochondroses are a group of conditions affecting children and adolescents that are characterized by disturbance of endochondral ossification in which both chondrogenesis and osteogenesis are deranged after a previously normal growth process. The condition can occur in any bone that grows by endochondral ossification and the exact cause is in general undefined; many theories have been proposed, but none has proven satisfactory. Since certain conditions show osteonecrosis, the conditions have been placed among vascular disorders of bone. Other investigators include the group among overuse injury syndromes since many are common among athletes [60]. Still others classify the group with degenerative diseases since degeneration occurs in these conditions followed by ossification in one or more of the ossification centers [61]. Accordingly, the osteochondroses are viewed as conditions with variable features including but not limited to osteonecrosis, traumatic changes and degenerative changes. The actual expression will depend on the spe-

Table 5.4. Osteochondroses

Involved bone	Disease	Probable nature of condition
Capital femoral epiphysis	Legg-Calvé-Perthes disease	Osteonecrosis
Metatarsal head(s)	Freiberg's disease	Osteonecrosis or stress fracture
Carpal lunate	Kienböck's disease	Osteonecrosis
Tarsal navicular	Kohler's disease	Developmental/ osteonecrosis
Capitellum of humerus	Panner's disease	Traumatic
Phalanges of hand	Thiemann's disease	Familial or traumatic
Tibial tuberosity	Osgood-Schlatter disease	Avulsion injury
Proximal tibial epiphysis	Blount's disease	Disturbance of growth/trauma
Vertebra	Scheuermann's disease	Degenerative
Patella	Sinding-Larson-Johansson disease	Trauma or stress
Calcaneus (apophysis of os calcis)	Sever's disease	Variation in ossification
Ischiopubic Synchondrosis	Van Neck's disease	Variation in ossification
Fifth metatarsal base	Iselin's disease	Variation in ossification
Iliac crest apophysis	Buchman's disease	Variation in ossification
Symphysis pubis	Pierson's disease	Unclear
Head of humerus	Hass disease	osteonecrosis
Heads of metacarpals	Mauclaire disease	Unclear
Lower ulna	Burns' disease	Unclear

cific form of the disease (Table 5.4). Legg-Calvé-Perthes disease and osteochondritis dissecans have been included in this group by some investigators. Legg-Calvé-Perthes disease is discussed above and osteochondritis dissecans is presented in Chap. 4.

The group may be categorized into (1) intra-articular conditions such as Kohler's disease, Freiberg's disease and Panner's disease; (2) physeal conditions such as Scheuermann's disease; (3) non-articular conditions affecting any other skeletal site, such as Osgood-Schlatter disease, which affects the tibial tuberosity. In general osteochondroses resolve spontaneously and are self-limited [62].

Abnormally increased uptake on a bone scan in a classic area of involvement for each condition should raise the possibility of aspecific condition. Without knowledge of the specifics of each of these conditions, the uptake will be interpreted as non-specific and the condition may pass undiagnosed.

5.4.8.1
Freiberg's Disease

This condition was originally described as osteonecrosis of the second metatarsal head, but it is now known also to affect the first and third (and possibly other) metatarsal heads. The condition presents usually in late adolescence and may lead to degenerative joint disease as a late complication, in a manner similar to several other osteochondroses.

5.4.8.2
Kohler's Disease

Osteonecrosis of the tarsal navicular leads to specific changes on radiographs, namely flattening, sclerosis and irregular rarefaction, the features of this condition which was originally described by Kohler in 1908. The condition has an excellent outcome and rarely affect children [63]. Recently, cases of the disease have been described in the patella [64]. Scintigraphically a focus of increased uptake is seen at the site of the tarsal navicular bone.

5.4.8.3
Osgood-Schlatter Disease

This condition affects the tibial tuberosity at the site of insertion of the patellar tendon. It affects boys more often than girls and is bilateral in approximately 25% of cases. The disease was believed to be due to repetitive overuse stress leading to ischemic necrosis; however, more recently it has been proved to be due to avulsion of the secondary ossification center due to repetitive tensile extension forces from the quadriceps applied to the apophyseal cartilage of the tibial tuberosity. This will lead to avulsion of segments of the anterior cartilage and/or anterior bone of the tuberosity [65].

References

1. Mankin HJ (1992) Non-traumatic necrosis of bone (osteonecrosis). N Engl J Med 326:1473–1479
2. Jones JP (1992) Intravascular coagulation and osteonecrosis. Clin Orthop 277:41–53
3. Greyson ND, Tepperman PS (1984) Three phase bone studies in hemiplegia with reflex sympathetic dystrophy and the effect of disuse. J Nucl Med 25:423–429
4. McAffe JG, Roba RC, Majid M (1995) The musculoskeletal system. In: Wagner HN (ed) Principles of nuclear medicine, 2nd edn. Saunders, Philadelphia, pp 986–1020
5. Graham J, Wood SK (1976) Aseptic necrosis of bone following trauma. In: Davidson JK (ed) Aseptic necrosis of bone. Excerpta Medica, Amsterdam
6. Enneking WF (1997) Classification of non-traumatic osteonecrosis of the femoral head. In: Urbaniak JR, Jones JP Jr (eds) Osteonecrosis: etiology, diagnosis and treatment. American Academy of Orthopaedic Surgeons, Rosemont, IL, 269–275
7. Ficat RP (1985) Idiopathic bone necrosis of the femoral head: early diagnosis and treatment. J Bone Joint Surg 67B:3–9
8. Gardeniers JWM (1993) ARCO (Association Research Circulation Osseous) Committee on Terminology and Classification. ARCO News 5:79–82
9. Hungerford DB, Lennox DW (1985) The importance of increased intraosseous pressure in the development of osteonecrosis of the femoral head: implications for treatment. Orthop Clin North Am 16:635–654
10. Jones JP Jr (1993) Osteonecrosis. In: McCarty DJ, Koopmann WJ (eds) Arthritis and allied conditions: a textbook of rheumatology, 12th edn. Lea and Febiger, Philadelphia, pp 1677–1696
11. Malizos KN, Soucacos PN, Beris AE (1995) Osteonecrosis of the femoral head: hip salvaging with implantation of a vascularized fibular graft. Clin Orthop 314:67–75
12. Marcus ND, Enneking WF, Massam RA (1973) The silent hip in idiopathic aseptic necrosis: treatment by bone-grafting. J Bone Joint Surg 55A:1352–1366
13. Markesmithl DC, Miskovsky C, Sculco TP et al (1996) Core decompression for osteonecrosis of the femoral head. Clin Orthop 323:226–233
14. Merle d'Aubigne R, Postel M, Mazabraud A et al (1965) Idiopathic necrosis of the femoral head in adults. J Bone Joint Surg 47B:612–633
15. Mont MA, Hungerford DS (1995) Current concepts review: non-traumatic avascular necrosis of the femoral head. J Bone Joint Surg 77A:459–474
16. Ohzono K, Saito M, Sugano N et al (1992) The fate of non-traumatic avascular necrosis of the femoral head: a radiologic classification to formulate prognosis. Clin Orthop 277:73–78
17. Smith SW, Meyer RA, Connor PM et al (1996) Interobserver reliability and intraobserver reproducibility of the modified Ficat classification system of osteonecrosis of the femoral head. J Bone Joint Surg 78A:1702–1706
18. Sotereanos DG, Plakseychuk AY, Rubash HE (1997) Free vascularized fibula grafting for the treatment of osteonecrosis of the femoral head. Clin Orthop 344:243–256
19. Steinberg ME, Hayken GD, Steinberg DR (1984) A new method for evaluation and staging of avascular necrosis of the femoral head. In: Arlet J, Ficat RP, Hungerford DS (eds) Bone circulation. Williams and Wilkins, Baltimore, pp 398–403
20. Steinberg ME, Hayken GD, Steinberg DR (1995) A quantitative system for staging avascular necrosis. J Bone Joint Surg 77B:34–41
21. McCrae F, Shouls J, Dieppe P, Watt I (1992) Scintigraphic assessment of osteoarthritis of the knee joint. Ann Rheum Dis 51:938–942
22. Boegard T, Rudling O, Dahlstrom J, Dirksen H, Petersson IF, Jonsson K (1999) Bone scintigraphy in chronic knee pain: comparison with magnetic resonance imaging. Ann Rheum Dis 58:20–22
23. MacLeod MA, Houston AS (1997) Functional bone imaging in the detection of ischemic osteopathies. Clin Nucl Med 22:1–5
24. Fragniere B, Chotel F, Vargas Barreto B, Berard J (2001) The value of early postoperative bone scan in slipped capital femoral epiphysis. J Pediatr Orthop 10:51–55
25. Tsao AK, Dias LS, Conway JJ, Straka P (1997) The prognostic value and significance of serial bone scintigraphy in Legg-Calvé-Perthes disease. J Pediatr Orthop 17:230–239
26. De Sanctis N, Rondinella F (2000) Prognostic evaluation of Legg-Calvé-Perthes disease by MRI, part II. Pathomorphogenesis and new classification. J Pediatr Orthop 20:463–470

27. Aaron RK(1998) Osteonecrosis: etiology, pathophysiology, and diagnosis. In: Callaghan JJ, Rosenberg AG, Rubash HE (eds) The adult hip. Philadelphia, Lippincott-Raven, pp 451–466

28. Lavernia CJ, Sierra RJ, Grieco FR (1999) Osteonecrosis of the femoral head. J Am Acad Orthop Surg 7:250–261

29. Jin-Sook R, Jae KS, Dae MH, Sung K, Myung S, Jae C, Soo P, Duck H, Hee L (2002) Bone SPECT is more sensitive than MRI in the detection of early osteonecrosis of the femoral head after renal transplantation. J Nucl Med 43:1008–1011

30. Kubota T, Ushijima Y, Okuyama C, Kubo T, Nishimura T (2001) Tracer accumulation in femoral head during early phase of bone scintigraphy after renal transplantation. J Nucl Med 42:1789–1794

31. Kawai K, Maruno H, Watanabe Y, Hirohata K (1980) Fat necrosis of osteocytes as a causative factor in idiopathic osteonecrosis inheritable hyperlipemic rabbits. Clin Orthop Relat Res 153:273

32. Collier BD, Carrera GF, Johnson RP, Isitman AT, Hellman RS, Knobel J et al (1985) Detection of femoral head avascular necrosis in adults by SPECT. J Nucl Med 26:979–987

33. Maillefert JF, Toubeau M, Piroth C, Piroth L, Brunotte F, Tavernier C (1997) Bone scintigraphy equipped with a pinhole collimator for diagnosis of avascular necrosis of the femoral head. Clin Rheumatol 16:372–377

34. Staudenherz A, Hofmann S, Breitenseher M, Schneider W, Engel AE, Imhof H, Leitha T (1997) Diagnostic patterns for bone marrow edema syndrome and avascular necrosis of the femoral head in dynamic bone scintigraphy. Nucl Med Commun 18:1178–1188

35. Hasegawa Y, Matsuda T, Iwasada S, Iwase T, Kitamura S, Iwata H (1998) Scintigraphic evaluation of transtrochanteric rotational osteotomy for osteonecrosis of the femoral head. Comparison between scintigraphy, radiography and outcome in 34 patients. Arch Orthop Trauma Surg 117:23–26

36. Ahlback S, Bauer GC, Bohne WH (1968) Spontaneous osteonecrosis of the knee. Arthritis Rheum 11:705–733

37. Shim SS, Leung BA (1986) Blood supply of the knee joint. A microangiographic study in children and adults. Clin Orthop 208:119–125

38. Laprade RF, Noffsinger MA (1990) Idiopathic osteonecrosis of the patella: an unusual cause of pain in the knee. J Bone Joint Surg 72A:1414–1418

39. Lotke PA, Ecker ML(1988) Current concepts review. Osteonecrosis of the knee. J Bone Joint Surg 70A:470–473

40. Kelman GJ, Williams GW, Colwell CW Jr, Walker RH (1990) Steroid-related osteonecrosis of the knee: two case reports and a literature review. Clin Orthop 257:171–176

41. Steinberg ME (1990) Classification of avascular necrosis: a comparative study. Acta Orthop Belg 65 [Suppl 1]:45–46

42. Motohashi M, Morii T, Koshino T (1991) Clinical course and roentgenographic changes of osteonecrosis in the femoral condyle under conservative treatment. Clin Orthop 266:156–161

43. Sakai T, Sugano N, Ohzono K, Matsui M, Hiroshima K, Ochi T (1998) MRI evaluation of steroid- or alcohol-related osteonecrosis of the femoral condyle. Acta Orthop Scand 69:598–602

44. Bjorkengren AG, Airowaih A, Lindstrand A et al (1990) Spontaneous osteonecrosis of the knee: value of MR imaging in determining prognosis. AJR 154:331–336

45. Zizic TM(1991) Osteonecrosis. Curr Opin Rheum 3:481–489

46. Narvaez J, Narvaez JA, Rodriguez-Moreno J, Roig-Escofet D (2000) Osteonecrosis of the knee: differences among idiopathic and secondary types. Rheumatology 39:982–989

47. LaPorte DM, Mont MA, Mohan V, Jones LC, Hungerford DS (1998) Multifocal osteonecrosis. J Rheumatol 25:1968–1974

48. Mont MA, Jones LC, LaPorte DM, Collaborative Osteonecrosis Group (1999) Symptomatic multifocal osteonecrosis. A multicenter study. Clin Orthop 369:312–326

49. Shimizu (1999) Steroid-induced multiple bone necroses: an analysis of 2000 joints in 250 patients. Presentation at the annual meeting of the American Academy of Orthopaedic Surgeons, Anaheim, California

50. Sugano N, Nishii T, Haraguchi K, Yoshikawa H, Ohzono K (2001) Bone scintigraphy for osteonecrosis of the knee in patients with non-traumatic osteonecrosis of the femoral head: comparison with magnetic resonance imaging. Ann Rheum Dis 60:14–20

51. Burt RW, Matthews TJ (1982) Aseptic necrosis of the knee: bone scintigraphy. AJR 138:571–573

52. Minoves M, Riera E, Constansa JM, Bassa P, Setoain J, Domenech FM (1998) Multiple aseptic bone necrosis detected by Tc-99m MDP bone scintigraphy in a patient with systemic lupus erythematosus on corticosteroid therapy. Clin Nucl Med 23:48–49

53. Smith JA (1996) Bone disorders in sickle cell disease. Hematol Oncol Clin North Am 10:1345–1346

54. Kim SK, Miller JH (2002) Natural history and distribution of bone and bone marrow infarction in sickle cell hemoglobinopathies. J Nucl Med 43:896–900

55. Keeley K, Buchanan GR (1982) Acute infarction of long bones in children with sickle cell anemia. J Pediatr 101:170–175

56. Elgazzar AH, Abdel-Dayem HM (1999) Imaging of skeletal infections: evolving considerations. In: Freeman LM (ed) Nuclear medicine annual. Lippincott Williams and Wilkins, Philadelphia, pp 157–191

57. Skaggs DL, Kim SK, Green NW, Harris D, Miler JH (2001) Differentiation between bone infarct and acute osteomyelitis in children with sickle-cell disease with use of sequential radionuclide bone-marrow and bone scans. J Bone Joint Surg (Am) 83:1810–1813

58. Sisayan R, Elgazzar AH, Webner P, Religioso DG (1996) Impact of bone scintigraphy on clinical management of a sickle cell patient with recent chest pain. Clin Nucl Med 21:523–526

59. Resnick D, Niwayama G (1998) Osteonecrosis: diagnostic techniques and complications. In: Resnick D, Niwayama G (eds) Diagnosis of bone and joint disorders, 2nd edn. Saunders, Philadelphia

60. Dapie T, Anticevic D, Capin T (2000) Overuse injury syndromes in children and adolescents. Arch Za Higijenu Rada J Tokisologyu 52:483–489

61. Swischuk LE, John SD, Allberg S (1998) Disk degenerative disease in childhood: Sheuermann's disease; Schmorl's nodes and limbus vertebra: MRI findings in 12 patients. Pediatr Radiol 28:334–338

62. Resnick D (1989) Bone and joint imaging. Saunders, Philadelphia, pp 979–999

63. Sharp RJ, Calder JD, Saxby TS (2003) Osteochondritis of the navicular: a case reprint

64. Pinar H, Giil O, Boya H, Ozcan C, Ozcan O (2002) Osteonecrosis of the primary ossification center of the patella (Kohler's disease of the patella). Report of three cases knee Surg Sports Traumatol Anthrosc; 10:141–143

65. Hirano A, Fukubayashi T, Ishii T, Ochiai N (2002) Magnetic resonance imaging of Osgood–Schlatter disease: the course of the disease. Skeletal Radiol 31:334–342

66. Elgazzar AH (2001) The pathophysiologic basis of nuclear medicine. Springer, Berlin Heidelberg New York

Neoplastic Bone Diseases

6

Benign and malignant primary bone tumors are rare, while metastatic disease is a common occurrence. The efficacy of the several currently available imaging modalities in the detection, staging, and follow-up of patients with skeletal neoplasia varies. Evaluation of bone tumors involves a multi-modality approach. Standard radiographs play an impor-

tant role in the diagnosis of both primary and metastatic tumors. Computed tomography (CT) scan and magnetic resonance imaging (MRI) are often complementary and are particularly useful in primary bone tumors. CT scan is especially useful in evaluating the cortex. MRI is superior in evaluating the extent of several primary tumors and detecting bone marrow lesions. The role of bone scintigraphy in preoperative evaluation of primary tumors is limited. Bone scintigraphy, on the other hand, is an excellent cost-effective screening modality in detecting metastatic disease in patients with skeletal and extra-skeletal malignancies. In breast, lung, and head and neck tumors bone scan is rarely positive for metastasis in patients with low stage disease. Metaiodobenzylguanidine (MIBG) scintigraphy is valuable in children with neuroblastoma. Bone scintigraphy and other radionuclide modalities are valuable in the long-term follow up of several cancers and in estimating the prognosis. The therapeutic response of malignant bone disease can particularly be assessed using Tl-201, Tc-99m methoxyisobutylisonitrile (MIBI) and PET.

6.1
Introduction

Primary bone tumors are rare while metastatic bone tumors are common and have a significant impact on decision-making regarding choice of therapy and its modification. The evaluation of bone tumors, whether they are primary or metastatic, involves several imaging modalities. Standard radiographs, computed tomography (CT) scanning, magnetic resonance imaging (MRI) and several functional modalities can all be used in a complementary way depending on the strengths and limitations of each of those modalities. Functional nuclear medicine modalities generally have a limited role, in the imaging of primary bone tumors, but are very useful in the initial detection of metastatic disease, the follow-up of the response to therapy and in estimating the prognosis. Various radiopharmaceuticals such as Tc-99m diphosphonates, I-123 or I-131

Table 6.1. Radiopharmaceuticals for tumor imaging

Isotope	Characteristics	Uptake mechanism at tumor area
Tc99m MDP, Tc99m HDP	Diphosphonate	Adsorption to hydroxyapatite crystals by reactive bone formation
Tc99m MIBI (technetium 99m-2-methoxyisobutylisonitrile)	Lipophilic agent	Accumulates preferentially within living malignant cells due to the higher transmembrane electrical potential as a consequence of the higher metabolic rate than in the surrounding normal cells.
Thallium-201	Potassium analogue	Adenosine triphosphatase pump
Gallium-67	Ferric ion analogue	Simple diffusion of unbound tracer facilitated by the increased permeability of tumor cells compared to normal cells. Binding of iron binding globulins which are present in higher concentration within interstitial fluid of the tumor.
F-18 FDG	Analog of glucose labeled with positron emitting radiotracer	Facilitated diffusion of FDG which is similar to glucose will be over utilized by these cells compared to normal tissue. This is caused by preferential anaerobic metabolism, an increase in number of glucose transporter molecules, increased activity of hexokinase isoenzymes and decreased activity of the glucose-6-phosphatase enzyme resulting in the metabolic trapping of FDG in malignant cells and increased uptake.
C-11 methionine	Amino acid analog labeled with positron emitting radiotracer	Increased amino acid metabolism by tumor cells. Used to evaluate amino acid uptake and protein synthesis, providing an indicator of tumor viability.

MIBG, thallium-201, Tc99m MIBI and positron emission tomography (PET) scanning are all used for bone tumor imaging (Table 6.1). With the advances in MRI and PET imaging and their applications, the role of each of the morphological and functional imaging modalities is constantly changing along with recommendations of when to use each. The use of nuclear medicine modalities in a correlative imaging approach in primary and metastatic bone tumors and the current recommendations for effective utilization of imaging in bone tumor diagnosis and management will be discussed below.

6.2
Pathophysiology

6.2.1
Primary Bone Tumors

The various primary bone tumors are generally classified, based on their cell of origin, into osteogenic, chondrogenic, collagenic and myelogenic tumors (Fig. 6.1).

6.2.1.1
Osteogenic Tumors

Osteogenic tumors originate from a bone cell precursor, the osteoblast, and are characterized by the formation of bone or osteoid tissue. These tumors include osteoid osteoma, osteosarcoma and osteoblastoma. *Osteoid osteoma* is a benign osteogenic tumor predominantly affecting children and is characterized by its small size (less than 2 cm), self-limited growth, and the

tendency to cause extensive reactive changes in the surrounding bone tissue. The lesion classically presents with severe pain at night that is dramatically relieved by non-steroidal antiinflammatory drugs (NSAIDs). The tumor has been shown to express very high levels of prostaglandins, particularly PGE2 and PGI2. The high local levels of these prostaglandins are presumed to be the cause of the intense pain seen in patients with this lesion. Studies have shown strong immunoreactivity to cyclo-oxygenase-2 (COX-2) in the nidus of the tumor but not in the surrounding reactive bone. COX-2 is one of the mediators of the increased production of prostaglandins by osteoid osteomas and may be the cause of the secondary changes shown by MRI [1, 2]. The usual sites of involvement (Fig. 6.2) include the bones of the lower extremities, pelvis and spine. *Osteoblastoma* is a tumor related to osteoid osteoma and has an almost identical histological appearance but the nidus is larger in size measuring more than 2 cm. It is commonly seen in the spine and can occur in any other location. Looking at the appendicular skeleton, the lower extremity is the most common location for osteoblastoma where 35 % of the lesions occur.

Osteogenic sarcoma is an osteogenic tumor with sarcomatous tissue. It is the most common malignant bone-forming tumor. It is more common in males than females (ratio of 3:2) due to their longer periods of skeletal growth. Sixty percent of cases occur before the age of 20 years, corresponding to the peak period of skeletal growth. A secondary peak incidence is found between 50 and 60 years of age, mainly in patients with a history of prior radiation therapy years earlier [3]. The bones with the highest growth rate are most frequently affected, characteristically the long tubular

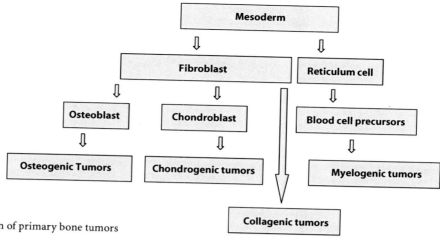

Fig. 6.1. Origin and classification of primary bone tumors

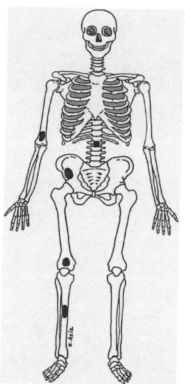

Fig. 6.2. Usual sites of involvement of osteoid osteoma

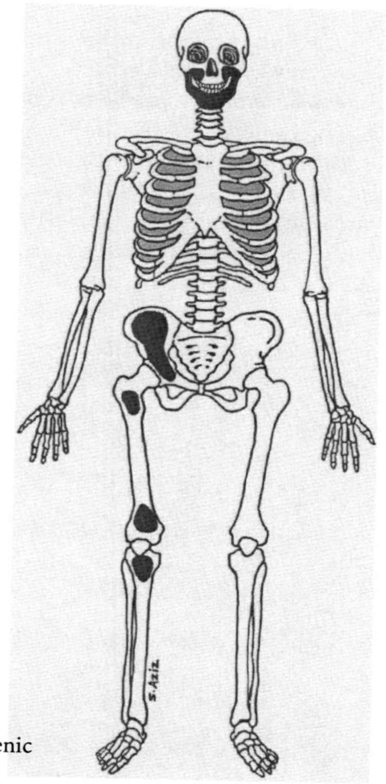

Fig. 6.3. Usual sites of involvement of osteogenic sarcoma

bones, especially in the metaphyseal region (Fig. 6.3). Additionally, within a specific bone the frequency of tumor occurrence corresponds to the sites of greatest growth rate. Therefore the distal femur and proximal tibia are the most frequently involved sites where 50% of the tumors occur. Approximately 15–20% of patients with osteosarcoma present with visible macrometastatic disease. Most metastatic lesions are found in the lung and other sites are the bones, pleura, pericardium, kidney, adrenal gland, and the brain [4, 5]. Approximately 1–3% of patients with osteosarcoma have

tumors in the multiple bony sites at the time of diagnosis. Whether these tumors arise synchronously, or are metastatic lesions from a primary tumor site is not clear [6]. Bone marrow involvement in osteosarcoma, however, is rare [7, 8].

6.2.1.2
Chondrogenic Tumors

These tumors either produce cartilage, primitive cartilage or a cartilage-like substance. *Chondroma* is a benign tumor composed of hyaline cartilage and may occur centrally within the trabecular bone, in which case it is called enchondroma, or it may occur subperiosteally, in which case it is called periosteal chondroma. The tumor is usually solitary. *Osteochondroma* is the most common benign tumor of bone. It is a developmental anomaly resulting from a displaced portion of growth plate underneath the periosteum. The bone and cartilage cap grow by endochondral ossification which explains the uptake of Tc-99m MDP by the cartilage cap as well [9]. This tumor can be solitary, or multiple, which can be familial. It can involve any bone in the body but it is common in the long bones and pelvis. The most common malignant chondrogenic tumor is *chondrosarcoma*. Two types of this malignant tumor are known: (1) primary chondrosarcoma occurring mainly in patients aged 50–70 years and (2) secondary chondrosarcoma which is derived from the benign chondrogenic tumor enchondroma and occurs more frequently in patients aged 20–30 years. The ilium, femur and humerus (metaphysis or diaphysis) are the most common sites (Fig. 6.4). It is extremely rare in the spine, craniofacial bones and small bones of the hands and feet (Fig. 6.5). The neoplasm consists of hyaline cartilage with bands of anaplastic cells and fibrous tissue, The tumor may infiltrate the joint spaces located near the end of the long bone. The tumor also can occur in the soft tissue.

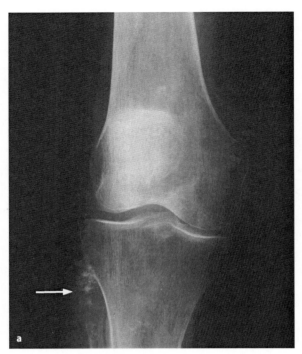

Fig. 6.5a, b. Standard radiograph (**a**) of chondrosarcoma of the right fibula of a 39-year-old man. There is irregular calcification at the site of the tumor in the upper end of the fibula (*arrow*)

6.2.1.3
Collagenic Tumors

Collagenic tumors are the primary bone tumors that produce fibrous connective tissue. *Fibrosarcoma* is a malignant collagen forming spindle cell tumor that occurs in a wide range of ages but it occurs most frequently in patients between 30–40 years (Table 6.2). It occurs slightly more commonly among females. A secondary form may occur following Paget's disease, radiation therapy and long-standing osteomyelitis. The tumor is located most frequently in the metaphysis of the femur or tibia (Fig. 6.6), although every bone of the skeleton can be involved. It begins in the marrow cavity and in-

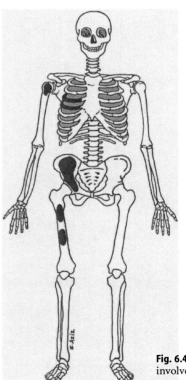

Fig. 6.4. Usual sites of involvement of chondrosarcoma

Table 6.2. Malignant bone tumors and patient age

Age	Tumor
1–30	Ewing's sarcoma Osteosarcoma
30–40	Fibrosarcoma and malignant fibrous histiocytoma Malignant giant cell tumor Reticulum cell sarcoma Parosteal sarcoma
40+	Metastases Myeloma Chondrosarcoma

Adapted from [197]

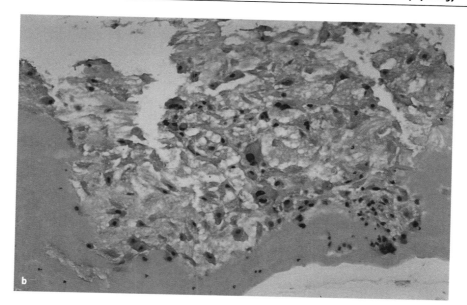

Fig. 6.5 (Cont.) b A photomicrograph of chondrosarcoma illustrating numerous bizzare tumor cells with large nuclei but cells retain some recognizable cartilogenous appearance

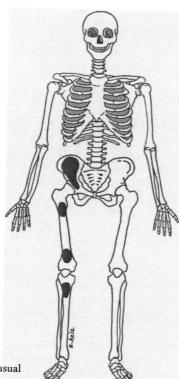

Fig. 6.6. Fibrosarcoma, usual sites of involvement

filtrates the trabeculae. Histological examination typically reveals collagen, malignant fibroblasts and occasionally giant cells.

6.2.1.4
Myelogenic Tumors

Myelogenic tumors are the group of bone tumors that originate from various bone marrow cells. *Myeloma* originates from the plasma cells of the reticuloendothelial element of the bone marrow and may be solitary, or multifocal. It is a highly malignant tumor that occurs more commonly in patients above 40 years of age with a peak in the eighth decade of life. It occurs more frequently in males and blacks. The tumor has a poor prognosis and radiation and chemotherapy have limited success. It mainly affects the spine, pelvis, ribs, skull and proximal bones of the extremities (Fig. 6.7). Patients are known to develop renal failure, anemia, thrombocytopenia and urine that contains Bence Jones protein. Bone pain is common and may progress over time during the course of the disease and pathological fractures may also take place. *Ewing's sarcoma* is another malignant tumor originating from the bone marrow and is most frequently encountered between the ages of 5–15 years and is rare after the age of 30 (Table 6.2). It is more common in males and in whites. It is characterized by a chromosomal translocation between chromosomes 11 and 22. Typically it occurs in the diaphysis of the long bones such as the femur and tibia and in flat bones such as the pelvis (Fig. 6.8); however, any bone may be affected. After originating from marrow, Ewing's sarcoma spreads through the bone cortex to form a tissue mass which does not contain osteoid. The tumor metastasizes early into the lung, other bones, bone marrow, lymph nodes, liver, spleen and the central nervous system. The prognosis is often poor, particularly if the tumor involves the pelvic rather than the long bones.

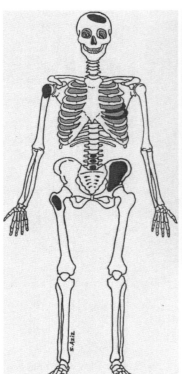

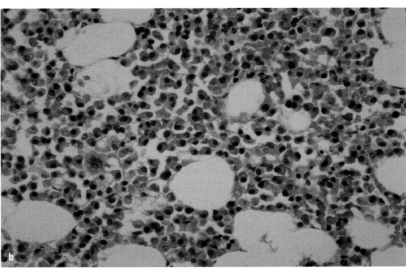

Fig. 6.7a, b. Myeloma. **a** Usual sites of involvement. **b** A photomicrograph of a histologic section of myeloma showing well differentiated myeloma cells that are easily recognizable as plasma cells but with more prominent nuclei

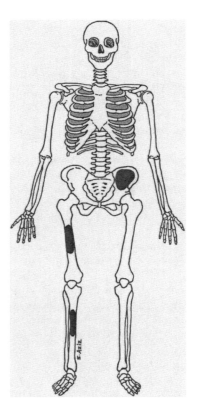

Fig. 6.8. Ewing's sarcoma, usual sites of involvement

Giant cell tumors are difficult to classify although many practitioners include them with the myelogenic tumors since they are believed to originate from the fibrous tissue of the bone marrow. The tumor occurs in patients between 10–70 years of age, although it is more commonly seen in patients between 20–40 years-old. Females are affected more often than males. The tumor occurs mainly around the knee, in the radius, and in the humerus (Fig. 6.9). It has a high regional recurrence rate often extending locally into adjacent soft tissues; but distant metastases occur more rarely. It consists particularly of osteoclast-like giant cells and anaplastic stromal cells with a minor component of osteoid and collagen [10].

Chordoma is a rare, slowly growing, primary bone neoplasm arising from notochordal remnants in the midline of the neural axis and involves the adjacent bone. It occurs in adults usually in the 6th and 7th decades of life. The main malignant potential of chordomas rests on their critical locations adjacent to important structures, their locally aggressive nature, and their extremely high rate of recurrence. The tumor rarely metastasize. CT and MRI are essential for an accurate evaluation. Myelography is used to determine intraspinal extension. Since the tumor may cause significant bone destruction when aggressive, it can be seen as a cold lesion on bone scan although it typically causes increased uptake.

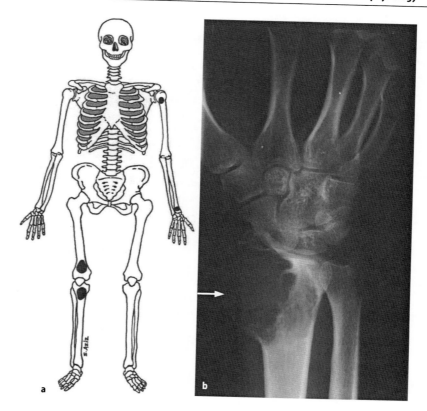

Fig. 6.9a, b. Giant cell tumor. **a** Sites of involvement. **b** A standard radiograph of a giant cell tumor of the distal radius with significant osteolysis

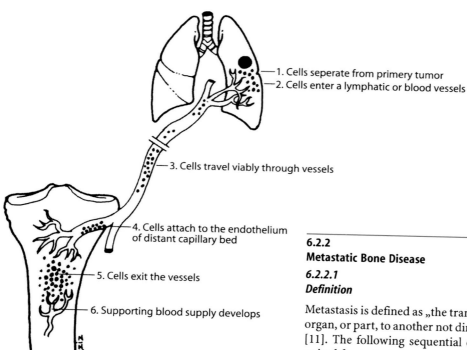

—1. Cells seperate from primery tumor
—2. Cells enter a lymphatic or blood vessels

—3. Cells travel viably through vessels

—4. Cells attach to the endothelium of distant capillary bed

—5. Cells exit the vessels

—6. Supporting blood supply develops

Fig. 6.10. Sequential events generally required for metastatic spread of tumors

6.2.2
Metastatic Bone Disease
6.2.2.1
Definition

Metastasis is defined as „the transfer of disease from one organ, or part, to another not directly connected with it" [11]. The following sequential events are generally required for metastatic spread of tumors (Fig. 6.10).

1. Separation of neoplastic cells from primary tumors
2. Access of separated cells to an efficient lymphatic channel or blood capillary

3. Survival of cells during the transport
4. Successful attachment of cells to the endothelium of a distant capillary bed
5. Exit of cells from the vessel at the new site
6. Successful development of a supporting blood supply for the cells at the site

6.2.2.2
Methods of Tumor Cell Transport

The pathophysiology of skeletal metastases includes two major events, transport of viable tumor cells to bone and interaction of these cells with osseous tissue. Other than **direct extension**, tumor cells are transported to produce metastases by:

Lymphatic Spread

This method of spread is relatively unimportant to the transport of tumor cells to the skeleton. Metastases in regional draining lymph nodes may, however, secondarily involve the adjacent bones.

Hematogenous Spread

This is a major route for the dissemination of malignant cells to distant bones, which occurs via the arterial or venous systems, particularly the vertebral plexus of veins of Batson [12]. The relative roles of the arterial and venous systems in the spread of the tumor to the bone are difficult to define. Metastases occur predominantly in the axial skeleton (specially the spine) and may be present in the absence of pulmonary, and other organ, involvement. This is a combination of findings which supports the significance of Batson's vertebral plexus in tumor spread. This vertebral plexus of veins consists of an intercommunicating system of thin-walled veins with low intra-luminal pressure. These veins frequently do not have valves and communicate extensively with veins in the spinal canal and with the caval, portal, intercostal, pulmonary and renal venous systems [13]. Hematogenous bone metastasis in humans generally begins in the medullary cavity and then involves the cortex.

Intraspinal Spread

This route for transporting malignant cells allows the secondary deposits in the spinal canal to develop in patients with intracranial tumors. This occurs by subarachnoid-spread occurring secondary to fragmentation of a tumor bathed with cerebrospinal fluid; shedding of portions of the tumor at the time of the surgery; ependymal breaching by the primary intracranial tumor; or by fissuring occurring secondary to hydrocephalus [13].

6.2.2.3
Bone Response to Metastases

The osseous response to metastatic lesions includes:
1. Bone resorption where there is increased bone resorption secondary to malignant disease. Osteoclast, tumor cells, tumor cell extract, monocytes and macrophages may all be involved in the process [14, 15].
2. Bone formation which occurs in two types:
   A. Stromal bone formation, which occurs earlier, and is quantitatively a less important mechanism of bone formation associated with metastasis. In this type of bone formation ossification occurs in areas of fibrous stroma within the tumor. This occurs only in those skeletal metastases, which are associated with the development of fibrous stroma such as those of carcinoma of the prostate. Highly cellular tumors have little, or no, stroma and are not associated with this type of bone formation.
   B. Reactive bone formation which occurs in response to bone destruction. Immature woven bone is deposited and is subsequently converted to lamellar bone. In highly anaplastic, rapidly growing tumors, lymphomas, myeloma or leukemias, reactive bone formation may be only minor or insignificant [16].

6.2.2.4
Distribution of Bone Metastasis

The distribution of skeletal metastases varies with the type of primary malignant tumor. However, metastases typically involve the axial skeleton (80%), which is a region rich in red bone marrow (Fig. 6.11). Factors favoring the predominant involvement of the red marrow include a large capillary network, a sluggish blood flow and the suitability of this tissue for the growth of tumor emboli. It is estimated that the blood flow to cancellous bone containing marrow is 5–13 times higher than that to cortical bone [17]. In the appendicular skeleton, the pelvic bones are the most commonly involved. In decreasing order of occurrence, the usual locations of bone metastases are the vertebral column, pelvic bones, ribs, sternum, femoral and humeral shaft and the skull (Figs. 6.12). Less common sites of skeletal metastases (Fig. 6.13) include the scapula, mandible, patella and the bones of the extremity distal to the elbow and knees [18]. Within the spine, metastases involve the lumbar region most commonly followed by the thoracic and cervical areas. Within the vertebra, metastases are more common in the vertebral body (Fig. 6.14) followed by the posterior elements [19]. The explanation for the involvement of the spine as the most common site for the occurrence of metastases include the

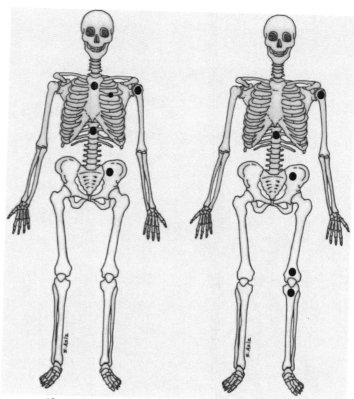

Fig. 6.11. Distribution of metastases according to age

After age 25 years   Before age 25 years

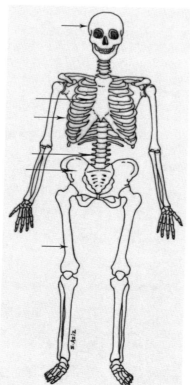

Fig. 6.12. Usual locatio
bone metastases

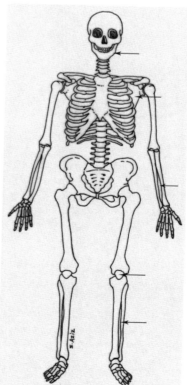

Fig. 6.13. Uncommon l
tions of bone metastas

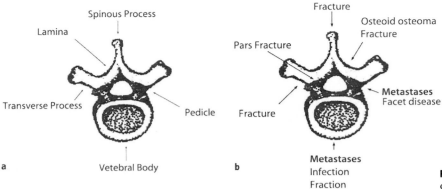

Fig. 6.14. a A diagram illustrating parts of the vertebra. **b** Pathologies affecting the different parts of the vertebra. Within the vertebra, metastases are more common in the vertebral body and the posterior elements

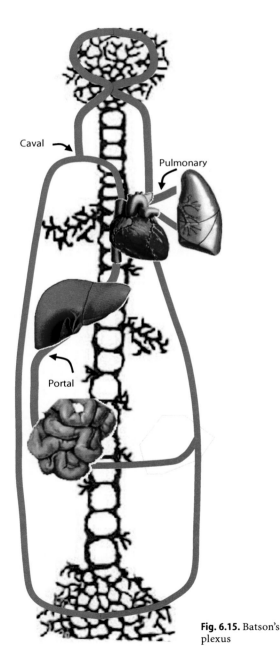

Fig. 6.15. Batson's plexus

Batson's venous plexus which provides direct communication between the spine and numerous other locations in the body (Fig. 6.15) and the large amount of bone mass and bone marrow. A possible explanation for the low frequency of metastases in the distal portion of the extremities is the blood supply, which is largely limited to the arterial provision and the relative absence of red bone marrow (this is a suitable medium for the growth of metastatic tumor cells).

6.2.2.5
Classification of Bone Metastases

Bone metastases can be classified according to several factors including the number of lesions, location, calcium contents and patterns of bone response. The skeleton may at times respond to the various metastatic tumor foci in a predictable manner; however, this is not always the case and sometimes bone metastases show, for example, either purely osteoblastic lesions, or mixed osteoblastic/osteolytic lesions in some sites, and purely osteolytic lesions in other sites. Based on the pattern of bone response, metastases can be classified from the radiographs into purely osteolytic (Table 6.3), purely osteoblastic (Table 6.4) or mixed osteolytic osteoblastic (Table 6.5).

Table 6.3. Tumors producing primarily osteolytic bone metastases

Renal
Thyroid
Ewing's sarcoma
Uterine carcinoma
Gastrointestinal cancers
Hepatoma
Wilm's tumor
Melanoma
Malignant pheochromocytoma
Squamous cell carcinoma of skin
Myeloma

Table 6.4. Tumors producing primarily osteoblastic bone metastases

Prostate
Medulloblastoma
Medullary carcinoma of thyroid
Carcinoid
Osteogenic sarcoma
Neuroblastoma
Nasopharyngeal carcinoma

Table 6.5. Tumors producing primarily mixed osteoblastic/osteolytic bone metastases

Breast
Lung
Urinary bladder
Pancreatic
Testicular
Cervical
Ovarian

6.2.2.6
Sources of Bone Metastases

Certain tumors are known to be common sources of bone metastases. The following primary tumors are the most common to metastasize in the bone: prostate, breast, lung, thyroid and kidney. Bladder and uterine carcinomas are less common sources. In children, skeletal metastases originate from neuroblastoma, Ewing's sarcoma and osteosarcoma. In adult males, carcinoma of the prostate accounts for 60% of bone metastases while in females, breast cancer accounts for 70% of such metastases.

6.2.2.7
Sequelae of Skeletal Metastases

Local Consequences

Bone Destruction
Both direct, and indirect, mechanisms of bone destruction are involved in the bone loss associated with tumor invasion of bone [20].

Direct stimulation of bone loss: tumors cause increased osteoclastic activity and consequently bone destruction through secretion of tumor-derived substances that directly stimulate osteoclasts. These substances include parathyroid hormone related protein, transforming growth factor alpha, transforming growth factor beta and prostaglandins

Indirect stimulation of bone loss by tumors occurs, on the other hand, by substances secreted by the tumor that stimulate first the immune cells which in turn release osteoclast stimulating cytokines such as tumor necrosis factor (TNF) and interleukin-1 (IL-1) which increase the osteoclastic activity and cause bone destruction (Fig. 6.16)

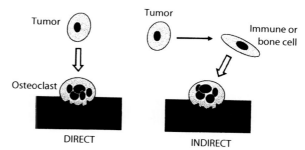

Fig. 6.16. Direct and indirect destruction of bone by metastases

Pathological Fractures
Metastases cause weakening of the involved bones and may lead to fractures in the vertebrae (compression fractures) or long bones, most commonly affecting the proximal portion of the femur [13].

Periosteal New Bone Formation
In general, a periosteal reaction due to metastases is minimal (if present) compared to significant new bone formation in association with primary bone tumors.

Soft Tissue Extension
Soft tissue masses may infrequently present regionally in association with metastases.

This occurs particularly with rib lesions in association with myeloma and in the pelvis in association with colon cancer.

Bone Expansion
Bone expansion may occur with both osteolytic and osteoblastic lesions. Carcinomas of prostate, kidney and thyroid and hepatocellular carcinoma are particularly known to cause expansile metastatic lesions (Fig. 6.17).

Generalized or Metabolic Consequences

Malignant Hypercalcemia
Malignant hypercalcemia occurs in up to 20% of cancer patients and can be associated with metastases due to destruction of the bone but also with primary tumors in the absence of skeletal metastases.

Lung cancer is the most frequent tumor to cause hypercalcemia comprising 36% of malignancies causing hypercalcemia followed by breast cancer (25%) and hematological malignancies as myeloma and lymphoma (14%) [20]. Deposition of calcium in various soft tissues also occurs in cancer patients. This metastatic calcification was first described by Virchow in 1855 and is associated with metastatic neoplasms but is not limited to cancer as it can also occur in chronic renal disease, hemodialysis, parathyroid tumors, hyperparathyroidism, and others. The calcific process principally affects the blood vessels, peri-articular soft tissue, lungs, stomach, kidneys, and the myocardium.

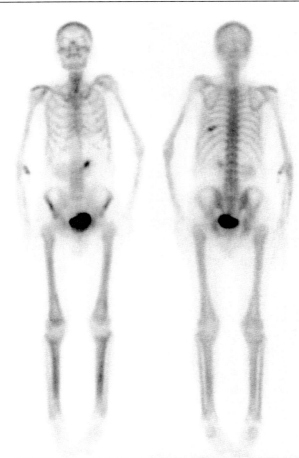

R ANTERIOR L   L POSTERIOR R

Fig. 6.17. Whole body scan of a 60-year-old man with lung cancer. Expanded metastatic lesion of the left 9th rib posteriorly is seen. The scan shows also hypertrophic osteoarthropathy with diffusely increased uptake in the bones of the extremities

Hypocalcemia
An unidentified humoral substance capable of stimulating osteoclasts in some cancer patients with skeletal metastases is proposed to be the underlying mechanism behind the presence of hypocalcemia in up to 16% of cancer patients. It also occurs as one of the metabolic manifestations of tumor lysis syndrome [21].

Oncogenic Osteomalacia
In some patients with skeletal metastases, depressed levels of 1,25-dihydroxy vitamin D3, hypocalcemia and hypophosphatemia are recognized and can be associated with a generalized weakness, and pain of bones and muscles (oncogenic osteomalacia). Oncogenic osteomalacia, is characterized by hypophosphatemia (which occurs secondary to inappropriate phosphaturia), reduced concentrations of serum calcitriol, and defective bone mineralization. Removal of tumors results in complete reversal of these biochemical defects [22].

6.3
Scintigraphy of Primary Bone Tumors

6.3.1
Overall Role

Morphological imaging modalities play a major role in evaluating the local extent of the primary tumors of bone. MRI has become the examination of choice for local staging (Fig. 6.18) (Table 6.6) while standard radiographs are the initial and most specific technique for the diagnosis of such tumors. Using several radiotracers including Tc-99m MDP, thallium-201 (Fig. 6.19), Tc-99m MIBI (Fig. 6.20), gallium-67 and F-18 fluorodeoxyglucose (FDG) (Fig. 6.21), scintigraphy helps in the diagnosis, grading and the evaluation of the response to chemotherapy of the primary bone tumors. Bone scintigraphy has a limited role in local staging but is still the modality of choice in detecting distant metastases.

Fig. 6.18a, b. MRI images of a patient with osteogenic sarcoma of the distal left femur with clear delineation of its extent. MRF is the current modality of choice for local staging of such primary tumor

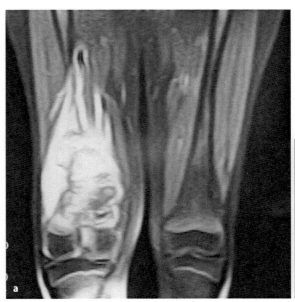

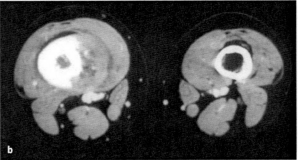

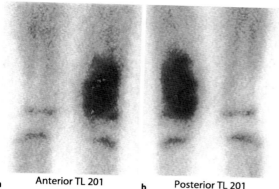

a   Anterior TL 201   **b**   Posterior TL 201

Fig. 6.19a–d. T1-201 in a bone tumor (a 13-year-old boy with a mass in his left thigh). Note the intense T1-201 uptake (**a–b**) bone which corresponds to the tumor as seen on Tc99m MDP bone scan (**c, d**)

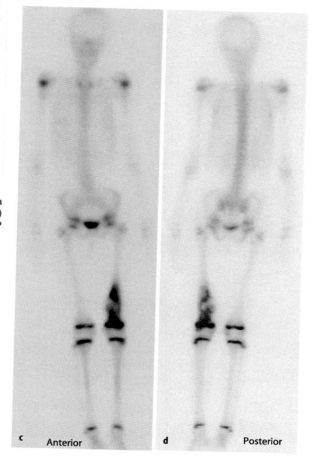

c   Anterior   **d**   Posterior

Table 6.6. Uses of MRI in malignant bone disease

1. Local staging of primary bone tumors
2. Suspected vertebral metastases or equivocal vertebral lesions on bone scan.
3. Patients with neurologic symptoms suggesting vertebral involvement or when spinal cord compression is suspected.
4. Solitary bone lesions.

Bone scintigraphy may detect metastatic and other lesions as small as 2 mm [23]; however, the sensitivity depends on the nature of the lesion as well as its location. The specificity, however, for malignancies including metastases is low. Thallium-201, Tc-99m MIBI and F-18 FDG can help in differentiating malignant from benign bone lesions [24–28]. Thallium-201 and F-18 FDG imaging showed a positive correlation between the grade of the tumor and the retention of thallium-201 and the degree of FDG uptake by a single tumor type [28]. Sequential Tl-201 scintigraphy before, and after treatment, is useful in assessing the degree of response of the tumor to chemotherapy. The early prediction of the chemotherapeutic effect by ^{201}Tl scintigraphy during treatment will affect the management of patients who do not respond to therapy. Thallium-201 is also used for the detection of the early recurrence of tumors [29]. PET is increasingly used to evaluate the response to therapy [30] (Table 6.7) and is considered to be the modality of choice for this purpose (when available). In a recent study [31] 17 patients with primary

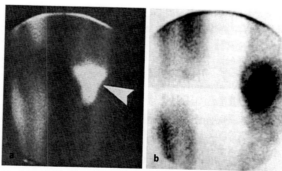

Fig. 6.20. Tc99m MIBI in a bone cancer. Osteogenic sarcoma of the left proximal tibia. MIBI image (**a**) show increased uptake in the tumor region corresponding to tumor uptake on Tc99m MDP bone image (**b**). (From [27] with permission)

bone tumors (11 osteosarcomas, 6 Ewing's sarcomas) treated with chemotherapy before surgery were studied using FDG-PET studies. PET showed a decrease of more 30% decrease in tumor to non-tumor ratios (T:NT) in all patients who had good responses as sub

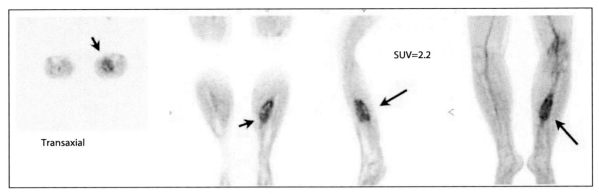

Fig. 6.21. F-18 fluorodeoxyglucose study in a patient with an osteogenic sarcome of the left tibia (*arrow*)

Table 6.7. Role of PET in malignant bone disease

1. Evaluate response to therapy of primary or metastatic bone disease.
2. Detection of recurrence of primary bone malignancies.
3. Early differentiation of progression and flare of metastatic bone disease seen on bone scan.
4. Solitary bone-lesion on bone scan.
5. Question detection of metastatic bone disease.

sequently determined histologically. Patients with poor responses had increasing or unchanged T:NT ratios or decreasing ratios of less than 30% [31].

PET also has a role in detecting the distant metastases of primary bone tumors. However, the accuracy may be dependent on tumor type and location In a study looking at the detection of osseous metastases in 70 patients with histologically proved malignant primary bone tumors (32 osteosarcomas, 38 Ewing's sarcomas) FDG-PET was compared to Tc-99m MDP bone scintigraphy. Among 54 proven osseous metastases (49 from Ewing's sarcomas, five from osteosarcomas), FDG-PET had a sensitivity of 90%, a specificity of 96% and an accuracy of 95% compared to 71%, 92% and 88% for bone scintigraphy. For Ewing's sarcoma patients, the sensitivity, specificity and accuracy of FDG-PET and bone scan were 100%, 96% and 97% and 68%, 87% and 82% respectively. None of the five osseous metastases from osteosarcoma were detected using FDG-PET, but all were detected using bone scintigraphy. The study suggests that the sensitivity, specificity and accuracy of FDG-PET in the detection of osseous metastases from Ewing's sarcomas are superior to those of bone scintigraphy while FDG-PET seems to be less sensitive than bone scintigraphy in the detection of osseous metastases from osteosarcoma [32, 33]. The standardized uptake value (SUV) of F-18 FDG-PET was determined by Aoki et al. [34] in 52 primary bone le-

sions, 19 malignant and 33 benign prior to tissue diagnosis. Overall, there was a statistically significant difference in SUV between benign (2.18) and malignant (4.34) lesions in general. However, there was no statistically significant difference in SUV between certain benign lesions including fibrous dysplasias, chondroblastomas, sarcoidosis, and Langerhans cell histiocytosis and those of chondrosarcoma and osteosarcoma [34]. Another study of 40 patients with primary bone lesions showed a considerable overlap of SUV values between benign and malignant lesions, although the values in malignant lesions were in general significantly higher than those in benign lesions [35].

6.3.2
Scintigraphy of Specific Tumors
6.3.2.1
Osteoid Osteoma

This benign tumor is most common in children, particularly boys. Typically it presents in the lower extremities, pelvis, or less commonly in the spine. Characteristically these lesions are intracortical and diaphyseal in location, although they occasionally involve the metaphysis. On standard radiographs, the characteristic appearance is a small (less than 1.5–2 cm), cortically based radiolucency (nidus) surrounded by marked sclerosis and cortical thickening, combined with the classic clinical history of pain, worse at night, that is relieved by aspirin. Using CT, an area of increased bone density surrounding a lucent nidus is typical of this tumor (Figs. 6.22, 6.23). Scintigraphically there is a focal area of increased flow, increased blood pool activity and increased delayed uptake (Figs. 6.24) [36]. A specific scintigraphic pattern of a double intensity may be seen as a more intense uptake corresponding to the nidus and a peripheral area of less intense activity. The nidus of the tumor must be removed during surgery to avoid re-growth. Single photon emission computed tomography (SPECT) may help to localize an osteoid osteoma before surgery and a gamma

Fig. 6.22. Bone scan of osteoid osteoma. There is slightly increased blood pool activity (**a**) and an intensely increased uptake on the whole body (**b**) and spot image (**c**) in the area of the tumor located in the right tibia

Fig. 6.23. A representative cut of a CT scan of osteoid osteoma of the left tibia of an 18-year-old patient. Note the values of CT in demonstrating the nidus (*arrow*)

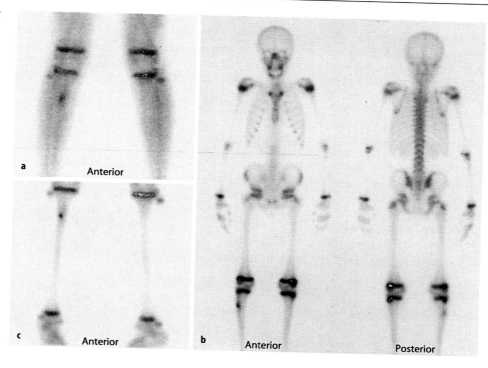

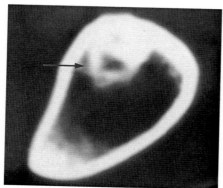

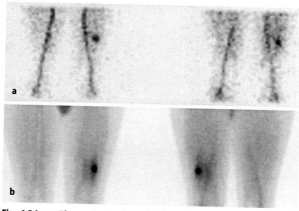

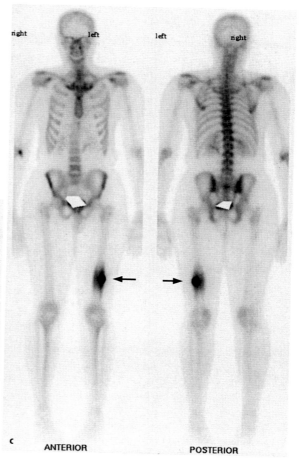

Fig. 6.24a–c. Flow (**a**) blood pool (**b**) and delayed (**c**) images of a patient with osteoid osteoma of the left femur showing intense flow and blood pool activity and on delayed images the specific pattern of double intensity (*arrow*)

probe is a useful operating room tool for localizing this tumor. The symptoms of osteoid osteoma are cured by removing the nidus. 'En-bloc' resection is often not successful because the nidus is hard to find and remove totally. Since the nidus is best localized with CT [37], surgery under CT control using standard equipment usually available in the operating room has been recently used successfully for CT-guided removal of the nidus [38]. MRI also shows intramedullary high intensity areas in the nidus on T2-weighted images and this was suggested to be due to high level of COX-2 expression in neoplastic osteoblasts in the nidus [2]. Intra-articular osteoid osteomas present special problems. Joint effusion and lymphoproliferative synovitis, similar to that seen in rheumatoid arthritis, are often seen with these lesions and may suggest an arthritic condition.

6.3.2.2
Osteoblastoma

As stated earlier this tumor is related to osteoid osteoma and most commonly affects spine and lower extremities. Scintigraphically, osteoblastoma shows an intense uptake similar to osteoid osteoma. Radiographically, a pattern of lysis with, or without, a rim of surrounding sclerosis is characteristic. Extensive surrounding sclerosis is usually absent; however, the surrounding inflammatory changes are often identified using MRI.

6.3.2.3
Osteochondroma

This tumor can appear as sessile/pedunculated (exostosis) or asessile. The lesions, particularly the pedunculated, have a central core of cancellous bone surrounded by a shell of cortical bone and covered by a cap of hyaline cartilage. It can be familial, and multiple, forming the entity of hereditary multiple exostoses that is dis-

covered in childhood. We have encountered a case of this condition where the patient had more than 300 lesions, which show variable degree of uptake on bone scintigraphy (Fig. 6.25). Standard radiographs and CT scanning usually are enough to detect the lesions; however, bone scanning is particularly useful in detecting multiple lesions and also following up patients who have hereditary disease since there is a risk of malignant transformation in up to 30% of cases [39]. MRI delineates and assesses the thickness of cartilage cap and is useful in planning tissue biopsy of the lesions. A cartilage cap 1.5 – 2 cm thick in a skeletally mature per-

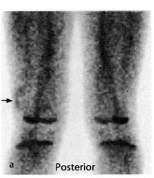

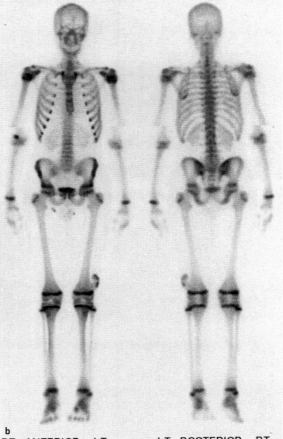

Fig. 6.26. Solitary osteochondroma in the left distal femur in a 14-year-old athletic boy who complained of pain and swelling in the left distal thigh for 1 week before he was referred for a bone scan. There is increased blood pool activity (**a**) and delayed uptake (**b**) in the pedunculated lesion that was proved to be osteochondroma after surgery

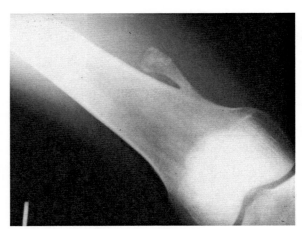

Fig. 6.25. Radiographic appearance of a pedunculated osteochondroma originating from the distal end of the femur

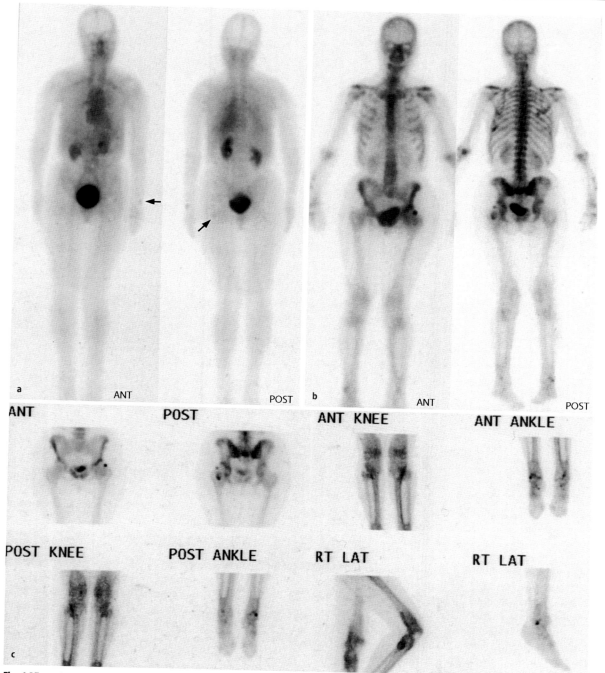

Fig. 6.27a–c. Bone scan of a patient with multiple osteochondromas. Note the numerous small foci of increased uptake in the cervical spine, ribs, pelvis, bones of the lower extremity and right forearm seen on whole body (**b**) and spot images (**c**). On whole body blood pool images (**a**), some lesions show increased blood pool activity (*arrows*)

son is highly suggestive of malignant transformation. Scintigraphically a variable degree of uptake is seen (Figs. 6.26, 6.27) which may reflect the lesion's activity; however, active peripheral lesions, particularly if small, may not show enough uptake to be detected on bone scans [40 – 42].

6.3.2.4
Osteogenic Sarcoma

Scintigraphically, osteogenic sarcoma presents as an area of intense uptake (Fig. 6.28). Rarely, the tumor may present as a cold lesion [43, 44]. CT and, particu-

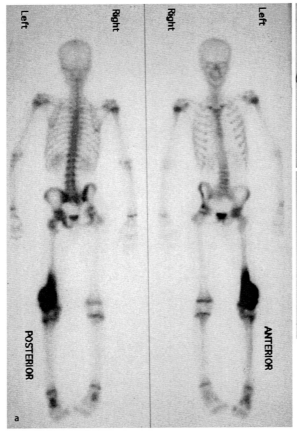

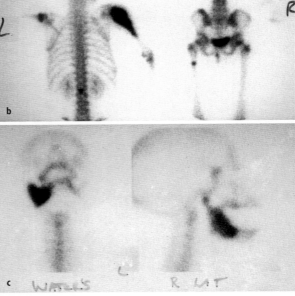

Fig. 6.28a–c. Osteogenic sarcoma. The tumor presents scintigraphically with intense uptake. **a** Osteogenic sarcoma of the distal femur; **b** osteogenic sarcoma of the humerus (with metastases); **c** osteogenic sarcoma of the mandible

larly, MRI are superior to bone scanning in evaluating the extent of the tumor. Bloem [45], evaluated the relative value of MRI, CT, Tc-99m bone scintigraphy and angiography prospectively in the local-tumor staging of 56 patients with a primary bone sarcoma. MRI was significantly superior to CT and scintigraphy in defining intraosseous tumor lengths and as accurate as CT in demonstrating the cortical bone and joint involvement. Additionally MRI was superior to CT in demonstrating involvement of skeletal muscle. Bone metastases are extremely rare at the time of presentation. McKillop et al. [46] have investigated the value of bone scanning at the time of presentation and during follow-up. The authors found only one patient out of 55, with bone metastases. On the other hand, during follow-up bone metastases developed in a further 20 patients who also developed abnormal bone scans; with (approximately half of them) asymptomatic. The authors concluded that the initial bone scan yield although small is justified at the time of presentation because the results may profoundly alter the treatment of the patient and is indicated for all patients (routinely) during follow-up even if they are asymptomatic.

Bone scintigraphy is useful in detecting tumor recurrence. In a study of 27 patients (6 osteosarcomas, 21 Ewing's sarcomas), [41] FDG-PET examination was performed for the diagnosis, or exclusion, of recurrent disease. Conventional imaging techniques consisted of MRI of the primary tumor site, thoracic CT, and Tc-99m MDP bone scintigraphy. The reference methods were the histopathological analysis and/or the clinical and imaging follow-up. In 25 examinations, reference methods revealed 52 sites of recurrent disease The sensitivity, specificity and accuracy of FDG-PET in the detection of recurrences from osseous sarcomas were high (96%, 81% and 82% respectively) but showed only a small advantage in the detection of osseous and soft-tissue recurrences compared with conventional imaging [47].

To follow up the response of the tumor to therapy, PET has proved useful [30, 31, 48]. Tc-99m-MIBI and thallium-201 are also useful for this purpose and predict the prognosis. Studies have suggested that P-glycoprotein (Pgp) expression is a prognostic factor for patients with osteosarcoma. Some investigators have found a relationship between the wash-out rate of Tc-99m MIBI and the Pgp score, with a significant difference in wash-out rate being observed between patients with high, and patients with low, Pgp expression [49]. Others have found that Tc-99m MIBI imaging is not an effective predictor of prognosis since the Tc-99m MIBI half-life and uptake ratio showed no correlation with histological necrosis following induction chemotherapy and did not correlate with P-glycoprotein expression [50]. Using thallium-201, the pattern of doughnut uptake was found to be a predictor of lower event-free survival in patients with extremity osteogenic sarcoma, but does not correlate with the histological response to therapy [51].

The initial glucose metabolism of primary osteosarcoma, as assessed by F-18 FDG-PET using tumor to non-tumor ratios, provides prognostic information related to the grading and biological aggressiveness. High F-18 FDG uptake correlates with poor outcome and F-18 FDG uptake may be complementary to other well-known factors in judging the prognosis in osteosarcoma [52–54].

6.3.2.5
Myeloma

Traditional staging of myeloma depends partially on the extent of the disease evaluated by full skeletal survey. The tumor presents on radiographs as osteolytic areas due to demineralization of bone by the tumor (Fig. 6.29). Tc-99m MDP, Tc-99m-MIBI and thallium-201 have all been used to image multiple myeloma and the bone mineral density can be measured using dual energy X-ray absorptiometry [55, 56]. Bone scanning is generally viewed to be unreliable for staging, although in a recent study reviewing the literature (comparing the usefulness of conventional skeletal radiography and bone scans in diagnosing the osteolytic lesions of myeloma) it has been shown that bone scintigraphy, (considered by many to have no role in the detection of osteolytic lesions of myeloma), is in fact more sensitive than radiography in the detection of lesions in the ribs, scapula, and spine [57]. Radiographs, however, are also known to underestimate the extent of bone and bone marrow involvement [58]. Although cold areas are commonly seen on bone scans, increased uptake is the most common scintigraphic pattern [59, 60]. This should not contradict the fact that myeloma is the most

Table 6.8. Causes of cold lesions on bone scintigraphy

1. Radiation therapy
2. Osteomyelitis
3. Infarction
4. Tumors
   Myeloma
   Renal cell carcinoma
   Thyroid carcinoma
   Histiocytosis X
   Eosinophilic granuloma
   Neuroblastoma
   Osteogenic carcinoma (rare)
   Metastases of osteogenic sarcoma
5. Artifacts: barium, belts or other metal objects

common tumor to cause cold lesions on bone scanning (Table 6.8). Regarding the use of Tl-201, Watanabe et al. studied 19 patients with multiple myeloma with both Tl-201 and bone scintigraphy. The authors found that the combination of Tl-201 and bone scintigraphy was more accurate than bone scintigraphy alone in detecting lesions of multiple myeloma [60].

Alexandrakis studied 28 patients with multiple myeloma using Tc-99m MIBI in comparison with Tc-99m MDP, standard radiographs, CT scan and MRI. Tc-99m MIBI scintigraphy was found to detect bone marrow lesions in myeloma patients that could not be detected using other imaging methods and it was able provide prognostic information related to the disease activity and multi-drug resistance. This was because the intensity of Tc-99m MIBI uptake correlated well with disease activity as determined by lactate dehydrogenase (LDH), C-reactive protein (CRP), β2-microglobulin, and serum ferritin [61]. MRI has been found to be more accurate than other modalities in assessing the tumor sites [62, 63] and CT scanning has an established role in the evaluation of regional disease [64]. A common limitation of both MRI and CT, however, is the frequent inability to differentiate the active disease from necrosis, bone fracture and other benign disease [65]. Recently Durie et al. [66] used whole body FDG-PET in 66 patients with multiple myeloma and found it very useful in identifying active disease, patients with remission and those with relapse. The authors found it particularly useful in evaluating non-secretory myeloma and found that detected residual, or recurrent, disease after therapy especially extra medullary is a poor prognostic factor. Finally, the staging, follow-up and determination of the prognosis of patients with myeloma depends on the use of multiple modalities that are complementary. Bone scintigraphy is not highly accurate in detecting myeloma sites, although it can be useful in certain locations. Standard radiography is known to underestimate the extent of the disease. Tl-201 and Tc-99m MIBI have no clear role in this tumor. CT scan and MRI are the most useful but cannot determine the activity of the disease and PET has a promising role in this tumor.

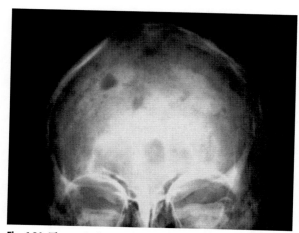

Fig. 6.29. The typical osteolytic myeloma lesions on a standard radiograph

6.3.2.6
Ewing's Sarcoma

As with other primary bone tumors, morphological imaging modalities, including CT and MRI, are the principal imaging modalities for assessing the local extent of this tumor. Bone scanning is, however, indicated when metastases need to be excluded (Fig. 6.30). The detection of the osseous metastases of Ewing's sarcoma, therapy monitoring and the diagnosis of recurrences are potentially useful clinical indications for FDG-PET [67]. FDG-PET has been reported to detect more lesions of metastatic Ewing's sarcoma than bone and gallium scans, especially for those with bone marrow involvement [68, 69]. Tc-99m MIBI has also been used in this tumor to provide an imaging assessment of multiple-drug resistance. The presence, or absence, of Tc-99m MIBI uptake at diagnosis, or after therapy, has been found to have no prognostic significance. Tc-99m MIBI was present in the two tumors that were P-glycoprotein positive and in only one of four tumors that were P-glycoprotein negative. Tc-99m MIBI imaging does not appear to be useful in Ewing's sarcoma [70].

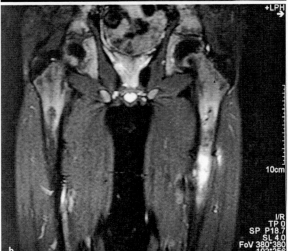

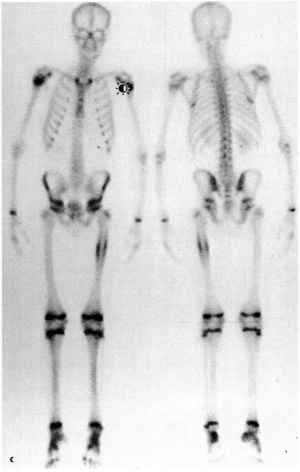

Fig. 6.30a–c. Ewing's sarcoma of the left femur seen on standard radiograph (**a**), MRI (**b**), and bone scan (**c**). MRI shows heterogenous signal intensity at the metaphysis and diaphyseal region of the left femur with no soft tissue component. Note that the value of MRI is in assessing the local tumor extent compared to bone scanning, which, however, showed no additional lesions to suggest of distant metastases

6.4
Scintigraphy and Correlative Imaging of Metastatic Bone Disease

Bone is the third most common site of metastatic disease. Skeletal metastases are clinically significant because of the associated symptoms, complications such as the pathological fracture and their significant impact on staging, treatment, quality of life and prognosis. Therefore, detection of bone metastases is an important part of treatment planning. The frequency with which metastases are detected varies considerably with the type of primary tumor and with the methodology used for detection. In general, four main modalities are routinely utilized clinically: standard radiography, CT scanning, scintigraphy and MRI [71]. Additionally, PET is increasingly evaluated for the detection of bone metastases and the initial experience is promising. Bone scanning, however, is the most widely used and the most practical and cost-effective screening technique for assessing the entire skeleton for bone metastases. This is in addition to it being a very sensitive modality for detecting the disease. However, a variable false-negative rate occurs in certain locations such as the spine and in lesions confined to bone marrow [72]. In a study of 18 patients with known malignant tumors and suspected bone metastases, whole-body bone marrow MRI detected 91% of the confirmed malignant lesions, whereas bone scintigraphy detected 85% [73]. Detection of vertebral metastases was shown to depend on the size of the lesion and their location. Lesions less than 2 cm in diameter and intramedullary lesions are not likely to be detected compared to sub-cortical and transcortical lesions since cortical involvement is likely to be the cause of positive findings on bone scanning of vertebral metastases [74].

In a comparative study, the diagnostic accuracy of whole-body MR imaging, skeletal scintigraphy and FDG-PET for the detection of bone metastases in children was determined. Thirty-nine patients aged between 2 and 19 years who had Ewing's sarcoma, osteosarcoma, lymphoma, rhabdomyosarcoma, melanoma, or Langerhans' cell histiocytosis were studied. Twenty-one patients exhibited 51 bone metastases. The sensitivities for the detection of bone metastases were 90% for FDG-PET, 82% for whole-body MR imaging, and 71% for skeletal scintigraphy. False-negative lesions were different for the three imaging modalities, mainly depending on the lesion location. Most false-positive lesions were diagnosed using FDG-PET [75].

A recent study showed that FDG-PET has a better specificity, but a lower sensitivity for detecting malignant bone metastases when compared with bone scanning. Twenty-four patients with biopsy-proven malignancies and suspected bone metastases, had whole body FDG-PET and bone scan. In 39 bone lesions with discordant findings between FDG-PET and bone scanning, the final diagnosis revealed eight metastatic with positive FDG-PET findings. They were not detected on bone scanning indicating that no false positive findings occurred using PET. On the other hand, 11 metastatic and 20 benign bone lesions (with positive bone scan findings) were not detected using FDG-PET [76]. Another study of 56 patients with malignant lymphoma, whole body FDG-PET was shown to have a high positive predictive value and was more sensitive and specific than bone scintigraphy in 12 patients with bone metastases [77].

A prospective study of 44 patients with prostate, lung or thyroid carcinomas showed a sensitivity of 83% for bone scanning in detecting malignant and benign osseous lesions in the skull, thorax and extremities and a sensitivity of 40% in the spine and pelvis. F-18 FDG-PET was more sensitive in detecting osseous lesions and detected all the lesions that were detected by bone scanning. With bone scans, the sensitivity in detecting osseous metastases appears highly dependent on the anatomical localization of these lesions, whereas the detection rates of osteoblastic and osteolytic metastases were similar [78]. Higher detection rates and more accurate differentiation between the benign and malignant lesions with F-18 PET suggests that F-18 PET should be used for the detection of bone metastases when possible [78]. Accordingly, PET is a promising modality for the detection of metastases that will prove useful especially in tumors known to produce atypical patterns of metastases. The higher spatial resolution of PET compared to gamma cameras and the routinely included tomography are characteristics that increase the sensitivity of this modality in detecting metastases.

6.4.1
Scintigraphic Patterns of Bone Metastases on Bone Scans
6.4.1.1
Typical Pattern

The most common and typical pattern (Table 6.9) of bone metastases is that of multiple randomly distributed foci of increased uptake (Fig. 6.31), these are usually found in the axial skeleton and follow the distribution of the bone marrow including the shoulder girdle.

Table 6.9. Patterns of bone metastases on bone scan

1. Typical pattern: multiple, randomly distributed lesions
2. Atypical patterns:
   Solitary lesion
   Cold lesions
   Diffuse pattern
   Equilibrium
   Flare pattern
   Symmetric

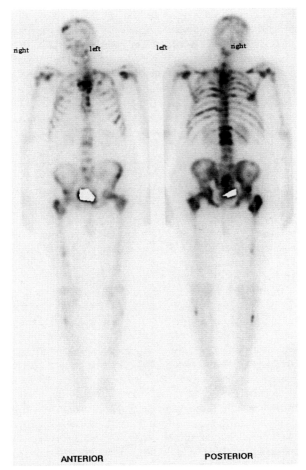

ANTERIOR   **POSTERIOR**

Fig. 6.31. The most common and typical pattern of bone metastases is that of multiple-randomly distributed foci with increased uptake.

Table 6.10. Causes of multiple hot spots on bone scan mimicking metastases

 1. Tuberculosis
 2. Atypical mycobacteria
 3. Coccidioidomycosis
 4. Tertiary syphilis
 5. Brucellosis
 6. Sarcoidosis
 7. Multiple fractures
 8. Multiple infarcts
 9. Multifocal osteomyelitis
10. Mast cell disease
11. Paget's disease
12. Spondyloarthritis
13. Multiple pseudo-fractures secondary to osteomalacia

There is relatively less extensive involvement of the ribs. Metastases present in the peripheral bones of the extremities are rare [79]. Certain pathologies other than metastases, particularly hematogenously disseminated infections of bone [80–84], can cause a pattern that may mimic metastases (Fig. 6.32) (Table 6.10).

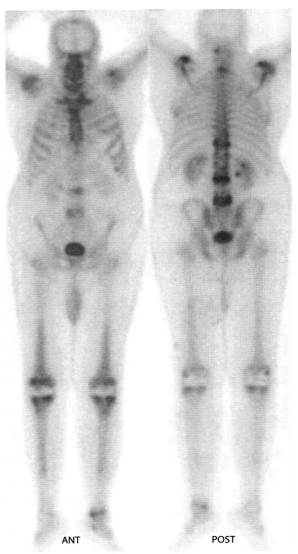

ANT   **POST**

Fig. 6.32. A whole body bone scan of a patient with brucellosis with a scintigraphic abnormalities of multiple foci of increased uptake. The foci in the spine and ribs in this case can be confused for bone metastases. (From [198] with permission)

6.4.1.2
Atypical Patterns

Solitary Lesion

In cancer patients solitary metastasis occurs in the axial and appendicular skeleton to varying degrees. These lesions are commonly asymptomatic and are not suspected clinically. Less than half of these lesions are present on radiographs. These facts further emphasize the importance of obtaining a scan of the entire skeleton in cancer patients. The incidence of malignancy (Table 6.11) in solitary lesions varies with the location and may also be linked to the type of the primary tumor [24, 78, 85–99]. The incidence is highest in the verte-

Table 6.11. Incidence of malignancy in solitary bone lesions in cancer patients [24, 87–99]

Author	Year	Incidence of malignancy
Shirazi [87]	1974	54%
Corcoran [88]	1976	64%
Rappaport [89]	1978	19%
Brown [90]	1983	39% (pediatric)
Tumeh [91]	1985	10% (Ribs)
Matsumoto [92]	1987	39% (Ribs)
Kwai [93]	1988	76% (sternal)
Boxer [94]	1989	20%
Brown [95]	1989	55%
Elgazzar [24]	1989	28%
Coakley [96]	1995	43% (Spine)
Baxter [97]	1995	41% (Ribs)
Hashimi [98]	1999	21% (Skull)
Tomada [99]	2001	23%

brae and low in the skull and extremities. Within the vertebral column, the location is also linked to the probability of malignancy. A recent study using bone scintigraphy in 109 patients yielded the following probability intervals for the intraosseous malignant lesions distributed in the lumbar spine: pedicle 88–100%; vertebral body 36–57%; spinous process 19–81% and facet joints 0.8–21%. The authors concluded that lesions affecting the pedicle are a strong indicator for malignancy, whereas involvement of the facet joints is usually related to benign disease. Lesions affecting the vertebral body, or the spinous process, do not show a clear tendency towards being either malignant or benign. However, in this study in contrast to other studies, a significant probability of malignancy (>36%) was observed in lesions exclusively affecting the vertebral body [86]. When the solitary rib lesion is elongated it carries a higher incidence of malignancy. A solitary hot spot in the skull is rare and is predominantly benign in nature. Retrospective evaluation of bone scans over 10 years was performed to determine the incidence of a solitary hot spot in the skull. A review of the reports of bone scans in 9968 patients yielded 37 (0.37%) patients with a solitary hot spot in the skull. In the group of 27 patients with extra-skeletal malignancy, the hot spot was secondary to metastasis in four patients and of a non-metastatic origin in 15. In the remaining eight patients, the cause was indeterminate. Two of the four metastatic foci were located along the suture lines [98]. The authors indicated that the location of a hot spot along the suture lines may not always be a normal variation and can represent a solitary bone metastasis. Regarding the primary tumor type, although the incidence of malignancy in solitary bone lesion in patients with lung cancer presence was reported to be higher, others found no significant difference [86, 100]. Tomoda reviewed 1167 consecutive bone scans of patients with a history of lung, breast or prostatic cancer. There were 185 bone scans (lung 121, breast 36, prostate 28)

showing solitary hot spot. Of the solitary hot spots, 42 lesions (23%) were malignant: 30 (25%) lung cancer cases, eight (22%) breast cancer cases, and four (14%) prostatic cancer cases. The difference in the frequency of bone metastasis according to the site of primary tumor was not significant [99].

A wide array of imaging modalities is available for etiologic classification of solitary lesions of bone. The standard radiograph, remains the initial imaging modality of choice and is an influential factor in determining whether further imaging is required. Although uptake on bone scanning is non-specific, certain patterns are known to occur in certain lesions and have a higher specific diagnostic value. Osteoid osteoma may show a specific pattern of double intensity, bone islands should show no significant uptake and giant cell tumors may show a characteristic pattern of the 'doughnut sign' [101]. Bone scanning is useful in distinguishing bone islands from other sclerotic lesions, particularly malignancies, since any significant uptake should raise the suspicion of malignancy, or other aggressive lesions other than bone islands [102]. MRI is the examination of choice for staging solitary tumors of bone [103]. However, differentiation between benign and malignant etiologies remains largely unanswered by these three modalities. FDG-PET provides a more accurate differentiation between such lesions [78]. A recent study using FDG-PET examined 83 patients with 37 histologically proven malignancies and 46 benign lesions. The study looked at the standardized uptake value (SUV); global influx (Ki); computation of the transport constants K1-k4 with consideration of the distribution volume (VB) according to a 2-tissue-compartment model and the fractal dimension based on the box-counting procedure (parameter for the inhomogeneity of the tumors) were all determined. The mean SUV, the vascular fraction VB, K1-K4 and Ki were significantly higher in the malignant compared with benign lesions. Using the SUV alone, there was some overlap, which limited the diagnostic accuracy. The SUV alone showed a sensitivity of only 54%, a specificity of 91%, and a diagnostic accuracy of 74%. The fractal dimension was superior and showed a sensitivity of 71%, a specificity of 82%, and an accuracy of 77%. The combination of the SUV, fractal dimension, VB, K1-k4, and Ki revealed the best results with a sensitivity of 76%, a specificity of 97%, and an accuracy of 88%. The authors recommended the use of the full F-18 FDG kinetics to classify a bone lesion as malignant or benign [104].

Elgazzar et al. [24], evaluated 28 patients with solitary bone lesions found on Tc-99m MDP scans. Using 2 mCi of thallium-201 chloride, visual assessment and lesion-to-background ratio determination, they found a significant uptake with a mean lesion-to-background ratio of 4.2 in malignant lesions and a mean lesion-to-

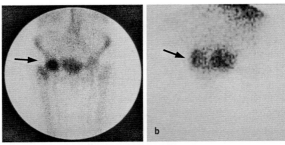

Fig. 6.33a, b. Solitary bone lesion in the right femoral head in a patient with Non Hodgkins lymphoma as seen on the static bone scan spot view of the pelvis (**a**). Increased T1-201 uptake is seen in the lesion (**b**)

background ratio of 1.37 in benign lesions (Fig. 6.33). Using early and delayed imaging and determination of retention of Tl-201 by the lesion is more accurate than using early imaging only for the etiologic classification of lesions since it decreases the overlap between malignant and certain benign conditions such as tuberculosis [29]. Despite these limitations when PET is not available, T1-201 can be considered the 'PET of the poor'. Tc-99m MIBI may also be used similarly to help differentiate benign from malignant lesions when PET is not an option.

Cold Lesions

Aggressive tumors may cause cold lesions on bone scan (Fig. 6.34). This is seen commonly in multiple myeloma and renal cell carcinoma [105]. Other tumors include primary tumors as osteolytic osteogenic sarcoma, fibrosarcoma and chordoma, and metastatic lesions of

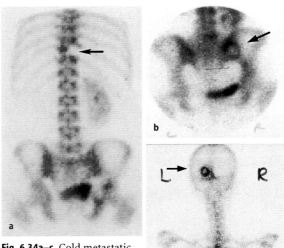

Fig. 6.34a–c. Cold metastatic lesions at different locations. Some lesions have no surrounding rim of increased activity (**a**) and some have (**b, c**)

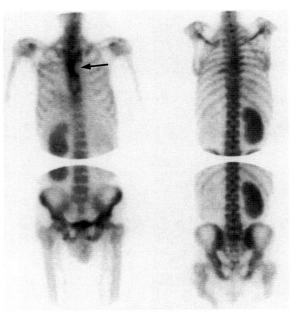

Fig. 6.35. Cold lesions of the sternum in a patient with renal cell carcinoma. Note the location and asymmetry of the lesions which are features to differentiate such metastatic lesion from normal variants as shown in figure 1.34

breast and lung cancers, lymphoma, neuroblastoma and osteogenic sarcoma. A high number of counts, higher intensity images and review of the images on computer screens are essential for the better detection of cold lesions on bone scanning. A cold lesion in the sternum constitutes a special problem since a highly variable normal appearance of the sternal area makes interpretation of the possible cold lesion difficult using planar bone imaging. A normal variant of a photopenic area in the lower sternum is not uncommon and is reported in 2–31% of patients [106]. These normal variants occur especially in the area above the xiphoid process of the sternum in which an oval photopenic area on anterior planar images may be seen. This finding is most likely caused by localized incomplete fusion. The variant is seen more clearly on SPECT images. Differentiation from malignancy appears to be related to lesion symmetry, location, midline, and evenly distributed radioactivity surrounding the edge of the photopenic area [106]. Malignant lesions typically occur at the sternal lateral edges and may be surrounded by non-uniform activity (Fig. 6.35).

Equilibrium Pattern

Hot lesions may show a relatively normal appearance with time (reflecting a point of equilibrium between osteoblastic activity and the bone destruction by the tumor). It appears that skeletal lesions may evolve through phases involving increased uptake, an equilibrium and then a decreased uptake. The second phase can result in minimal abnormalities of focal, non-uniform, minimally increased uptake or even near normal patterns that can be missed on scans. This phenomenon has been particularly observed and studied in rib lesions [107].

Flare Pattern

Successful treatment of metastatic disease may be accompanied by an initial apparent deterioration of some lesions on the bone scan, followed by improvement. New sites of activity can be seen along with the more typical change of increasing intensity of pre-existing lesions following chemotherapy. These apparently new lesions probably represent very small lesions, small cold lesions, or lesions in the equilibrium phase that existed but could not be seen on earlier studies. The healing process that occurs as a response to chemotherapy, or hormonal therapy, in the areas of metastases is behind the increasing activity on the follow-up scan of pre-visualized lesions as well as the visualization of presumably pre-existing, previously undetected very small lesions [108]. This phenomenon occurs in the metastatic disease of many tumors, particularly breast, lung, and prostate metastases. It can be seen for up to 8 months, or even longer, after chemotherapy but usually by 3 months the distinction between progression and this pseudo-progression can be made on the follow-up bone scan in most cases [109, 110].

Practically it may difficult to wait for 3 months to evaluate the efficacy of therapy using bone scans after the start of chemotherapy or endocrine therapy. Measuring type 1 carboxy-terminal telopeptide (ICTP), a bone resorption marker, has been suggested to help monitor the patients' responses to combination chemotherapy and may prevent the prolonged ineffective therapy, or unnecessary changes in therapy as a result of the flare phenomenon [111]. F-18 FDG was used to evaluate the bone metastases before, and after, endocrine therapy in a patient with metastatic bone disease of the prostatic carcinoma as seen on bone scans. PET demonstrated heterogeneous FDG uptake in the bones with regions of metastases and up to a 4.79-fold increase of SUV. Bone pain improved 2 weeks after receiving 500 mg diethylstilbesterol diphosphate daily as well as luteinizing hormone-releasing hormone analogue. Serum prostate specific antigen (PSA) decreased after 2 months. Bone scanning after treatment showed little, or no, change compared to that before treatment (with more uptake at lumbar vertebral lesions). Repeat PET showed decreases in fluorodeoxyglucose uptake compared with the pretreatment scan indicating a favorable response to treatment [112]. The information on the response to chemotherapy or hormonal therapy is provided more rapidly by PET than bone scanning,

providing the opportunity exists early to select a more effective therapy in cases of unfavorable response.

Diffuse Pattern

With advanced metastatic disease, the entire axial skeleton may be involved by a large number of tumor cells causing increased extraction of radiopharmaceutical. This pattern may be interpreted as normal depending on the display intensity and should also be differentiated from other causes of diffusely increased uptake in the skeleton (superscan) such as hyperparathyroidism, and other metabolic bone diseases and Paget's disease (Table 6.12).

A superscan secondary to metastases shows increased uptake that is usually confined to the axial skeleton while in case of metabolic disorders it also involves the skull, mandible and a variable length of the long bones. A preferential increase of uptake at the costochondral junctions and sternum are additional features of metabolic disease superscan [113].

Symmetrical Pattern

Metastases may unusually present as symmetrical lesions. Certain tumors are known to produce this pattern (Table 6.13), particularly in pediatric neuroblastoma. The pattern has also been reported in other tumors such as lung cancer [114, 115].

Table 6.12. Causes of diffuse increase of skeletal uptake on bone scan

Advanced metastatic bone disease
Primary and secondary hyperparathyroidism
Hypertrophic osteoarthropathy
Renal osteodystrophy.
Acromegaly
Aplastic anemia
Hyperthyroidism
Leukemia
Waldenström's macroglobulinemia
Myelofibrosis
Hypervitaminosis D
Paget's disease

Table 6.13. Tumors known to produce symmetrical bone metastases

Neuroblastoma
Retinoblastoma
Embryonal rhabdomyosarcoma
Breast carcinoma
Lung carcinoma (rare)

6.4.2
Scintigraphic Evaluation of Metastases of Certain Tumors
6.4.2.1
Metastases of Breast Cancer

Breast cancer is a common source of skeletal metastases. Patients with advanced breast cancer frequently have bone metastases [116–118]. The average incidence of metastases is, however, low, with incidences of less than 5% in stages 1 and 2 disease (the range varies from 0% to 40%. In clinical stage 3, the incidence of bone metastases is 20–45%. Thus, routine scanning during this stage is necessary, which may not be the case during the early clinical stages [119–121]. This was confirmed in a recent study of 250 patients with breast cancer, which showed metastases in 3% of patients with pathological T1–2 N0–1 disease, compared to 30% of patients with pathological stage T3–4 or N2 disease [122]. Bone pain is an appropriate indication for scanning, either at diagnosis or follow-up, because the documentation of metastases allows instituting the appropriate definitive therapy, or palliation [123]. However, pain has not been found to be an extremely accurate marker for metastatic disease [124, 125]. Shutte found evidence of metastases in only 60% of patients with persistent bone pain [125].

Radiologically, the tumor usually produces purely osteolytic or mixed osteolytic/osteoblastic lesions (Table 6.5). Rarely, breast cancer gives rise to osteoblastic lesions. Standard radiographs are less sensitive and impracticable to screen for metastases compared to bone scintigraphy. This has been re-confirmed in a recent study of 100 patients presenting with metastatic breast cancer, 67 of whom had skeletal metastases. Sixteen (24%) of these 67 patients had radiographically occult metastases [126]. Using bone scintigraphy metastases are almost always hot in appearance. The bone metastases develop most rapidly during the first 2 years [118, 120, 127] and it is appropriate to obtain frequent follow-up scans, perhaps every 6 months during this period. However, in its published guidelines about breast cancer surveillance, the American Society of Clinical Oncology (ASCO) indicated that data are insufficient to recommend routine bone scans, chest radiographs, blood counts, tumor markers, liver ultrasonograms, or CT scans in early clinical stages of the disease [128]. Initial, and follow-up, bone scans provide prognostic information by showing the extent of metastatic disease and evaluating the effectiveness of hormonal and other standard breast cancer therapies [129].

Among patients with breast cancer who have metastatic bone disease, the response to therapy and ultimate prognosis are often closely linked. Metastatic breast cancer with the disease limited to the bone has a better prognosis than when other distant sites are involved. This appears to be the case both in terms of the initial metastatic involvement and later disease recurrence [130–132]. Coleman et al. [133] recently reviewed the follow-up results for 367 patients with breast cancer who had a first occurrence of metastatic disease solely in the skeleton. The authors found that the 139 patients in whom the disease remained confined to the skeleton had a median survival 6 months longer than the patients who later developed metastases in other visceral locations. The extent of bone metastases at the initial relapse also appears to be of prognostic importance. This is because the subset of patients with breast cancer, with initial bone involvement at only one or two sites, has a survival advantage over patients with more extensive metastases at the time of initial positive scintigraphic findings [129].

In a report of 101 patients with bone metastases, who were studied with serial bone scans and radiography during treatment [134], patients whose scans showed disease regression had the longest survival, followed by those with a stable scintigraphic and radiographic pattern; the shortest survival was for those with disease progression. The importance of adequate follow-up and appreciation of scintigraphic flare was stressed by Vogel et al. [135] in reviewing data from a Scandinavian hormonal therapy trial, in which 29% of patients had evidence of flare on the scans performed 8 or 16 weeks after initiation of treatment. As the increased bone uptake seen in the flare phenomenon is usually associated with a response to therapy and healing, it is obviously important that the relevance of the finding be appreciated to avoid an effective therapy being discontinued.

Bone scintigraphy has been reported to be false-negative for vertebral metastases among patients with estrogen-receptor negative or highly proliferative tumors. In these patients, MRI has proven more useful, and is therefore recommended as the optimal radiological modality for post-operative follow-up [137].

F-18 FDG-PET has been used to detect breast cancer metastases (Fig. 6.36) and is being still investigated. It appears to be a powerful tool that has potential in detecting bony metastases with a high sensitivity and specificity and may have a greater role in the future. Data indicate that it may have the ability to demonstrate the very early bone reactions when small bone marrow metastases are present. The ability to perform the early detection of bone metastases would have a significant effect on clinical management [138, 139]. Schirrmeister studied 17 patients with 64 bone metastases detected on PET-FDG. Only 29 metastases were detected in 11 patients with bone scanning [140]. In a study of 51 female patients with breast cancer who had PET together with a bone scan within one month the sensitivity, specificity and accuracy of the bone scan for the detection of bone metastases were 78%, 81% and 80%, respectively. PET had a sensitivity, specificity and accuracy of 78%, 98% and 94%, respectively [139].

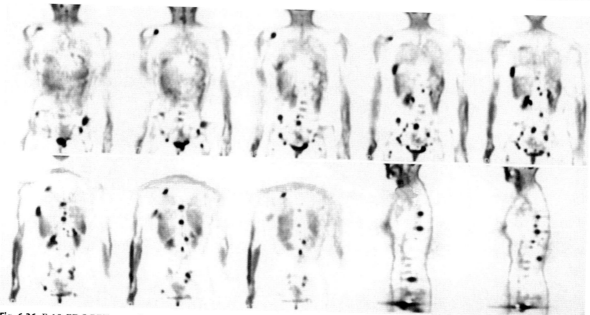

Fig. 6.36. F-18-FDG PET scan showing metastatic bone disease in a patient with recurrent breast cancer

Another study of 34 patients with carcinoma of the breast compared PET of the bones to bone scanning. The area under the receiver-operating characteristic curve was 1.00 for PET and 0.82 for bone scanning ($p < 0.05$). The PET scan changed the treatment recommendation for 4 of the patients, compared to what would have been recommended if only information from the bone scanning was available [140].

6.4.2.2
Metastases of Prostate Cancer

Metastatic bone disease is found to exist in 8–35% of patients with prostatic carcinoma at the time of diagnosis [110, 141, 142]. Bone pain has low predictive value in detecting metastatic disease [143]. Bone scans have been shown to be vastly superior to radiographs, and more accurate than acid phosphatase determinations, in the detection of bony metastasis [141, 144, 145]. Jacobson reviewed the bone scan patterns of benign and malignant uptake in 432 patients with newly diagnosed prostate carcinoma in relation to prostate-specific antigen (PSA) levels determined within 4 months of scintigraphy. The metastatic disease prevalence increased from 1% for PSA levels of < 20 ng/ml to 58% for PSA levels of < 100 ng /ml. The majority (69%) of the patients with limited skeletal metastases had PSA levels of < 100 ng /ml while almost all patients (89%), with extensive skeletal involvement had PSA levels of < 100 ng/ml. Among those with limited metastatic disease, most (13/16; 81%) had at least one lesion in the pelvis or sacrum; the next most common sites were in the thoracic and lumbar spine (38%) [146]. A case of extensive bone metastases and normal PSA level has also been reported recently [147]. Other studies have shown different results. In the series of Wymenga et al. [148], the results of bone scans were related retrospectively to levels of serum PSA and alkaline phosphatase (ALP) in 363 patients with newly diagnosed prostate cancer. One hundred eleven patients had a positive bone scan. Bone scan was positive in 19 of 144 (13%) patients with a PSA level of < 20 ng/ml. On the other hand, the bone scan was positive in 51% of patients with a PSA level of < 20 ng/ml. A threshold level of 100 U/l for ALP gave a better accuracy. Therefore, elevated ALP values correlated better with an abnormal bone scan than did PSA levels; ALP levels of < 90 U/l indicated a 60% chance for the presence of bone metastases. The authors recommended newly diagnosed and untreated prostate cancer patients to undergo bone scintigraphy if there is bone pain, or if the ALP levels are < 90 U/l. Contrary to other recent reports that discourage the routine use of a bone scan when the serum PSA level is < 20 ng/ml, this study indicated a greater chance of a positive bone scan in patients with low PSA levels [148]. A total of 446 patients with newly diagnosed prostate cancer were also reviewed by Rydh et al. [149]. Among 214 patients with PSA levels < 20 ng/ml, nine showed a positive bone scans. The incidence of bone metastases was particularly low among patients with PSA levels < 20 ng/ml who have small and well-differentiated tumors[149].

Follow-up bone scintigraphy has been shown to be quite valuable in assessing the response to therapy

[141]. Fitzpatrick reported that the bone scan demonstrates changes in response to therapy before either acid or alkaline phosphatase, prostate size, or symptomatology demonstrate alterations [142].

Prognostic information can be obtained from the bone scan since patients with a positive scan at the time of diagnosis generally do not survive as long as those with negative scans [150].

PET has been investigated in the detection of prostatic- cancer bone metastases and is again promising. C-11-Acetate, a new tracer for the detection of prostate cancer with PET, was evaluated in 22 patients with prostate cancer who underwent PET imaging after intravenous administration of 20 mCi (740 MBq) of C-11-acetate. Eighteen of the 22 patients were also studied with F-18 FDG-PET. Standardized uptake values for each tumor were investigated for tracer activity 10–20 min after C-11-acetate administration and 40–60 min after F-18 FDG administration. Adenocarcinoma of the prostate showed a variable uptake of C-11-acetate with SUVs ranging from 3.27 – 9.87. In contrast, SUVs for F-18 FDG ranged from 1.97 – 6.34. Visually, C-11-acetate accumulation in the primary prostate tumors was positive in all patients, whereas F-18 FDG accumulation was positive in only 15 of 18 patients. Bone metastases in two patients were C-11-acetate avid [151]. In another study, F-18 FDG and L-methyl-C-11-methionine (C-11-methionine) PET were compared in patients with metastatic prostate cancer. The C-11-methionine PET identified significantly more lesions than F-18 FDG. The sensitivities of F-18 FDG-PET and C-11-methionine PET were 48 % and 72, respectively [152].

6.4.2.3
Metastases of Lung Cancer

Lung cancer metastasizes to the bone via three possible routes: lymphatic spread to the mediastinal nodes with direct extension to the bone; lymphatic spread to para-aortic nodes with subsequent direct extension to bone, and invasion of pulmonary veins; and then by transport of tumor through the arterial circulation to any part of the skeleton including bones of appendicular skeleton. The lesions are predominantly osteolytic, or mixed, although osteoblastic lesions can occur in the minority of cases, particularly with small cell and adenocarcinoma [13]. The detection of bone metastases is important in the management of patients with lung cancer because bone metastasis has a major impact on the choice of treatment modality and the prognosis [14].

There are controversies regarding the use of routine preoperative bone scanning in patients with lung cancer although knowledge of the metastases could save the patient from a major surgery and significant cost. Bone scanning is generally sensitive in detecting metastases of lung cancer although it has been shown to be false-negative not infrequently in metastases of the spine. A study of 110 patients with lung cancer compared bone scanning to PET for the detection of bone metastases. Using clinical and radiological correlation, or clinical evolution as the gold standard, the comparison of PET to bone scan demonstrated the following: a sensitivity 90 % for each; a specificity 98 % vs. 61 %; positive predictive value 90 % vs. 35 %; and negative predictive value 98 % vs. 96 % [153]. In a recent study, 54 patients with small cell lung cancer, or locally advanced non-small cell lung cancer, were prospectively examined with planar bone scan, SPECT of the vertebral column, and F-18 FDG-PET. Among 12 patients with vertebral metastases, planar bone scintigraphy was abnormal in six, while SPECT detected metastases in 11 and F-18 FDG-PET detected all. Accordingly, FGD-PET was the most accurate for screening for bone metastases (Fig. 6.37) and SPECT imaging improves the accuracy of vertebral metastases [154]. Park et al, studied the effects of abnormal bone scan findings on the prognosis of patients with lung cancer. The overall survival of patients with abnormal bone uptake was not significantly different from those without abnormal uptake. However, the patients with more than two abnormal bone uptakes had a significantly shorter survival than those with no abnormal uptake [155].

6.4.2.4
Metastases of Renal Cell Carcinoma

Renal cell carcinoma often presents with distant metastases with the most common sites being the lung, liver and bone [156]. Radiologically, the metastatic lesions are predominantly osteolytic and in some cases expansile. They are produced through: (1) lymphatic channels to para-aortic, hilar, paratracheal and/or mediastinal nodes with subsequent invasion of bone, (2) invasion of renal veins transporting tumor cells to the inferior vena cava, right atrium and then pulmonary vessels to be disseminated to bones [157 – 159].

As with many other tumors, bone scanning is currently considered a sensitive tool for detecting the bone metastases of primary renal cell carcinoma. Scintigraphically, the metastases are seen predominantly as foci of increased uptake, although cold lesions are common (Fig. 6.38) and found in approximately 8 % of metastatic lesions of this tumor. The utility of performing whole-body bone scintigraphy as part of a routine staging workup for patients with renal cell carcinoma is currently being debated. In patients with renal cell carcinoma several groups have proposed that bone scanning should be limited to those with bone pain or elevated ALP levels. However, the proportion of patients with the various disease stages in whom the diagnosis may be missed based on such indications is not currently clear. In addition, ALP as an indicator for the use

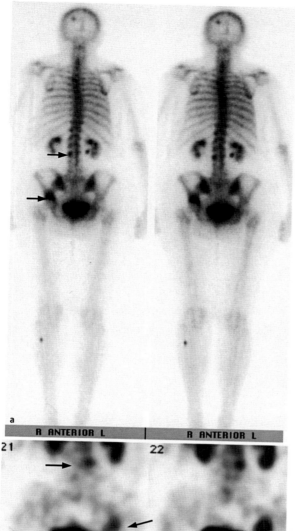

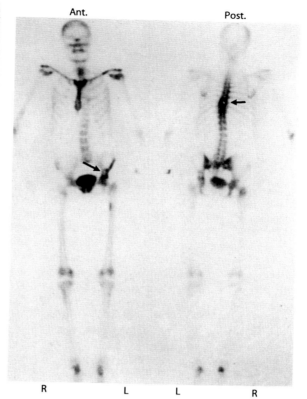

Fig. 6.38. Renal-cell carcinoma metastasis. There are multiple foci of increased and decreased uptake

Fig. 6.37a, b. a Whole body bone scan of a patient with non-squamous cell lung cancer showing bone metastases involving the skull, L-3 and right acetabular region. Coincidence SPECT using F18 FDG (**b**) was requested to further evaluate the nature of the L-3 vertebral lesion to permit the proper planning of radiation therapy. The L-3 lesion as well as the right acetabular lesion show intense uptake suggesting malignancy

bone scanning is controversial and the profile of renal cell carcinoma has changed in recent years because of early detection. The incidence of stage T1a disease with the tumor measuring 4 cm or less in diameter is increasing due to earlier diagnosis. Accordingly, the incidence of bone metastases is also increasingly seen [160–162] with longer follow-up periods. In general, the incidence of bone metastases in the early stages of the tumor is low and bone scan was even suggested to be emitted from mark up of patients with this tumor

[163]. A number of groups have recommended pre-operative bone scanning in renal cell carcinoma cases only when bone pain is present [164–166]; however, pain is not a reliable predictor of bone metastases. Others have reported that ALP is a better predictor of outcome than bone scans for renal cell carcinoma [166, 167]. In a study by Koga et al. [168], bone metastases were detected in 34 out of 205 patients (17%) at the time of diagnosis. Bone scans had 94% sensitivity and 86% specificity. Of the 124 patients with clinically localized, stages T1–2 N0 M0 disease bone metastases were found in six patients (5%), whereas 28 of 81 (35%) with locally advanced or metastatic disease had bone metastasis, including 12 (35%) who complained of bone pain. Accordingly, if a bone scan is omitted in patients who are free of bone pain, more than a half of those with bone metastasis could be missed [168].

Since the early detection of bone metastasis using bone scanning and surgical resection may improve survival, and also since bone scanning is helpful for localizing the site of biopsy, or surgical removal in such cases, it is recommended that a pre-operative bone scan is obtained. FDG-PET appears to have a potential role in accurately detecting the renal cell carcinoma metastases. In a recent study Tc-99m MDP bone and FDG-PET were compared in 18 patients with renal cell carcinoma [169]. Among 52 lesions, 40 were proven to be metastases and 12 were proven to be benign. FDG-PET accurately diagnosed the 40 malignant lesions while bone scanning accurately diagnosed only 31 of metastatic lesions.

6.4.2.5
Metastases of Thyroid Cancer

Bone scintigraphy is considered to lack sensitivity in detecting bone metastases from thyroid cancer due to the nature of such metastases as having no, or only a slight, osteosclerotic bone reaction. The anatomical distribution of bone metastases was reported by Schirrmeister [170] as follows: spine, 42%; skull, 2%; thorax, 16%; femur, 9%; pelvis, 26%; humerus and clavicle, 5%. The sensitivity of bone scanning was 64–85% and the specificity was 95–81%. The combination of bone scintigraphy and whole body iodine 131 scan was 100% sensitive in detecting metastatic bone disease [170]. In addition to I-131 and bone scintigraphy, Tl-201, Tc-99m MIBI and FDG-PET have a complementary role in identifying bone metastases of this tumor, particularly in those patients with negative bone and I-131 scans and elevated thyroglobulin levels since they can detect lesions not otherwise detected by a single modality [25, 171]. FDG-PET and thallium-201 were compared in a study of 32 patients with well-differentiated thyroid cancer in combination with I-131 with results in detecting metastases that are 94% concordant. Thus, a combination of I-131 and FDG-PET or Tl-201 was recommended as the method of choice for detecting metastatic lesions after total thyroidectomy [172].

6.4.2.6
Metastases of Other Tumors

Gynecological Tumors
Bone metastasis in cervical cancer is generally rare except in patients with a clinical suspicion of the metastatic disease. In a study of 38 patients with cervical cancer and suspicion of metastasis, 12 were confirmed as having metastasis and all were also detected by bone scanning (100% sensitivity) [173]. Currently, bone scanning is not routinely used pre-operatively but it is the investigation of choice for screening patients with symptoms suggestive of metastasis in all stage of the disease. Bone scanning also offers an additional advantage of reviewing the kidney size to look for ureteric involvement and subsequent hydronephrosis [172].

Lymphomas

The bone is affected in up to 20% of patients with Hodgkin's lymphoma and in up to 25% in those with non-Hodgkin's lymphoma. Furthermore, 3–5% of non-

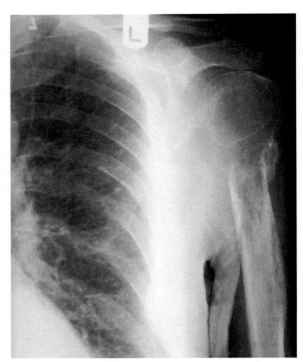

Fig. 6.39. Standard radiograph illustrating a primary bone lymphoma which appears as a destructive lesion in the neck of the left humerus

Hodgkin's lymphomas are primary tumors of bone (Fig. 6.39) [174–178] Routine bone scintigraphy, however, is of limited value in the clinical assessment of untreated patients with Hodgkin's disease [178]. On the other hand, scintigraphy has an important role in following up bone lymphomas and predicting the outcome after therapy. Recently a study reconfirmed the value of Ga-67 in evaluating the response to therapy in 44 patients with lymphoma and bone involvement and found it superior to CT, since 61% of successfully treated patients showed negative Ga-67 scans compared to 21% for negative CT findings [179].

Bone marrow involvement in non-Hodgkin's lymphoma, and in Hodgkin's disease, is of great therapeutic and prognostic significance. PET scanning may prove to be valuable in this regard. In a series of 50 patients, PET was compared to bone marrow biopsy. The latter is the gold standard for bone marrow involvement. The results for PET were: sensitivity 81%, specificity of 76%, positive predictive value of 62%, and negative predictive value of 90% [180].

Gastrointestinal Tumors

Gastrointestinal malignancies do not commonly metastasize to the bone although the frequency has increased in recent years due to the longer survival of patients. Gastric carcinoma is relatively common in the

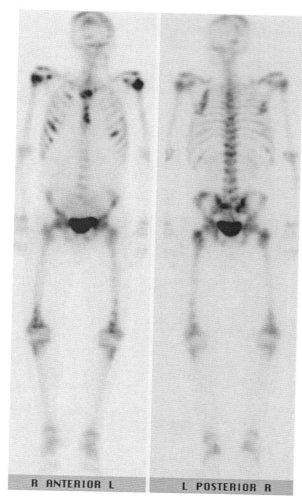

Fig. 6.40. A whole body bone scan of a 20-year-old male with gastric carcinoma metastasizing to bone

Asian population and the incidence of bone metastases could be as high as 45% among patients with stage III disease [181]. (Fig. 6.40). In such a group of patients with high pre-test probability of metastases, bone scanning may be considered routinely pre-operatively.

Nasopharyngeal Carcinoma

The routine use of bone scanning in detecting metastases is controversial although as many as 23% of newly diagnosed cases showed bone metastases [182]. SPECT bone scanning was found in a small series of patients to be more sensitive that CT scanning in assessing the skull base involvement by nasopharyngeal carcinoma [183].

Neuroblastoma

Howman-Giles found 29 out of 63 patients (46%) with neuroblastoma with bone metastases [114] including

nine symmetrical metastases. Bone scanning has been used to assess the metastatic disease of bone. I-123 MIBG has the advantage of showing both skeletal and extraskeletal tumor sites and has been suggested to replace bone scanning in detecting bony involvement by the tumor [184]. MIBG was found overall to be less sensitive than bone scanning in detecting bone metastases by some investigators [185]; however, in most investigators' experience the extent of metastatic bone and bone marrow lesions is defined most accurately by MIBG [186–188]. Hadj-Djiiani et al. reported 30 sites of metastases in eight patients with neuroblastoma imaged by both I-123 MIBG and bone scans, 12 were detected only by MIBG while seven were only seen by bone scan. Overall, however, MIBG identified more lesions than bone scanning. Interestingly the highest incidence of false-negatives on both modalities were histologically proven ganglioneuroblastoma [189]. Currently both modalities are commonly used routinely as they provide combined complementary information. Bone scanning provides relatively better resolution and accordingly better localization of the lesions, while MIBG may detect different lesions in bones as well as extraosseous lesions.

Kaposi's Sarcoma

Four forms of Kaposi's sarcoma are known. The chronic, or classic, form primarily affects men older than 50 years and is associated with a second malignancy, usually of the lymphoreticular or hematopoietic system. The second form, the lymphadenopathic from, predominantly affects young African children. The third form is the transplantation-associated. This affects less than 0.5% of patients who receive renal transplants, but has also been reported after other organ transplants and in association with immunosuppressive therapy. The fourth form of Kaposi's sarcoma is the HIV-related form, which affects young patients and may manifest clinically in any location.

Bone involvement has been reported in all four forms and develops during the more advanced stages of the disease. A patient who presents initially with Kaposi sarcoma of the bone invariably has extra skeletal tumors as well. Bone scanning, Tl-201 and Ga-67 are all used for the diagnosis and combined Ga-67 and Tl-201 can differentiate the tumor from others. The most common scintigraphic pattern is thallium positive and gallium negative images; however, this is not consistent, particularly in the presence of a concomitant infection [190–192].

Carcinoid Tumor

A recent retrospective study evaluated a group of patients with carcinoid tumors and bone metastases

[193]. All bone metastases occurred in 55 patients with mid-gut carcinoids. Plain radiography did not contribute to the diagnosis of bone metastases since it showed a sensitivity of 44 % while , MRI was the most sensitive (100 %). Bone scintigraphy showed a sensitivity of 90 % and octreotide scintigraphy 60 %. In nine patients, both octreotide and bone scintigraphy were performed and of 45 bone lesions, 22 (49 %) were visualized by both modalities, 13 (29 %) were visualized with octreotide scintigraphy but not with bone scintigraphy, and 10 (22 %) were visualized with bone scintigraphy but not with octreotide scintigraphy [193].

6.5
Follow-up of Malignant Bone Disease

Scintigraphy has a great value in assessing the response of metastatic bone disease to therapy [194]. Although several radiotracers including F-18 FDG (Fig. 6.46) are used for this purpose, bone scintigraphy is still a good modality for the follow-up of metastatic bone disease of many tumors. A favorable response is indicated when a decreasing number of scintigraphically observed lesions or decreasing activity is seen (Fig. 6.41) [195]. It may also show a decreasing activity in the primary extraosseous tumor if it shows tracer uptake initially such as neuroblastoma (Fig. 6.42). Patients with stable scans have survived up to twice as long as those with scintigraphic evidence of progressive bone disease [118]. Citrin et al. [195] found that 7 months were required for a bone scan to show a favorable response but only 4 months to show a progression of disease [195]. He therefore advocates a follow-up scan 3–6 months after instituting therapy. Progression is confirmed if the number of lesions increases, or the activity of the known lesions dramatically increases (Fig. 6.43). Increasing activity, however, must be applied with great caution because of the potential pitfall of the flare effect, which causes transient increases of activity of the

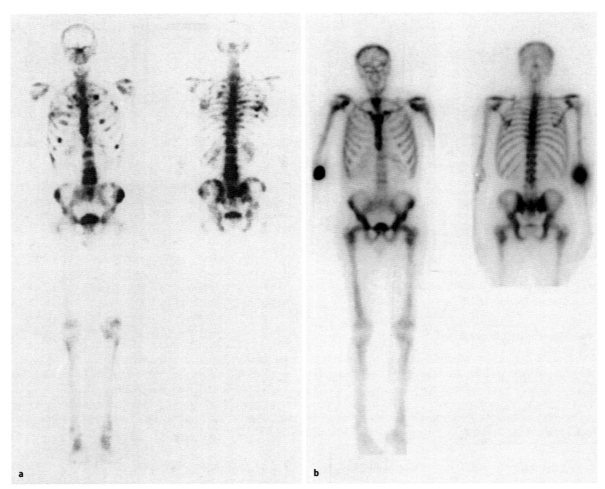

a   b

Fig. 6.41. a Tc99m MDP bone scan of a patient with prostatic carcinoma illustrating widespread bone metastases. **b** Follow-up scan illustrating improving in response to hormonal therapy for 1 year

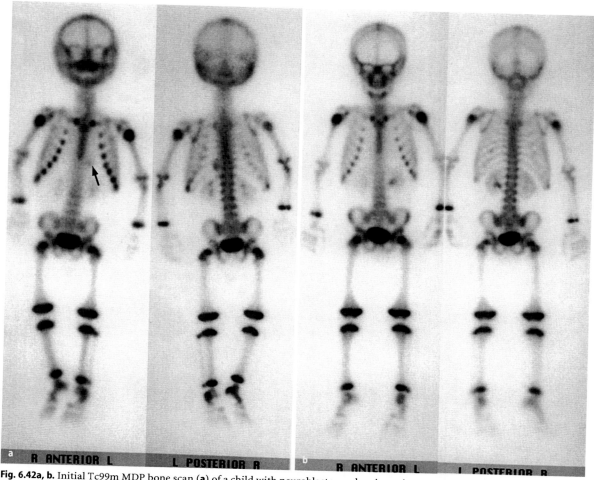

Fig. 6.42a, b. Initial Tc99m MDP bone scan (**a**) of a child with neuroblastoma showing primary tumor uptake (*arrow*). Follow-up scan (**b**) showing improvement of the primary tumor uptake after therapy

pre-existing lesions, following the institution of effective therapy. This is presumably due to reactive bone formation due to the healing accompanying the therapy [196]. PET can readily solve the problem of flare, when available, by showing a decreasing activity in the post-therapy scan without waiting 3 months, or some-times longer, to obtain the same result from bone scintigraphy delaying possible change in treatment strategies. Tl-201, Tc99m MIBI and particularly PET imaging are also useful in assessing the response to therapy by primary bone tumors (Figs. 6.44).

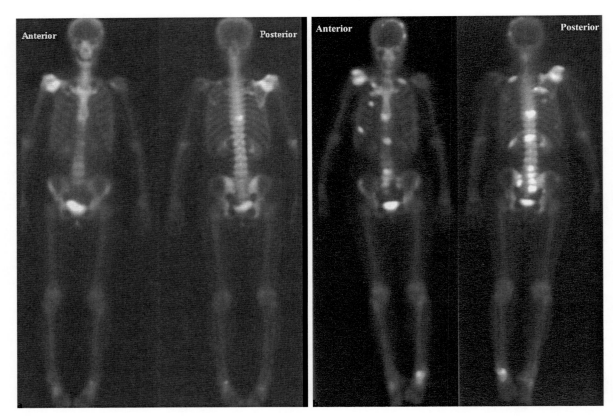

Fig. 6.43a, b. Initial (**a**) and follow-up (**b**) bone scans of a patient with breast cancer showing progressive metastatic bone disease

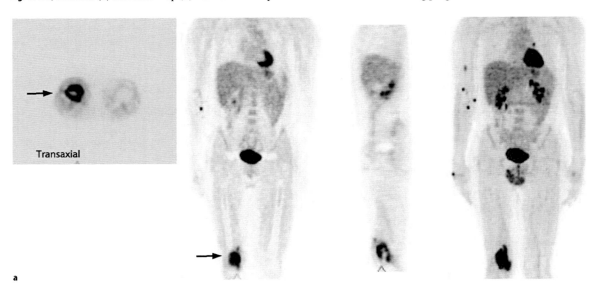

Fig. 6.44a, b. F-18-FDG PET study of a patient with osteogenic sarcoma of the distal right femur showing intense increased uptake

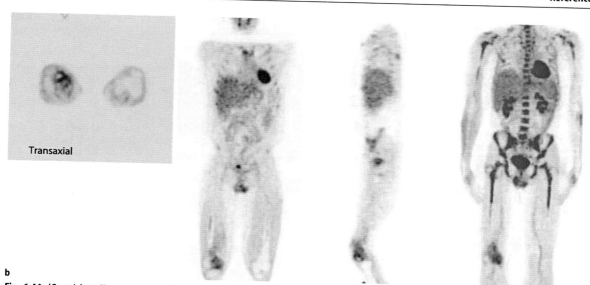

b

Fig. 6.44. (Cont.) b Follow-up scan obtained after chemotherapy showing a significant decrease of the initial uptake indicating good response to therapy

References

1. Mungo DV, Zhang X, O'Keefe RJ, Rosier RN, Puzas JE, Schwarz EM (2002) COX-1 and COX-2 expression in osteoid osteomas. J Orthop Res 20:159–162
2. Kawaguchi Y, Hasegawa T, Oka S, Sato C, Arima N, Norimatsu H (2001) Mechanism of intramedullary high intensity area on T2-weighted magnetic resonance imaging in osteoid osteoma: a possible role of COX-2 expression. Pathol Int 51:933–937
3. Dablin DC, Conventry MB (1967) Osteogenic sarcoma: a study of 600 cases. J Bone Joint Surg (Am) 49:101–110
4. Link NP, Eiber F (1997) Osteosarcoma. In: Pizzo PA, Poplack DG (eds) Principles and practice of pediatric oncology, 3rd edn. Lippincott-Raven, Philadelphia, pp 889–920
5. Uribe-Botero G, Russel W, Sutow W et al (1997) Primary osteosarcoma of bone: A clinicopathologic investigation of 243 cases, with necropsy studies in 54. Am J Clin Pathol 67:427–435
6. Parham DM, Pratt CB, Parvey LS et al (1985) Childhood multifocal osteosarcoma: clinicopathologic and radiologic correlates. Cancer 55:2653–2658
7. Gunawardena S, Chintagumpala M, Trautwein L et al (1999) Multifocal osteosarcoma: an unusual presentation. J Pediatr Hematol Oncol 21:58–62
8. Elhasid R, Vlodavsky E, Nachtigal A, Keidar Z, Postovsky S, Ben Arush M (2001) Pediatric tumors. J Clin Oncol 19:276–278
9. McCarthy EF (1997) Histopathologic correlates of a positive bone scan. Semin Nucl Med 27:309–320
10. Huvos AG (1991) Bone tumors; diagnosis, treatment and prognosis, 2nd edn. Saunders, Philadelphia
11. Dorland's illustrated medical dictionary, 27th edn. (1988) Saunders, Philadelphia
12. Batson OV (1995) The function of the vertebral veins and their role in the spread of metastases. Clin Orthop Relat Res 312:4–9
13. Resnick D, Niwayama K (1998) Skeletal metastases. In: Resnick D, Niwayama K (eds) Diagnosis of bone and joint disorders, 2nd edn. Saunders, Philadelphia, pp 3945–4010
14. Hanagiri T, Kodate M, Nagashima A, Sugaya M, Dobashi K, Ono M, Yasumoto K (2000) Bone metastasis after a resection of stage I and II primary lung cancer. Lung Cancer 27:199–204
15. Resnick D, Niwayama K, Galasko CSD (1981) Bone metastasis studied in experimental animal. Clin Orthop Relat Res 155:269
16. Galasko CSD (1982) Mechanisms of lytic and blastic metastatic disease of bone. Clin Orthop Relat Res 20:20–27
17. Tondevold E, Eliasen P (1982) Blood flow rates in canine cortical and cancellous bone measured with Tc 99m, labeled human albumin microspheres. Acta Orthop Scand 53:7–11
18. Esther RJ, Bos GD (2000) Management of metastatic disease of other bones. Orthop Clin North Am 31:647–759
19. Gates GF (1998) SPECT bone scanning of the spine. Semin Nucl Med 28:78–94
20. Garrett IR (1993) Bone destruction in cancer. Semin Oncol 20:4–9
21. Arrambide K, Toto RD (1993) Tumor lysis syndrome. Semin Nephrol 13:273
22. Jan de Beur SM, Streeten EA, Civelek AC, McCarthy EF, Uribe L, Marx SJ, Onobrakpeya O, Raisz LG (2002) Localisation of mesenchymal tumors by somatostatin receptor imaging. Lancet 359:761–763
23. Ell PJ, Dixon HJ, Abdullah AZ (1980) Unusual spread of juxtacortical osteosarcoma. J Nucl Med 21:190–191
24. Elgazzar AH, Malki AA, Abdel-Dayem HM, Sahweil A, Razzak S, Jahan S, Elsayed M, Omar YT (1989) Role of thallium 201 in the diagnosis of solitary bone lesions. Nucl Med Commun 10:477–485
25. Elgazzar AH, Fernendaz-Ulloa M, Silberstein EB (1993) Thallium 201 as a tumor imaging agent: current status and future consideration. Nucl Med Commun 14:96–103
26. Van der Wall H, Murray IP, Huckstep RL, Philips RL (1993) The role of thallium scintigraphy in excluding malignancy in bone. Clin Nucl Med 18:551–557
27. Caner B, Kitapcl M, Unlu M et al (1992) Technetium 99m MIBI uptake in benign and malignant bone lesions: a comparative study with technetium 99m MDP. J Nucl Med 33:319–324

28. Pneumaticos SG, Chatziioannou SN, Moore WH, Johnson M (2001) The role of radionuclides in primary musculoskeletal tumors beyond the bone scan. Crit Rev Oncol Hematol 37:217–226

29. Sumiya H, Taki J, Higuchi T, Tonami N (2001) Nuclear imaging of bone tumors: thallium-201 scintigraphy. Semin Musculoskel Radiol 5:177–182

30. Schulte M, Brecht-Krauss D, Werner M et al (2000) Evaluation of neoadjuvant therapy response of osteogenic sarcoma using FDG PET. J Nucl Med 40:1637–1643

31. Franzius C, Sciuk J, Brinkschmidt C, Jurgens H, Schober O (2000) Evaluation of chemotherapy response in primary bone tumors with F-18 FDG positron emission. Clin Nucl Med 25:874–878

32. Franzius C, Sciuk J, Daldrup-Link HE, Jurgens H, Schober O (2000) FDG-PET for detection of osseous metastases from malignant primary bone tumors: comparison with bone scintigraphy. Eur J Nucl Med 27:1305–1311

33. Cook GJ, Fogelman I (2001) The role of nuclear medicine in monitoring treatment in skeletal malignancy. Semin Nucl Med 31:206–211

34. Aoki J, Watanabe H, Shinozaki T, Takagishi K, Ishijima H, Oya N, Sato T, Inoue T, Endo K (2001) FDG PET of primary benign and malignant bone tumors: standardized uptake value in 52 lesions. Radiology 219:774–777

35. Dimitrakopoulou-Strauss A, Heichel TO, Lehner B, Bernd L, Ewerbeck V, Burger C, Strauss LG (2001) Quantitative evaluation of skeletal tumors with dynamic FDG PET: SUV in comparison to Patlak analysis. Eur J Nucl Med 28:704–710

36. Smith FW, Gilday DL (1980) Scintigraphic appearance of osteoid osteoma. Radiology 137:191–195

37. Miller SL, Hoffer FA (2001) Malignant and benign bone tumors. Radiol Clin North Am 39:673–699

38. Buhler M, Binkert C, Exner GU (2001) Osteoid osteoma: technique of computed tomography-controlled percutaneous resection using standard equipment available in most orthopaedic operating rooms. Arch Orthop Trauma Surg 121:458–461

39. Moser RP Jr, Masewell JF (1987) An approach to primary bone tumors. Radiol Clin North Am 25:1049–1093

40. Woerthler K, Linder N, Gosheger G, Brinkschmidt C, Heindel W (2000) MR imaging of tumor-related complications. Eur Radiol 10:832–840

41. Brian WE, Mirra JM, Luck JV Jr (1999) Benign and malignant tumors of bone and joint: their anatomical and theoretical basis with an emphasis on radiology, pathology and clinical biology II. Juxtacortical cartilage tumors. Skeletal Radiol 28:1–20

42. Moody EB, Classman SB, Hansen AV, Lawrence SK, Delbeke D (1992) Nuclear medicine case of the day. AJR 158:1382–1386

43. Siddiqui AR, Ellis JH (1982) „Cold spots" on bone scan at the site of primary osteosarcoma. Eur J Nucl Med 7:480–481

44. Rossleigh MA, Smith J, Yeh SD, Huvos AG (1987) Case reports: a photopenic lesion in osteosarcoma. Br J Radiol 60:497–499

45. Bloem JL, Taminiau AHM, Eulderink F, Hermans J, Pauwels EKJ (1988) Radiologic staging of primary bone sarcoma: MR imaging, scintigraphy, angiography, and CT correlated with pathologic examination. Radiology 169:805–810

46. McKillop JH, Etcubanas E, Goris ML (1981) The indications for and limitations of bone scintigraphy in osteogenic sarcoma. Cancer 48:1133–1138

47. Franzius C, Daldrup-Link HE, Wagner-Bohn A, Sciuk J, Heindel WL, Jurgens H, Schober O (2002) FDG-PET for detection of recurrences from malignant primary bone tumors: comparison with conventional imaging. Ann Oncol 13:157–160

48. Abdel-Dayem HM (1997) The role of nuclear medicine in primary bone and soft tissue tumors. Semin Nucl Med 27:355–363

49. Burak Z, Ersoy O, Moretti JL, Erinc R, Ozcan Z, Dirlik A, Sabah D, Basdemir G (2001) The role of 99mTc-MIBI scintigraphy in the assessment of MDR1 overexpression in patients with musculoskeletal sarcomas: comparison with therapy response. Eur J Nucl Med 28:1341–1350

50. Gorlick R, Liao AC, Antonescu C, Huvos AG, Healey JH, Sowers R, Daras M, Calleja E, Wexler LH, Panicek D, Meyers PA, Yeh SD, Larson SM (2001) Lack of correlation of functional scintigraphy with (99m)technetium-methoxyisobutylisonitrile with histological necrosis following induction chemotherapy or measures of P-glycoprotein expression in high-grade osteosarcoma. Clin Cancer Res 7:3065–3070

51. Kaste SC, Billips C, Tan M, Meyer WH, Parham DM, Rao BN, Pratt CB, Fletcher BD (2001) Thallium bone imaging as an indicator of response and outcome in nonmetastatic primary extremity osteosarcoma. Pediatr Radiol 31:251–256

52. Franzius F, Bielack S, Flege S, Sciuk J, Heribert Jürgens H, Schober O (2002) Prognostic significance of ^{18}F-FDG and ^{99}Tc-mehylene diphosphonate uptake in primary osteosarcoma. J Nucl Med 43:1012–1017

53. Schulte M, Brecht-Krauss D, Heymer B et al (2000) Grading of tumors and tumorlike lesions of bone: evaluation by FDG PET. J Nucl Med 41:1695–1701

54. Kile AC, Nieweg OE, Hoekstra HJ, van Horn JR, Koops HS, Vaalburg W (1998) Fluorine-18-fluorodeoxyglucose assessment of glucose metabolism in bone tumors. J Nucl Med 39:810–815

55. Mariette X, Khalifa P, Ravaud P et al (1992) Bone densitometry in patients with multiple myeloma. Am J Med 93:595

56. Mariette X, Bergot C, Ravaud P et al (1995) Evolution of bone densitometry in patients with myeloma treated with conventional or intensive therapy. Cancer 76:1559

57. Murthy NJ, Rao H, Friedman AS (2000) Positive findings on bone scan in multiple myeloma. South Med J 93:1028–1029

58. Waxman AD, Steimsen JK, Levine AM et al (1981) Radiographic and radionuclide imaging in multiple myeloma: the role of gallium scintigraphy. Concise communication. J Nucl Med 22:232–236

59. Silberstein EB, McAfee JG, Spasoff AP (1998) Diagnostic patterns in Nuclear Medicine. Soc Nucl Med, Reston, pp 223–230

60. Watanabe N, Shimizu M, Kageyama M, Tanimura K, Kinuya S, Shuke N, Yokoyama K, Tonami N, Watanabe A, Seto H, Goodwin DA(1999) Multiple myeloma evaluated withTl-201 scintigraphy compared with bone scintigraphy. J Nucl Med 40:1138–1142

61. Alexandrakis MG, Kyriakou DS, Passam F, Koukouraki S, Karkavitsas N (2001) Value of Tc-99m sestamibi scintigraphy in the detection of bone lesions in multiple myeloma: comparison with Tc-99m methylene diphosphonate. Ann Hematol 80:349–353

62. Kusumoto S, Jinnai I, Itoh K et al (1997) Magnetic resonance imaging patterns in patients with multiple myeloma. Br J Hematol 99:649–655

63. Van de Berg BC, Lecouvet FE, Michaux L et al (1996) Stage I multiple myeloma: value of MR imaging of bone marrow in the determination of prognosis. Radiology 201:243–246

64. Kyle RA, Schreiman J, McLeod R (1985) Computed tomog-

raphy in diagnosis of multiple myeloma and its variants. Arch Intern Med 145:1451–1460

65. Vagler JB, Murphy WA (1988) Bone marrow imaging: state of the art. Radiology 168:676–686

66. Durie BG, Waxman AD, D'Angelo A, Williams CM (2002) Whole body f-18 FDG PET identifies high risk myeloma. J Nucl Med 43:1457–1463

67. Franzius C, Schulte M, Hillmann A, Winkelmann W, Jurgens H, Bockisch A, Schober O (2001) Clinical value of positron emission tomography (PET) in the diagnosis of bone and soft tissue tumors. 3rd interdisciplinary consensus conference „PET in Oncology": results of the Bone and Soft Tissue Study Group. Chirurg 72:1071–1077

68. Hung GU, Tan TS, Kao CH, Wang SJ (2000) Multiple skeletal metastases of Ewing's sarcoma demonstrated on FDG-PET and compared with bone and gallium scans. Kaohsiung J Med Sci 16:315–318

69. Connolly LP, Drubach LA, Ted Treves S (2002) Applications of nuclear medicine in pediatric oncology. Clin Nucl Med 27:117–125

70. Bar-Sever Z, Cohen IJ, Connolly LP, Horev G, Perri T, Treves T, Hardoff R (2000) Tc-99m MIBI to evaluate children with Ewing's sarcoma. Clin Nucl Med 25:410–413

71. Rybak LD, Rosenthal DI (2001) Radiological imaging for the diagnosis of bone metastases. Quart J Nucl Med 45:53–64

72. Ron IG, Striecker A, Lerman H, Bar-Am A, Frisch B (1999) Bone scan and bone biopsy in the detection of skeletal metastases. Oncol Rep 6:185–188

73. Steinborn MM, Heuck AF, Tiling R, Bruegel M, Gauger L, Reiser MF (1999) Whole-body bone marrow MRI in patients with metastatic disease to the skeletal system. J Comput Assist Tomogr 23:123–129

74. Taoka T, Mayr NA, Lee HJ, Yuh WT, Simonson TM, Rezai K, Berbaum KS (2001) Factors influencing visualization of vertebral metastases on MR imaging versus bone scintigraphy. Am J Roentgenol 176:1525–1530

75. Daldrup-Link HE, Franzius C, Link TM, Laukamp D, Sciuk J, Jurgens H, Schober O, Rummeny EJ (2001) Whole-body MR imaging for detection of bone metastases in children and young adults: comparison with skeletal scintigraphy and FDG PET. AJR 177:229–236

76. Kao CH, Hsieh JF, Tsai SC, Ho YJ, Yen RF (2000) Comparison and discrepancy of 18F-2-deoxyglucose positron emission tomography and Tc-99m MDP bone scan to detect bone metastases. Anticancer Res 20:2189–2192

77. Moog F, Kotzerke J, Reske SN (1999) FDG PET can replace bone scintigraphy in primary staging of malignant lymphoma. J Nucl Med 40:1407–1413

78. Schirrmeister H, Guhlmann A, Elsner K, Kotzerke J, Glatting G, Rentschler M, Neumaier B, Trager H, Nussle K, Reske SN (1999) Sensitivity in detecting osseous lesions depends on anatomic localization: planar bone scintigraphy versus F18 PET. J Nucl Med 40:1623–1629

79. Asthana S, Deo SV, Shukla NK, Raina V (2001) Carcinoma breast metastatic to the hand and the foot. Austr Radiol 45:380–382

80. Al-Mulhim F, Ibrahim EM, El-Hassan AY, Moharram HM (1995) Magnetic resonance imaging of tuberculous spondylitis. Spine 20:2287–2292

81. Elgazzar AH, Abdel-Dayem HM, Shible O (1991) Brucellosis simulating metastases on Tc99m MDP bone scan. Clin Nucl Med 16:162–164

82. Caglar M, Naldoken S (2000) Multiple brown tumors simulating bone metastases: a case of parathyroid adenoma coexisting with papillary carcinoma of the thyroid. Clin Nucl Med 25:772–774

83. Hadi A, Al-Nahhas A, Vivian G, Hickling P (2002) Tc-99m MDP and Tc-99m MIBI in the assessment of spondyloart-

hritis presenting as bone metastasis before treatment with infliximab. Clin Nucl Med 27:297–298

84. Reginato AJ, Falasca GF, Pappu R, McKnight B, Agha A (1999) Musculoskeletal manifestations of osteomalacia: report of 26 cases and literature review. Semin Arthritis Rheum 28:287–304

85. Puig S, Staudenherz A,Steiner B, Eisenhuber E, Leitha T (1998) Differential diagnosis of atypically located single or bouble spots in whole bone scanning. J Nucl Med 39:1263–1266

86. Reinartz P, Schaffeldt J, Sabri O, Zimny M, Nowak B, Ostwald E, Cremerius U, Buell U (2000) Benign versus malignant osseous lesions in the lumbar vertebrae: differentiation by means of bone SPET. Eur J Nucl Med 27:721–726

87. Shirazi RH, Rayudu GVS, Fordham EW (1974) Review of solitary 18-F bone scan lesions. Radiology 112:369–372

88. Corcoran RJ, Thrall JH, Kyle RW, Kaminski RJ, Johnson MC (1976) Solitary abnormalities in bone scans of patients with extraosseous malignancies. Radiology 121:663–667

89. Rappaport AH, Hoffer PB, Genant HK (1978) Unifocal bone findings by scintigraphy. Clinical significance in patients with known primary cancer. West J Med 129:188–192

90. Brown ML (1983) Significance of solitary lesion in pediatric bone scanning: concise communication. J Nucl Med 24:114–115

91. Tumeh SS, Beadle G, Kaplan WD (1985) Clinical significance of solitary bone lesions in patients with extraskeletal malignancies. J Nucl Med 26:1140–1143

92. Matsumoto K (1987) Bone metastasis from renal cell carcinoma. Gan To Kagaku Ryoho 14:1710–1716

93. Kwai AH, Stomper PC, Kaplan WD (1988) Clinical significance of isolated sternal lesions in patients with breast cancer. J Nucl Med 29:324–328

94. Boxer DL, Todd CE, Coleman R, Fogelman I (1989) Bone secondaries in breast cancer: the solitary metastases. J Nucl Med 30:1318–1320

95. Brown ML (1989) The role of radionuclides in the patient with osteogenic sarcoma. Semin Roentgenol 24:185–192

96. Coakley FV, Jones AR, Finlay DB, Belton IP (1995) The etiology and distinguishing features of solitary spinal hot spots on planar bone scans. Clin Radiol 50:327–330

97. Baxter AD, Coakley FV, Finlay DB, West C (1995) The etiology of solitary hot spots in ribs on planar bone scans. Nucl Med Commun 16:834–837

98. Hashmi R, Uetani M, Ogawa Y, Aziz A (1999) Clinical significance of a solitary hot spot in the skull. Nucl Med Commun 20:703–710

99. Tomoda Y, Ishino Y, Nakata H (2001) Assessmenet of solitary hot spots of bone scintigraphy in patients with extraskeletal malignancies. Jpn J Nucl Med 38:721–726

100. Aglar M, Ceylan E (2001) Isolated carpal bone metastases from bronchogenic cancer evident on bone scintigraphy. Clin Nucl Med 26:352–353

101. Veluvolu P, Collier BD, Isitman AT (1984) Scintigraphic skeletal doughnut sign due to giant cell tumor of the fibula. Clin Nucl Med 9:631–634

102. Greenspan A, Stadalnik RC (1995) Bone island: scintigraphic findings and their clinical applications. Canadian Assoc Radiol J 46:368–379

103. Sundaram M (1999) Magnetic resonance imaging for solitary lesions of bone: when, why, how useful? J Orthop Sci 4:384–396

104. Dimitrakopoulou-Strauss A, Strauss LG, Heichel T, Wu H, Burger C, Bernd L, Ewerbeck V (2002) The role of quantitative (18)F-FDG PET studies for the differentiation of malignant and benign bone lesions. J Nucl Med 43:510–518

105. Goris ML, Basso LV, Etcublanaas E (1980) Photopenic lesions in bone scintigraphy. Clin Nucl Med 5:299–301
106. Han JK, Shih WJ, Stipp V, Magoun S (1999) Normal variants of a photon-deficient area in the lower sternum demonstrated by bone SPECT. Clin Nucl Med 24:248–251
107. Sy WM, Westring DW, Weinberger G (1975) Cold lesions on bone imaging. J Nucl Med 16:1013–1016
108. Galasko CSB (1980) Mechanism of uptake of bone imaging isotopes by skeletal metastases. Clin Nucl Med 12:565
109. Pollen JJ, Witztum KF, Ashburn WL (1984) The flare phenomenon on radionuclide bone scan in metastatic prostate cancer. AJR 142:773
110. Fossa SD, Heilo A, Lindegaard M et al (1983) Clinical significance of routine follow up examination in patients with metastatic cancer of the prostate under hormone treatment. Eur J Urol 9:262–266
111. Koizumi M, Matsumoto S, Takahashi S, Yamashita T, Ogata E (1999) Bone metabolic markers in the evaluation of bone scan flare phenomenon in bone metastases of breast cancer. Clin Nucl Med 24:15–20
112. Nobuaki M, Hiroshi Y, Hidetoshi O, Noboru I, Tomio E, Keigo (1999) Fluorodeoxyglucose positron emission tomography scan of prostate cancer bone metastases with flare reaction after endocrine therapy. Am J Urol 16:608–609
113. Fukuda T, Inoue Y, Ochi H et al (1982) Abnormally high diffuse activity on bone scintigram: the importance of exposure time for its recognition. Eur J Nucl Med 7:275–277
114. Howman-Giles RB, Gilday DL, Ash J (1979): Radionuclide skeletal survey in neuroblastoma. Radiology 131:497–502
115. Reddy MP, Floresca J, Juweid M, Graham MM (2002) Unusual bilateral symmetrical osteolytic metastases visualized by bone scintigraphy. Clin Nucl Med 27:299–301
116. Clark DG, Painter RW, Sziklas JJ (1978) Indications for bone scans in preoperative evaluation of breast cancer. Am J Surg 135:667–670
117. Lee YN (1981) Bone scanning in patients with early breast carcinoma: should it be a routine staging procedure? Cancer 47:486–495
118. Baker RR (1978) Preoperative assessment of the patient with breast cancer. Surg Clin North Am 58:681–691
119. Fogelman I, McKillop JH (1991) The bone scan in metastatic disease. In: Rubess RD, Fogelman I (eds) Bone metastases: diagnosis and treatment. Springer, Berlin Heidelberg New York, pp 31–61
120. O'Connell MJ, Wahner HW, Ahmann DL et al (1978) Value of preoperative radionuclide bone scan in suspected primary breast carcinoma. Mayo Clin Proc 53:221–226
121. Elgazzar AH, Omar A, Higazi E, Abdel-Dayem HM, Omar YT (1990) Reevaluation of bone scanning in breast cancer. Eur J Nucl Med 16:S63
122. Curigliano G, Ferretti G, Colleoni M, Marrocco E, Peruzzotti G, De Cicco C, Paganelli G, Goldhirsch A (2001) Bone scan had no role in the staging of 765 consecutive operable T(1–2)N(0–1) breast cancer patients without skeletal symptoms (letter). Ann Oncol 12:724–725
123. Samant R, Ganguly P (1999) Staging investigations in patients with breast cancer: the role of bone scans and liver imaging. Arch Surg 134:551–553
124. Charkes ND, Malmud LS, Caswell T et al (1975) Preoperative bone scans. JAMA 233:516–518
125. Shutte H (1979) The influence of bone pain of the results of bone scans. Cancer 34:2039–2043
126. Whitlock JP, Evans AJ, Jackson L, Chan SY, Robertson JF (2001) Imaging of metastatic breast cancer: distribution and radiological assessment at presentation. Clin Oncol (R Coll Radiol) 13:181–188
127. Massie JD (1984) Bone scanning and metastatic disease. Proceedings of 35th annual meeting, South Eastern Chapter, Society of Nuclear Medicine, pp V1-V20
128. Smith TJ, Davidson NE, Schapira DV, Grunfeld E, Muss GE, Vogel VG III, Somerfield MR, for the American Society of Clinical Oncology Breast Cancer Surveillance Expert Panel (1999) American Society of Clinical Oncology 1998 update of recommended breast cancer surveillance guidelines. J Clin Oncol 17:1080–1082
129. Jacobson AF, Shapiro CL, Van den Abbeele AD, Kaplan WD (2001) Prognostic significance of the number of bone scan abnormalities at the time of initial bone metastatic recurrence in breast carcinoma. Cancer 91:17–24
130. Fogelman I, Coleman R (1988) The bone scan and breast cancer. In: Freeman LM, Weissman HS (eds) Nuclear medicine annual. Raven, New York, pp 1–38
131. Jacobson Af, Shapiro CL, Kaplan WD (1993) Bone metastases in patients with breast cancer: significance of scintigraphic patterns at presentation and follow-up. J Nucl Med 34:74P9 (abstract)
132. Yamashita K, Ueda T, Komatsubara Y et al (1991) Breast cancer with bone-only metastases visceral metastases-free rate in relation to anatomic distribution of bone metastasis. Cancer 68:634–637
133. Coleman RE, Smith P, Rubens RD (1998) Clinical course and prognostic factors following bone recurrence from breast cancer. Br J Cancer 77:336–340
134. Janicek MJ, Shaffer K (1995) Scintigraphic and radiographic patterns of skeletal metastases in breast cancer: value of sequential imaging in predicting outcome. Skeletal Radiol 24:597–600
135. Vogel CL, Schoenfelder J, Shemano I et al (1995) Worsening bone scan in the evaluation of antitumor response during hormonal therapy of breast cancer. J Clin Oncol 13:1123–1128
136. Nishimura R, Nagao K, Miyayama H, Yasunaga T, Asao C, Matsuda M, Baba K, Matsuoka Y, Yamashita H, Fukuda M (1999) Diagnostic problems of evaluating vertebral metastasis from breast carcinoma with a higher degree of malignancy. Cancer 85:1782–1788
137. Altehoefer C, Ghanem N, Hogerle S, Moser E, Langer M (2001) Comparative detectability of bone metastases and impact on therapy of magnetic resonance imaging and bone scintigraphy in patients with breast cancer. Eur J Radiol 40:16–23
138. Cook GJ, Fogelman I (1999) Skeletal metastases from breast cancer: imaging with nuclear medicine. Semin Nucl Med 29:69–79
139. Ohta M, Tokuda Y, Suzuki Y, Kubota M, Makuuchi H, Tajima T, Nasu S, Suzuki Y, Yasuda S, Shohtsu A (2001) Whole body PET for the evaluation of bony metastases in patients with breast cancer: comparison with 99Tcm-MDP bone scintigraphy. Nucl Med Commun 22:875–879
140. Schirrmeister H, Guhlmann A, Kotzerke J, Santjohanser C, Kuhn T, Kreienberg R, Messer P, Nussle K, Elsner K, Glatting G, Trager H, Neumaier B, Diederichs C, Reske SN (1999) Early detection and accurate description of extent of metastatic bone disease in breast cancer with fluoride ion and positron emission tomography. J Clin Oncol 17:2381–2389
141. Pollen JJ, Gerber K, Ashburn WL et al (1981) The value of nuclear bone imaging in advanced prostate cancer. J Urol 125:222–223
142. Fitzpatrick JM, Constable AR, Sherwood T et al (1978) Serial bone scanning: the assessment of treatment response in carcinoma of the prostate. Br J Urol 50:555–561
143. Spiers AS, Deal DR, Kasimis BS et al (1982) Evaluation of the bones and bone marrow in patients with metastatic

carcinoma of the prostate: radiologic, cytologic and cytogenetic findings. J Med 13:303–307

144. McGregor B, Tulloch AG, Quinlan MF et al (1978) The role in bone scanning in the assessment of prostatic carcinoma. Br J Urol 50:178–181

145. O'Donoghue, EP, Constable AR, Sherwood T et al (1978) Bone scanning and plasma phosphatases in carcinoma of the prostate. Br J Urol 50:172–177

146. Jacobson AF (2000) Association of prostate-specific antigen levels and patterns of benign and malignant uptake detected. On bone scintigraphy in patients with newly diagnosed prostate carcinoma. Nucl Med Commun 21:617–622

147. Yuksel M, Cermik TF, Kaya M, Salan A, Ustun F, Salihoglu YS, Yigitbasi ON, Berkarda S (2001) Extensive bone metastases in a patient with prostatic adenocarcinoma and normal serum prostate-specific antigen and prostatic acid phosphatase. Clin Nucl Med 26:962

148. Wymenga LF, Boomsma JH, Groenier K, Piers DA, Mensink HJ (2001) Routine bone scans in patients with prostate cancer related to serum prostate-specific antigen and alkaline phosphatase. BJU Int 88:226–230

149. Rydh A, Tomic R, Tavelin B, Hietala SO, Damber JE (1999) Predictive value of prostate-specific antigen, tumour stage and tumour grade for the outcome of bone scintigraphy in patients with newly diagnosed prostate cancer. Scand J Urol Nephrol 33:89–93

150. Lund F, Smith PH, Suciu S et al (1984) Do bone scans predict prognosis in prostatic cancer? A report of the EORTC protocol 30762. Br J Urol 56:58–63

151. Oyama N, Akino H, Kanamaru H, Suzuki Y, Muramoto S, Yonekura Y, Sadato N, Yamamoto K, Okada K (2002) 11C-acetate PET imaging of prostate cancer. J Nucl Med 43:181–186

152. Nunez R, Macapinlac HA, Yeung HW, Akhurst T, Cai S, Osman I, Gonen M, Riedel E, Scher HI, Larson SM (2002) Combined 18F-FDG and 11C-methionine PET scans in patients with newly progressive metastatic prostate cancer. J Nucl Med 43:46–55

153. Bury T, Bareeto A, Daenen F, Barthelemy N, Ghaye B, Rigo P (1998) Fluorine-18 deoxyglucose positron tomography for the detection of bone metastases in patients with non-small cell lung cancer. Eur J Nucl Med 25:1244–1247

154. Schirrmeister H, Glatting G, Hetzel J, Nussle K, Arslandemir C, Buck AK, Dziuk K, Gabelmann A, Reske SN, Hetzel M (2001) Prospective evaluation of the clinical value of planar bone scans, SPECT, and (18)F-labeled NaF PET in newly diagnosed lung cancer. J Nucl Med 42:1800–1804

155. Park JY, Kim KY, Lee J, Kam S, Son JW, Kim CH, Jung TH (2000) Impact of abnormal uptakes in bone scan on the prognosis of patients with lung cancer. Lung Cancer 28:55–62

156. Saitoh H (1981) Distant metastasis of renal adenocarcinoma. Cancer 48:1487

157. Galsko CSB (1980) Mechanism of uptake of bone imaging isotopes by skeletal metastases. Clin Nucl Med 12:565

158. Fogelman I, McKillop JH (1991) The bone scan in metastatic disease. In: Rubess RD, Fogelman I (eds) Bone metastases: diagnosis and treatment. Springer, Berlin Heidelberg New York, pp 31–61

159. Aktolun C, Berk F, Demir H (2001) Detection of cold bone metastasis by Tc-99m MIBI imaging. Ann Nucl Med 15:393–395

160. Aso Y, Homma Y (1992) A survey on incidental renal cell carcinoma in Japan. J Urol 147:340

161. Staudenherz A, Steiner B, Puig S, Kainberger F, Leitha T (1999) Is there a diagnostic role for bone scanning of pa-

tients with a high pretest probability for metastatic renal cell carcinoma? Cancer 85:153–155

162. Mundy GR (1997) Mechanism of bone metastases. Cancer [Suppl] 80:1546

163. Staudenherz A, Steiner B, Puig S, Kainberger F, Leitha T (1999) Is there a diagnostic role for bone scanning of patients with high protect probability for metastatic renal cell carcinoma? Cancer 85:153–155

164. Coleman RE (1997) Skeletal complication of malignancy. Cancer [Suppl] 80:1588

165. Bos SD, Piers DA, Mensink HA (1995) Routine bone scan and serum alkaline phosphatase for staging in patients with renal cell carcinoma is not cost-effective. Eur J Cancer 31A:2422

166. Seaman E, Goluboff ET, Ross S et al (1996) Association of radionuclide bone scan and serum alkaline phosphatase in patients with metastatic renal cell carcinoma. Urology 48:692

167. Atlas I, Kwan D, Stone N (1991) Value of serum alkaline phosphatase and radionuclide bone scans in patients with renal cell carcinoma. Urology 38:220

168. Koga S, Tsuda S, Nishikido M, Ogawa Y, Hayashi K, Hayashi T, Kanetake H (2001) The diagnostic value of bone scan in patients with renal cell carcinoma. Clin Urol 166:2126–2128

169. Wu HC, Yen RF, Shen YY, Kao CH, Lin CC, Lee CC (2002) Composing whole body 18-F-2-deoxyglucose positron emission tomography and technetium-99m methylene diphosphonate bone scan to detect bone metastases in patients with renal cell carcinomas – a preliminary report. Cancer Res Clin Oncol 50:503–506

170. Schirrmeister H, Buck A, Guhlmann A, Reske SN (2001) Anatomical distribution and sclerotic activity of bone metastases from thyroid cancer assessed with F-18 sodium fluoride positron emission tomography. Thyroid 11:677–683

171. Lorberboym M, Murthy S, Mechanick JF, Bergman D, Morris JC, Kim CK (1996) Thallium-201 and Iodine-131 scintigraphy in differentiated thyroid carcinoma. J Nucl Med 37:1487–1491

172. Shiga (2001) Comparison of FDG, I-131 & Tl-201 in the diagnosis of recurrent or metastatic thyroid CA. J Nucl Med 42:414

173. Kumar R, Gupta R, Khullar S, Padhy AK, Julka PK, Malhotra A (2000) Bone scanning for bone metastasis in carcinoma cervix. J Assoc Physic India 48:808–810

174. Ozdemirli M, Mankin HJ, Aisenberg AC et al (1996) Hodgkin's disease presenting as a solitary bone tumor: a report of four cases and review of literature. Cancer 77:79–88

175. Schmidt AG, Kohn D, Bernards J et al (1994) Solitary skeletal lesions as primary manifestations of non-Hodgkin's lymphoma. Arch Orthop Trauma Surg 113:121–128

176. Baar J, Burkes RL, Bell R et al (1994) Primary non-Hodgkin's lymphoma of bone. Cancer 73:1194–1199

177. Stroszczynski C, Oellinger J, Hosten N et al (1999) Staging and monitoring of malignant lymphoma of bone.: comparison of Ga-67 and MRI. J Nucl Med 40:387–393

178. Landgren O, Axdorph U, Jacobsson H, Johansson B, Grimfors G, Bjorkholm M (2000) Routine bone scintigraphy is of limited value in the clinical assessment of untreated patients with Hodgkin's disease. Med Oncol 17:174–178

179. Israel O, Meckel M, Bar-shalom R, Epelbaum R, Hermony N, Haim N, Dann E et al (2002) Bone lymphoma: Ga-67 scintigraphy and CT for prediction of outcome after treatment. J Nucl Med 43:1295–1303

180. Carr R, Barrington SF, Madan B, O'Doherty MJ, Saunders

CA, van der Walt J, Timothy AR (1998) Detection of lymphoma in bone marrow by whole-body positron emission tomography. Blood 91:3340–3346

181. Choi CW, Lee DS, Chung J et al (1993) Evaluation of bone metastases by tc99m MDP imaging in patients with stomach cancer. Clin Nucl Med 20:310–314

182. Sundram FX, Chua ET, Goh AS et al (1990) Bone scintigraphy in nasopharyngeal carcinoma. Clin Radiol 42:160–168

183. Yui N, Togawa T, Kinoshita F et al (1992) Assessment of skull base involvement of nasopharyngeal carcinoma by bone SPECT using three detector system. Jpn J Nucl Med 29:37–40

184. Piepsz A, Gordon I, Hahn K (1991) Pediatric nuclear medicine. Eur J Nucl Med 18:41–66

185. Gordon I, Peters AM, Gutman A, Morony S, Dicks-Mireaux C, Pritchard J (1990) Skeletal assessment of neuroblastoma. The pitfalls of I-123 MIBG scans. J Nucl Med 31:129–134

186. Gelfand MJ (1993) Metaiodobenzylguanidine in children. Semin Nucl Med 23:231–242

187. Gelfand MJ, Paltiel HJ, Elgazzar AH et al (1992) I-123 MIBG imaging in pediatric neural crest tumors. J Nucl Med 33:1072 (abstract)

188. Shulkin BL, Shapiro B, Hutchinson RJ (1992) Iodine-131 metaiodobenzylguanidine and bone scintigraphy in detection of neuroblastoma. J Nucl Med 33:1735–1740

189. Hadj-Djiiani NL, Lebtahi NE, Bischof Delaloye A, Laurini R, Beck D (1995) Diagnosis and follow up of neuroblasoma by means of iodine-123 metaiodobenzylguanidine scintigraphy and bone scan and the influence of histology. Eur J Nucl Med 22:322–329

190. Abdel-Dayem HM, Scott AM, Macpinlac HA et al (1994) Role of Tl-201 chloride and Tc99m sestamibi in tumor imaging. Nuclear medicine annual. Raven, New York

191. Abdel-Dayem HM (1994) Thallium and gallium scintigraphy in pulmonary kaposi sarcoma in HIV-positive patient. Letter to the editor. Clin Nucl Med 19:473

192. Gomez MA, Beiras JM, Gallardo FG, Verdejo AJ (1994) Thallium and gallium scintigraphy in pulmonary kaposi sarcoma in HIV-positive patient. Clin Nucl Med 19:467–468

193. Meijer WG, van der Veer E, Jager PL, van der Jagt EJ, Piers BA, Kema IP, de Vries EGE, Willemse PHB (2003) Bone metastases in carcinoid tumors: clinical features, imaging characteristics, and markers of bone metabolism. J Nucl Med 44:184–191

194. Muroff LR (1981) Optimizing the performance and interpretation of bone scans. Clin Nucl Med 6:68–76

195. Citrin DL, Hougen C, Zweibel W et al (1981) The use of serial bone scans in assessing response of bone metastases to systemic treatment. Cancer 47:680–685

196. Alexander JL, Gillespie PJ, Edelstyn GA (1976) Serial bone scanning using technician 99m diphosphonate in patients cyclical combination chemotherapy for advanced breast cancer. Clin Nucl Med 1:13–17

197. Helms CA (1995) Fundamentals of skeletal radiology, 2nd edn. Saunders, Philadelphia

198. Baqer MM, Qurtom MA, Al-Ajmi AJ, Collier BD, Elgazzar AH (2002) Multifocal brucellosis spondylodiscitis. Clin Nucl Med 27:842–843

Diagnosis of Joint Disorders

Although scintigraphy has a limited role in the diagnosis of rheumatic diseases it can provide important complementary information and familiarity with the scintigraphic patterns of different disease conditions of the joints and peri-articular structures is important. Scintigraphy, however, could be more useful in evaluating the activity of the disease processes. The scintigraphic pattern of different arthropathies varies depending on the type and phase of the condition. Some conditions affect mainly small or large joints, while others affect both in either symmetrical or asymmetrical fashion. Primary osteoarthritis and rheumatoid arthritis show a classically symmetrical uptake. When large joints as shoulders, hips or knees are only involved, it indicates certain conditions such as osteoarthritis, ankylosing spondylitis, calcium pyrophosphate dihydrate crystal deposition disease (CPPD), or joint infection. Other radionuclides used in the diagnosis and follow-up of these conditions include In-111- and Tc-99m-labeled poly- and monoclonal antibodies such as Tc-99m-labeled human polyclonal immunoglobulin G, Tc-99m-anti-E-selectin-Fab respectively, Tc-99m-hexamethylpropylene amine oxime (Tc-99m-HMPAO), Tc-99m-SC, Tc-99m-nanocolloid and F-18 fluoro-2-deoxy-D-glucose (FDG). The use of SPECT and pinhole techniques should be remembered since they add diagnostic value to the scintigraphic methods. F-18 FDG positron emission tomography has a potential to quantitatively assess the degree of arthritis activity.

7.1
Introduction

Studying arthritis can be difficult because of the wide variety of disease patterns, the significant overlap of the various types and the lack of a clear and unified classification of this group of disorders. This chapter provides an overview of the evaluation of the arthropathies and related joint disorders in a simplified version that is in no way complete but will help the reader in identifying the major scintigraphic and correlative imaging patterns along with the necessary pathophysiological features of the relevant joint disorders. The reader may refer to Chap. 1 for the basic anatomical and physiological basis of joint diseases.

Generally, several modalities are used to diagnose and follow up joint diseases. Standard radiographs remain the initial modality of choice among the morphological modalities. Scintigraphy is needed in certain situations to help in the differential diagnosis and to evaluate the activity of the diseases. Among the scintigraphic methods, bone scanning is the most helpful and cost effective technique. The value of bone scanning was illustrated by Duncan [1], who studied 136 bone scans. This is the most common diagnostic imaging service requested by Australian rheumatologists, The primary indications for scanning were to confirm a clinical diagnosis (38%), to exclude a diagnosis (34%), and to accurately localize the site of pain (17%). The common diseases that rheumatologists were attempting to confirm, or exclude, with bone scanning were inflammatory arthritis such as rheumatoid arthritis and the possibility of differentiating it from malignancy and fracture. Bone scans were successful in excluding a diagnosis in 87% and confirming a diagnosis in 80% of cases. In 32% bone scans altered the clinical diagnosis, and in 43% they changed the course of disease management. Bone scan results prevented further investigations in 60% [1]. Single-head and dual-head pinhole images were reported to further enhance the role of bone scintigraphy in joint diseases [2]. The added value of dual-head pinhole bone scintigraphy using two opposing pinhole-collimated detectors is to obtain a pair of magnified images of the bone and joint at the same time thereby reducing the scan time [3].

7.2
Classification

No unified classification for the many types of joint diseases is available.

Arthropathies, however, can be grouped into two main categories: inflammatory and non-inflammatory [4]. (Table 7.1). The inflammatory joint disease group is further classified into infectious and non-infectious. The infectious type is caused by bacteria, mycoplasmas, fungi, viruses or protozoa, while the non-infectious sub-group is caused by immune reactions such as rheumatoid arthritis and spondyloarthropathies, the deposition of crystals in, and around, the joint (e.g. gout which is caused by deposition of monosodium

Table 7.1. Main types of joint disease with major examples

A. Inflammatory joint disease
1. Infectious
Infectious arthritis
2. Non infectious
Rheumatoid arthritis
Crystal deposition arthropathies (gouty arthritis, CPPD)
Sacroiliitis
Neuropathic joint disease
Spondyloarthropathies
Ankylosing spondylitis
Psoriatic arthritis
Reactive arthritis (formerly Reiter's disease)
Inflammatory bowel disease-associated arthritis
B. Non-inflammatory joint disease
1. Primary osteoarthritis
2. Secondary osteoarthritis

urate crystals), or vasculitis such as Behçet's disease. Alternatively, the inflammatory joint disease group can also be sub-classified into an immuno-inflammatory sub-group including rheumatoid arthritis, infectious or crystal deposition arthritis associated with a connective tissue disease (e.g., systemic lupus erythematosus) and those associated with vasculitis such as Behçet's disease. The non-inflammatory joint disease is exemplified by the common osteoarthritis, or degenerative joint disease, which can be idiopathic (primary) or secondary. It should be noted that certain conditions such as neuroarthropathy and sacroiliitis have multiple overlapping pathogenic features which may be immunological, vascular and degenerative.

7.3
Rheumatoid Arthritis

This autoimmune disease causes inflammation of the connective tissue mainly in the joints. It is thought that micro-vascular injury and mild synovial cell proliferation initially occur along with obliteration of the small blood vessels. The synovial inflammatory response is triggered by immune complexes in the blood and synovial tissue through activation of plasma protein complement. This complement activation stimulates release of kinin and prostaglandins which cause the increase in vascular permeability in the synovial membranes and attracts leukocytes from the circulation to the synovial membrane. Inflammation eventually spread from the synovial membrane to the articular cartilage, joint capsule and the surrounding tendons and ligaments with resultant pain, loss of function and joint deformity (Fig. 7.1, Fig. 7.2). The small joints of the hands, joints in the feet, and the wrists, elbows, ankles and knees are the most commonly affected. Synovitis activity is the dominant clinical variable that determines the therapeutic approach in patients with rheumatoid arthritis. At present, the amount of painful and swollen joints assessed by physical examination is generally used to measure the degree of synovitis activity. A gold standard for the assessment of synovitis activity is not available [5].

Using bone scintigraphy, the disease presents symmetrically with increased perfusion and delayed uptake peri-articularly in the areas of the joints affected. These are commonly the small joints of the hands, joints in the feet, and the wrists, elbows, ankles and knees (Figs. 7.3, 7.4). In-111 and Tc-99m-labeled poly- and mono-clonal antibodies are also used to image rheumatoid arthritis. Tc-99m polyclonal human immunoglobulin-G (HIG) has been shown to be a successful agent in the depiction of active inflammation in rheumatoid arthritis [6]. Sahin compared the uptake behaviors of Tc-99m HIG and Tc-99m MDP in rheuma-

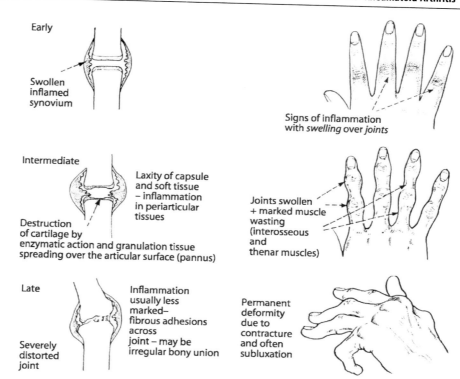

Fig. 7.1. The major pathological changes of rheumatoid arthritic joints (From "Illustrated Pathology" [65] with permission)

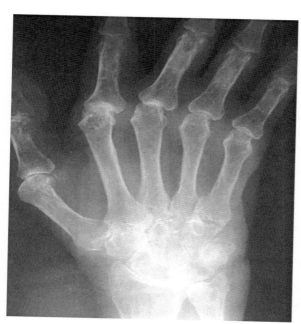

Fig. 7.2. Radiograph of a hand showing deformities associated with rheumatoid arthritis

toid arthritis. A total of 25 patients with rheumatoid arthritis and its variants presenting with active inflammation were included in this study. Target-to-background (T/B) ratios were obtained exclusively over the joint regions. Tc-99m HIG T/B ratios of the active joints in rheumatoid arthritis were significantly higher than those of the non-active joints and the control group of patients with well-diagnosed osteoarthritis. Tc-99m HIG T/B ratios in active joints showed a progressive increase between 2 and 24 h images. The T/B ratios in Tc-99m MDP bone scans were higher in all the active joints than in joints of non-active rheumatoid arthritis and those of controls but significant differences were only detected in wrist and elbow joints and the detection rate of active joint inflammation with Tc-99m HIG was higher than with Tc-99m MDP [7]. Monoclonal antibody which reacts with porcine E-selectin was evaluated to image rheumatoid arthritis. Tc-99m-labeled Fab fragment of 1.2B6 and Tc-99m HDP were used by Jamar et al. [8] in 10 patients. Images were obtained 4 h and 20–24 h after injection. Two normal volunteers were also imaged. The diagnostic accuracy, using joint tenderness or swelling as the clinical standard, was 88%, higher than that of Tc-99m-HDP (57%) as a result of the low specificity of the latter in rheumatoid arthritis. No uptake of Tc-99m-Fab was observed in the inactive or normal joints, whereas Tc-99m HDP was taken up by all joints to a varying degree, making the decision as to whether a particular joint is actively involved or chronically damaged very difficult. The authors concluded that Tc-99m-anti-E-selectin-Fab scintigraphy can be used successfully to image synovitis with better specificity than Tc-99m-HDP bone scanning [8].

Labeled leukocytes have been used to evaluate the activity of the disease and is a promising method for

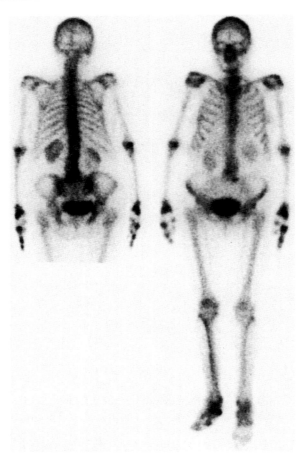

Fig. 7.3. Bone scan of a patient with rheumatoid arthritis. Note the symmetrical pattern of increased uptake

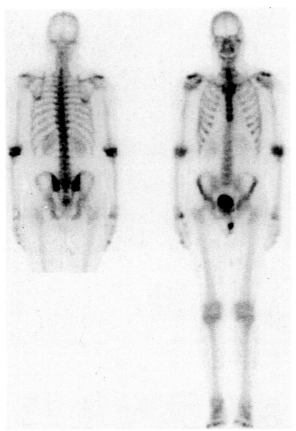

Fig. 7.4. Bone scan of a 34-year-old male known to have active rheumatoid arthritis. Note the symmetrical involvement of the particularly affected elbow joints

this purpose. In a recent study by Gaal and associates [9], the applicability of 99mTc-hexamethylpropylene amine oxime (99mTc-HMPAO)-labeled leukocyte joint scintigraphy in the assessment of disease activity was tested in 21 patients with rheumatoid arthritis. The degree of accumulation of 99mTc-HMPAO leukocytes showed no correlation with a patient's age and gender, duration of disease, use of disease modifying antirheumatic drugs or any laboratory parameters. However, a significant correlation was found between the global regional accumulation of the labeled leukocytes of the hands and feet, and the clinical assessment of joint activity [9].

7.4
Crystal Deposition Arthropathies

Apart from gout, there are several other types of calcium deposition that can lead to arthritis [10]. These include CPPD (pseudogout), calcium hydroxyapatite crystals, and calcium oxalate crystals (oxalosis).

7.4.1
Gouty Arthritis

Gout is a metabolic disorder that results in hyperuricemia and leads to the deposition of monosodium urate monohydrate crystals at various sites in the body, especially joint cartilage. It continues to be a health problem worldwide despite the availability of effective therapies. The disease is rare in children and pre-menopausal females and uncommon in males under 30 years of age. The prevalence is influenced by genetic factors, alcohol consumption, obesity, and hypertension. There is an association between hyperuricemia and cardiovascular disease which seems to be linked to insulin resistance [11]. It is closely linked to purine metabolism and kidney function. An accelerated rate of purine synthesis may occur in some individuals with overproduction of uric acid since the latter is a breakdown product of purine nucleotides [12]. In other individuals, the rate of breakdown, rather than synthesis, of purine nucleotides is accelerated, also resulting in high levels of uric acid. Uric acid is predominantly eliminated via the kidney. Urate excretion by the kidney may be sluggish due to a decrease in the glomerular filtration of urate or an acceleration of urate re-absorption. Urate crystals are deposited in the renal interstitium, causing impaired renal flow, and may also precipitate, resulting in renal stones. Uric acid crystallizes when it reaches certain concentrations in fluids, forming insoluble crystals that can precipitate in the connective tissue of different parts of the body. When this process involves the synovial fluid, it causes acute inflammation of the joint. Although the effect is the same, classic gouty arthritis is caused by deposition of monosodium urate crystals, while deposition of calcium pyrophosphate dihydrate crystal causes pseudogout [13].

Monosodium urate crystals deposition triggers an acute inflammatory response in the synovial membrane and other tissues of the joints. Leukocytes, particularly neutrophils, are attracted out of the circulation to phagocytize the crystals. Trauma is the most common aggravating factor. Therefore, the great toe is a common presenting site (50% of initial attacks); this is due to the chronic strain during walking.

Scintigraphically, there is increased flow, blood pool activity and delayed uptake in the areas of the joint involved. The ankle, knee and the first metatarsophalangeal joint are the joints most often affected [14, 15]. The most typical is, however, that of the metatarsophalangeal joint of the great toe, called podagra. Recently a case of gouty tophus of the patella was evaluated by positron emission tomography (PET) using a combination of an amino-acid analog emitter, L-[3-F-18]-alphamethyl tyrosine (FMT), which does not accumulate in malignancies and showed increased levels of metabolic activity and the glucose analog emitter, F-18 FDG, which essentially accumulates in malignancies did not show appreciable activity. This case report suggests that PET may be useful for the pre-operative evaluation of gouty tophus (Fig. 7.4), including detection and differentiation from malignant tumors [16].

7.4.2
Calcium Pyrophosphate Dihydrate Deposition Disease

Calcium pyrophosphate dihydrate deposition disease (CPPD) was described approximately 50 years ago when calcium pyrophosphate dihydrate crystals were identified in the synovial fluid of patients who had gout-like symptoms with no urate crystals identified. The term chondrocalcinosis and pyrophosphate arthropathy were also applied to the same disease. It generally occurs in elderly individuals and is said to affect 20–30% of people older than 65 years and 30–60% of those older than 85 years. In most cases it is relatively asymptomatic but it can occasionally cause severe disabling arthritis [10]. It may occasionally form tumor-like masses and in this case the term tophaceous pseu-

dogout is applied. Patients with gout have an increased chance of having CPPD as well. Up to 40% of the patients with gout concomitantly have CPPD.

7.5
Infectious Arthritis (see also Chap. 2)

In children, infectious (septic) arthritis usually occurs secondary to hematogenous seeding but it can also be produced by direct extension of osteomyelitis. More than half of the patients are younger than 2 years-old. A recent history of trauma is found in one third of patients and nearly 50% have recent otitis media or an upper respiratory tract infection. Infectious arthritis secondary to adjacent osteomyelitis can occur in joints where the metaphysis is within the capsule (hip or shoulder). It can be found in infants, because of the epiphyseal location of osteomyelitis. *Staphylococcus aureus* is the major causative agent followed by the *Streptococcus* species. In children less than 2 years old, *Haemophilus influenzae* is the main causative agent, although its incidence has decreased following the introduction of vaccination [17]. Patients present with fever, pain, limitation of movement and limp, and infants may demonstrate joint dislocation. The hip and knee are the most commonly affected joints in children, while the shoulder is more often affected in neonates. Rapid cartilage destruction and bone ischemia caused by increased intracapsular pressure lead to sequelae such as growth discrepancies, limitation of movement, and dislocation. Accordingly, the condition is an orthopedic emergency, and any de-

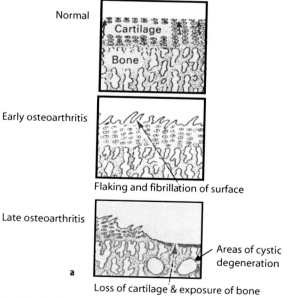

Fig. 7.5a, b. The major pathologic changes of osteoarthritis (from [65] with permission)

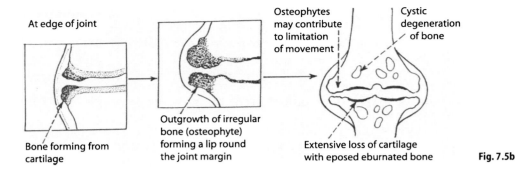

At edge of joint

Bone forming from cartilage

Outgrowth of irregular bone (osteophyte) forming a lip round the joint margin

Osteophytes may contribute to limitation of movement

Cystic degeneration of bone

Extensive loss of cartilage with eposed eburnated bone

Fig. 7.5b

lay in diagnosis often leads to catastrophic sequelae. Permanent loss of joint function occurs in up to 25–50% of patients [18–20]. The diagnosis can be made from clinical observation and joint aspiration. Combination of joint and blood cultures allows identification of the pathogen in two thirds of cases [17, 20]. Ultrasound allows the rapid identification of joint effusion and can act as a guide during aspiration. It should be noted that ultrasound cannot differentiate whether the joint effusion is the result of infection, or just inflammation, since the severity of effusion of the septic hip group may not be greater than the non-infectious synovitis [21]. Sonography can also be used to detect the extent of the infection, since it may reveal the periosteal elevation, sub-periosteal abscess and cortical erosion much earlier than radiographs if metaphyseal osteomyelitis has occurred [22]. In cases of equivocal ultrasonography and if the presence of osteomyelitis is to be evaluated, bone scanning is the modality of choice (see chapter 2).

7.6
Osteoarthritis

Osteoarthritis can be primary with no known predisposing factors (idiopathic) or it can be secondary due to several etiologies. Both primary and secondary forms of osteoarthritis have the same pathological characteristics (Fig. 7.5). Primary, or idiopathic, osteoarthritis is the most common type of non-inflammatory joint disease. Although it can affect any joint, the joints most commonly involved are the hand joints, wrists, lower cervical spine, lumbar spine, sacroiliac joints, hips, knees, ankles and foot joints (Fig. 7.6). Aging is an important risk factor although the cause of osteoarthritis is unknown. Premature cartilage degeneration due to an inherited genetic defect encoding for the structural components of the articular cartilage have been suggested as the etiology for this condition.

Primary osteoarthritis progresses with age. Secondary osteoarthritis occurs when the predisposing cause is known, e.g., following intraarticular fracture or other trauma (post-traumatic osteoarthritis); rheumatoid

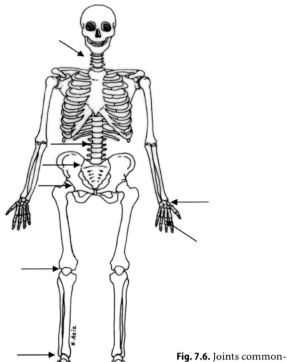

Fig. 7.6. Joints commonly involved with osteoarthritis

diseases; neurogenic and metabolic disorders; xenobiotic agents and recurrent hemarthrosis (as may occur among hemophiliac patients and following certain forms of osteochondrosis and osteonecrosis). The pain of osteoarthritis is caused by intracapsular tension, muscle spasm, abnormal stress on the bone and increased intra-osseous venous pressure.

The ability of the articular cartilage to repair is very limited. Intrinsic repair occurs in infants, as the chondrocytes are still able to proliferate. Extrinsic repair occurs by granulation tissue growing from the adjacent bone. The granulation tissue changes to fibrocartilage, which is inferior to normal cartilage in its mechanical properties.

The changes that occur to the articular cartilage in osteoarthritis involve a progression from fibrillation to

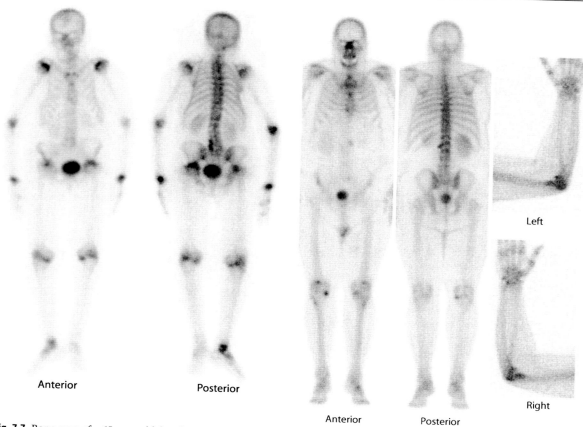

Fig. 7.7. Bone scan of a 65-year-old female with osteoarthritis complaining of generalized joint pains. Scan shows intensely increased uptake in the joints of the upper and lower extremities

Fig. 7.8. Bone scan in a patient with osteoarthritis. Moderately increased uptake is noted in knees, elbows, wrists, and spine. A focus of increased uptake in L-1 is extending to the left beyond the boundaries of the vertebra and is corresponding to an osteophyte seen radiographically

erosion, and then in the advanced stages it leads to the complete loss of cartilage. At this point the exposed bone is exposed to increased stress, becomes more compressed and shows subarticular sclerosis [23].

Thus, the pathological features of osteoarthritis include gradual loss of the articular cartilage, thickening and hardening (sclerosis) of the bone underneath the cartilage (sub-chondral sclerosis) and formation of osteophytes (spurs). As the articular cartilage erodes, the cartilage coated osteophytes often grow into the joint. Small pieces of osteophyte may break off and become liberated within the synovial cavity. These pieces, called joint mice, irritate the synovial membrane resulting in synovitis and joint effusion. In addition, the joint capsule may thicken and in some cases adhere to the underlying bone, causing limitation of movement.

The osteoarthritic changes can usually be seen on standard radiographs as well as other morphological modalities. Using bone scintigraphy, increased peri-articular uptake is commonly seen as an incidental finding in the commonly involved joints. The degree of uptake is proportional to the severity of the disease (Figs. 7.7, 7.8) [24].

7.7
Sacroiliitis

The sacroiliac joints may be involved in degenerative diseases, or septic processes, as well as in the different arthropathies. Infection involving the sacroiliac joint is an uncommon condition in which non-specific clinical features and delayed radiographic features may lead to incorrect diagnoses and delayed, or inappropriate, treatment. Sacroiliac infections occur due to the hematogenous spread of organisms, and a history of pre-existing infection is often present, particularly a cutaneous, pharyngeal, postpartum, urinary tract infection, or osteomyelitis elsewhere [25]. The most frequently isolated organisms include staphylococci [26, 27]. Whether the infection begins in the joint, or within the adjacent bone, is controversial. Nixon emphasizes that it is far more likely that infection begins in bone (ilium), where, similar to the metaphyses elsewhere, the vascular anatomy predisposes this site to blood-borne infection [27].

The role of imaging studies in the evaluation of patients with sacroiliitis is controversial. Planar and SPECT bone scintigraphy, Tc-99m SC and Tc-99m nanocolloid along with quantitative methods have all been used for the diagnosis. Diagnosis of sacroiliitis with bone scintigraphy may be difficult even with a quantitative approach. A combination of bone and bone marrow scintigraphy has been proposed as an alternative method that may have a role in characterizing patients with active sacroiliitis that has been found typically to show a decreased bone marrow uptake [28, 29]. A total of 31 patients who were clinically suspected to have sacroiliitis were studied using bone and bone marrow scans by Bozkurt et al. [28]. Both visual and quantitative assessment of MDP uptake and a visual assessment of the sulfur colloid uptake in the sacroiliac joints was performed. Increased Tc-99m-MDP uptake with decreased/normal sulfur colloid uptake was the most common scintigraphic pattern seen in the acute phase of sacroiliitis cases in which radiographic findings were normal or slightly changed. In at least eight patients bone marrow uptake of sulfur colloid was clearly decreased, supporting the diagnosis [28]. SPECT bone scan was found to have the best accuracy (97% sensitivity and 90% specificity) [30].

7.8
Neuroarthropathy (see also Chap. 2).

Neuroarthropathy is characterized by destructive joint changes. Loss of protective pain and proprioceptive sensation along with hyperemia secondary to loss of vasoconstrictive neural impulses are thought to result in atrophic neuropathy, most frequently occurring in the forefoot [31]. On the other hand, absence of sympathetic fibers in the presence of sensory fiber involvement tends to result in hypertrophic neuroarthropathy, which occurs most frequently in the mid- and hindfoot. Since the patient continues to walk and traumatize the foot, disuse osteoporosis is usually absent. Unrelenting trauma may also result in rapidly progressive destruction, sometimes with disintegration of one or more tarsal bones within a period of only a few weeks. In this rapidly progressive form of neuroarthropathy there is a greater degree of inflammatory reaction than in other types. A long history of diabetes mellitus with a combination of angiopathy, neuropathy and immunopathy predisposes the patient to pedal osteomyelitis, which may be difficult to differentiate from neuroarthropathy (particularly the rapidly progressive form). Metatarsal bones and the proximal phalanges are the most commonly involved sites [31–33].

The condition is characterized by cartilage destruction, bony collapse, synovial and capsular hypertrophy, and disorganization of the joints involved. Radiography shows diffuse soft-tissue swelling, joint space narrowing, subluxation, slanting joint deformity, and irregular destruction and exophytic derangement of bone. Scintigraphically, neuroarthropathy presents with an increased uptake to variable degrees on bone scan and gallium-67 scans which cannot differentiate the condition from osteomyelitis. Furthermore, the condition may cause false-positive results of labeled leukocyte scans, since the rapidly progressive neuroarthropathy may cause abnormal accumulation of labeled leukocytes simulating osteomyelitis. Simultaneous In-111 leukocyte and Tc-99m bone scanning is the most accurate technique for differentiating both conditions. Bone scanning using a pinhole collimator shows bizarre tracer uptake in and around the diseased joint, possibly showing fragmentation.

7.9
Spondyloarthropathies

This group of disorders were formerly called rheumatoid variants and are currently called seronegative HLA-B27-positive spondyloarthropathies. They share common clinical and radiographic features, with characteristic involvement of the sacroiliac joints, spine, and to various degrees, the peripheral joints, are linked to HLA B27 histocompatibility antigen. The group includes ankylosing spondylitis, psoriatic arthritis, reactive arthritis (Reiter's disease), enteropathic spondylitis (ulcerative colitis, Crohn's disease and Whipple's disease), and an entity known as undifferentiated spondyloarthropathy. Additionally, these disorders are also characterized by (1) absence of rheumatoid factors in the blood; (2) absence of subcutaneous nodules; (3) familial aggregation.

Although plain radiographs are the first line of imaging investigation, they are often unable to demon-

Table 7.2. Typical distribution of sacroiliitis

Unilateral	Asymmetrical	Symmetrical	
Ankylosing spondylitis	–	early, uncommon	+
Rheumatoid arthritis	+	+	+
Gouty arthritis	+	+	+
Psoriatic arthritis	+	+	+
Reactive arthritis (Reiter's disease)	+	+	+
Degenerative disease	+	+	+
Osteitis condensans	+	+	+
Brucellosis	+	+	+
Familial Mediterranean fever	+	+	–
Infectious arthritis	+	–	–
Enteropathic arthritis	–	–	+
Renal osteodystrophy	–	–	+

Modified from [64], with permission

Table 7.3. Classic scintigraphic findings of major joint diseases

Disease	Scintigraphic findings
Rheumatoid arthritis	Symmetrical uptake involving small and large joints
Gouty arthritis	Uptake of metatarsophalangeal joint of the great toe and large joints, commonly symmetrical
Ankylosing spondylitis	Symmetrical intense tracer uptake in both sacroiliac joints and spine
Osteoarthritis	Uptake of large joints, symmetrical in primary type
Reactive arthritis	Asymmetrical uptake of large and small joints and spine
Psoriatic arthritis	Asymmetrical uptake of large and small joints typically of upper extremity, including fingers, and spine
Infectious arthritis	Uptake involving a large joint
Enteropathic arthritis	Uptake of large joints (asymmetrical), sacroiliac joints (symmetrical) and spine

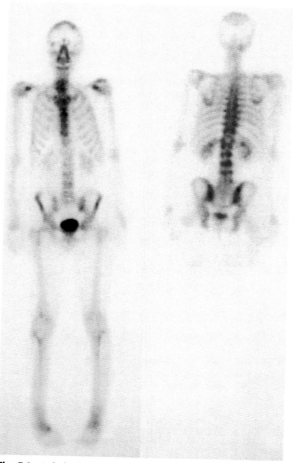

Fig. 7.9. Ankylosing spondylitis in a 32-year-old male with known ankylosing spondylitis and low back pain. There is increased uptake in sacroiliac joints and multiple vertebrae.

strate the early changes of sacroiliitis which are needed in order to establish the early diagnosis of seronegative spondyloarthropathy. The radiographic appearances of each of the inflammatory diseases involving the sacroiliac joints are similar. Differences in symmetry and severity may, however, suggest the correct diagnosis (Table 7.2).

Other imaging modalities, including conventional tomography, bone scintigraphy, computed tomography, and MRI, have improved the visualization of inflammatory changes in the sacroiliac joints [34].

7.9.1
Ankylosing Spondylitis

Stiffening and fusion (ankylosis) of the spine and sacroiliac joints causing, most frequently, low back pain and stiffness characterize this chronic inflammatory joint disease which is the most common type of the seronegative spondyloarthropathies. It predominantly affects the axial joints, particularly the sacroiliac joints, with a strong genetic predisposition associated with HLA-B27. Other joints such as the hips, knees and shoulders are involved in approximately 30% of patients. The condition usually affects males and begins in adolescence with inflammation of the fibrocartilage in cartilaginous joints (primarily in the vertebrae) along with infiltration of inflammatory cells (mainly macrophages and lymphocytes) into the fibrous tissue of the joint capsule, cartilage and periosteum. This process is followed by repair of cartilaginous structures by the proliferation of fibroblasts that secrete collagen, which later becomes organized into fibrous scar. This scar eventually undergoes calcifica-

tion and ossification leading to a loss of flexibility and fusion of joints [35].

Scintigraphically, the patterns vary according to the disease stage. In the early stages, scintigraphy reveals typical, but not always symmetrical, intense tracer uptake in both sacroiliac joints. Associated spinal lesions may, or may not, be present at this stage. Later, as the spine becomes involved (Fig. 7.9), pinhole scintigraphy reveals patchy uptake in the apophyseal joints, horizontal band-like uptake in the disco-vertebral junctions, and midline segmental uptake in the spinous processes and the interspinous ligaments [2].

7.9.2
Psoriatic Arthritis

The association of psoriasis with a specific type of arthritis is now well established and can be differentiated on the basis of spotty involvement, negative rheumatoid factor, the radiographic and scintigraphic findings, and sometimes a positive HLA-B27 antigen test. Distribution is asymmetrical, spotty, or sometimes unilateral, more regularly affecting the upper extremity joints, including fingers, typically with inflammatory involvement of the distal interphalangeal joints.

Yun et al. [36] described a patient with psoriatic arthritis in whom an increased level of F-18 FDG uptake was seen in the joints of the hands. The areas of increased activity correlated well with the regions of symptoms reported by the patient. This finding illustrates the potential use of F-18 FDG-PET to quantitatively assess the degree of arthritis activity [36].

7.9.3
Reactive Arthritis (Reiter's Disease)

The syndrome as described originally by Hans Reiter in 1916 comprises a triad: non-gonococcal urethritis, arthritis and conjunctivitis. Willkens et al. [37], defined the condition as an episode of arthritis lasting longer than 1 month in association with urethritis or cervicitis. The associated synovitis develops after a primary infection distant from the joint, mainly localized in the genitourinary (uroarthritis) or the gastrointestinal (enteroarthritis) tract [38]. The disease can also follow salmonellosis, shigellosis, and yersiniasis, in which case it can be described as post-enteric reactive arthritis. Because of the possible involvement of the spine and enthesis, and the HLA-B27 association, reactive arthritis is considered to be one of the spondylarthropathies. Recently, bacterial components, or viable bacteria, were found in the involved joints. Radiologically, the first signs to be observed in joints include peri-articular soft-tissue swelling, joint space narrowing, and osseous erosions in the absence of significant osteoporosis. Periosteal thickening may be noted in the pelvis, trochanters and heel. The spurs in the plantar and posterior aspects of the calcaneus and the 'sausage digit' deformity in the toes are other important signs. Asymmetrical, or even symmetrical, sacroiliitis may be seen.

Bone scintigraphy appears to be the method of choice for the panoramic mapping of the characteristic spotty, asymmetrical foci of the polyarthritis and spondylopathy (Table 7.3). In general, the grade of tracer uptake in a lesion appears roughly to parallel the activity of the inflammatory process. Particularly when augmented with the pinhole imaging, bone scintigraphy has proven to be more sensitive, and often more specific, than radiography in revealing the associated early enthesopathies, especially in the heel and knee [39].

7.9.4
Enteropathic Spondylitis

Enteropathic arthropathies are induced by, or associated with, inflammatory bowel diseases, including ulcerative colitis, Crohn's disease, Whipple's disease, intestinal bypass surgery and celiac disease. The exact cause-and-effect relationship between arthritis and the inflammatory bowel diseases has not been fully clarified, although both an immune mechanism and articular infection (either primary or secondary to intestinal infection) have been implicated. In recent years the importance of a genetic role in the evolution of enteropathic arthropathies has been discussed. Approximately 90% of patients with ulcerative colitis and Crohn's disease who develop spondylitis or sacroiliitis demonstrate HLA-B27 antigen [40]. The most common radiographic changes are peri-articular soft-tissue swelling and osteoporosis.

Whole-body bone scintigraphy is useful for the demonstration of the asymmetrical pattern of peripheral joint involvement and the occurrence of sacroiliitis and spondylitis (Table 7.3).

Pinhole scintigraphy can again show clearly the irregular spotty, or patchy, uptake in the peri-articular bones and joint space narrowing.

7.10
Other Arthropathies and Related Conditions
7.10.1
Behçet's Syndrome

This is an uncommon disorder characterized by the presence of recurrent oral and genital ulceration and relapsing iritis. It is named after Halushi Behçet, a Turkish dermatologist who described it in 1937. The disease is more common in Mediterranean countries and Japan. Diagnosis is made by the presence of recurrent aphthous oral ulcers along with two of the following:(1) recurrent genital ulcers, (2) uveitis, or retinal vasculitis (4) cutaneous pustules or erythema nodosum or cutaneous pathergy and synovitis. Patients with a European heritage (e.g., North America) seldom have a cutaneous pathergy; instead, an association with the following may be added: large vessel vasculitis, meningoencephalitis or cerebral vasculitis [41]. Arthritis occurs in nearly one-half to three-quarters of cases and is usually polyarticular. Sacroiliitis and spondylitis have rarely been noted and permanent changes are uncommon.

7.10.2
Costochondritis (Tietze's Syndrome)

This is a painful condition that is self-limited and short lived. It was first described by Tietze in 1921 [42] and is also termed costosternal syndrome. The condition is common and affects the costochondral junction, usually in young individuals. Although trauma and infection have been proposed, the etiology remains unknown. Although any rib can be affected, the first and second ribs are most commonly involved [43].

The radiographic study is unremarkable in most of the cases. Bone scintigraphy simply reveals increased tracer uptake without specific features [44], but pinhole scintigraphy, can demonstrate characteristic alterations [45]. During the active phase, intense tracer uptake may appear in the whole costal cartilage, which is enlarged, producing a 'drum stick' appearance. Later, in the chronic phase, the abnormal uptake becomes reduced in size and localized in the costochondral junction. The latter is now shrunken owing to the resolution of the inflammation and shows a 'comma-like' appearance

7.10.3
SAPHO Syndrome

SAPHO syndrome is characterized by synovitis, acne, palmoplantar pustulosis, hyperostosis, and osteitis. There is tenderness and swelling of the small and large joints of the feet, the ankles, knees, hips, sacroiliac joints, and shoulders. Bone scanning may be helpful in diagnosing arthritis associated with the SAPHO syndrome. Tc-99m MDP scanning can detect signs of arthritis not seen with other imaging methods. This is because the arthritis is inflammatory in nature and does not always cause the bone erosion that is able to be detected by morphological imaging. Such findings on bone scanning, along with presence of hydradenitis, can also lead to the correct diagnosis of SAPHO syndrome [46].

7.10.4
Synovitis (see also Chap. 4)
7.10.4.1
Transient Synovitis

Transient synovitis is a self-limited, non-specific, inflammatory joint disease of transient nature among children. Other terms for the condition of the hip are irritable hip syndrome, observation hip, transitory arthritis, transitory coxitis, and simple serous coxitis. Boys are affected much more often than girls since it is found most frequently in boys between 5–10 years of age. It preferentially affects the hip, or knee, and subsides without antibiotics. The etiology has not been firmly established but the most likely mechanisms include viral infection and a hypersensitivity reaction to infection occurring elsewhere in the body.

The basic radiographic abnormality is capsular distension, and in the majority of patients no abnormalities are detected. Using three-phase bone scanning, transient synovitis demonstrates diffusely increased joint activity on the blood flow and blood pool images. On the delayed images, there is diffusely increased tracer uptake in the subchondral layers of periarticular bones covered with the synovium. The increased tracer uptake in the subchondral bone in synovitis has been accounted for by the increased blood flow through the anastomotic vascular channels induced by hyperemia in the inflamed synovium [47]. The degree of uptake is minimal, barely delineating the femoral head and acetabular fossa. This may be so subtle so that it can hardly be recognized on planar images. Pinhole imaging, however, can identify subtle changes [48]. Other patterns include normal or decreased uptake [49, 50].

7.10.4.2
Synovitis in renal transplantation

Following a renal transplant, or during long repeated hemodialysis, acute or chronic synovitis may supervene [51]. Generally the articular inflammation is simple, but occasionally infection has been reported [52]. Radiographically, the inflamed joint capsule is distended, and the periarticular soft tissues are swollen when the process becomes chronic. The joint space is narrowed, and the peri-articular bones are diffusely osteoporotic (usually mild to moderate). Pinhole scintigraphic changes are much more similar to those noted in other types of synovitis, although they are usually mild unless complicated with an infection.

7.10.4.3
Pigmented Villonodular Synovitis

Pigmented villonodular synovitis (PVNS) is a chronic, inflammatory process of the synovium that causes synovial proliferation. A swollen joint with lobular masses of synovium occurs (Fig. 7.10), which causes pain and joint destruction. The condition affects individuals in their third to fourth decade of life and in most cases is mono-articular, predominantly affecting the knee (80%), followed by the hip and ankle. It is rarely polyarticular [53]. Scintigraphically, non-specific activity is seen peri-articularly [54–56]. Tl-201 has also been reported to accumulate in this condition [57].

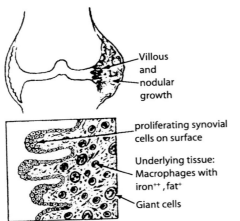

Fig. 7.10. Pathological changes of pigmented villonodular synovitis (from [65] with permission)

7.11
Periarticular Soft-Tissue Syndromes

Periarticular soft-tissue syndromes such as tenosynovitis, bursitis, and plantar fasciitis are characterized by local pain, tenderness, and swelling in the bursa, tendon sheath, or enthesis (the insertion of tendon, ligament, or capsule into the peri-articular bones). Individual lesions may present as bursitis, tenosynovitis, capsulitis, fibrosis, or calcification. Trauma and repeated physical irritation are the common causes of this painful inflammation in the peri-articular soft tissue structures. Idiopathic lesions are not rare. Standard radiography often plays a decisive role in the diagnosis of bursitis, tenosynovitis, and plantar fasciitis. Ultrasonography can play a crucial role in confirming the diagnosis of bursitis and in guiding needle aspiration. Bursitis shows abnormal amounts of fluid in the bursae and the associated synovial hypertrophy on ultrasound [58, 59]. In these conditions planar bone scanning may reveal increased tracer uptake in the regions of the involved bursa, tendon, or enthesis. However, the anatomical site of a lesion is extremely difficult to assess by planar imaging. In contrast, pinhole scintigraphy can reveal the anatomy of a lesion so that it points to the diagnosis of bursitis or tenosynovitis. It should be noted that, in bursitis and tenosynovitis, bone scintigraphy may reveal intense tracer uptake when secondary erosion, reactive osteitis, and sclerosis in the neighboring bone is present. These secondary bone alterations are seen in association with trochanteric bursitis, subdeltoid bursitis, supra-acromial bursitis, subacromial bursitis, sub-Achilles tenosynovitis and plantar fasciitis [60].

7.11.1
Septic Bursitis

This condition may result from penetrating trauma, extension from a nearby septic arthritis or bacteremia. The superficially located bursae (e.g., the bursae of the olecranon and patella) are more commonly involved than the deep bursae (e.g., the trochanteric bursae). This condition may be confused with septic arthritis [61]. Trochanteric bursitis most frequently occurs in elderly and obese patients, and its presentation may require a bone scan to exclude a traumatic cause for the pain. A history of frank trauma can usually only be elicited in about 25% of patients, although Allwright et al. [62] suggested that it might be caused by inflammation, or related to gluteal tendon insertion strain and associated periosteal reaction. In addition to the general features presented above, the authors described the characteristic scintigraphic findings of this condition on delayed images: a short linear band of moderate uptake confined to the superior and lateral aspects of the greater trochanter (Fig. 7.11).

7.11.2
Septic Tenosynovitis

This condition also results from penetrating injuries, or the spread of infection from a contiguous injury, and generally involves the flexor tendons of the hands and feet of diabetic patients. Early diagnosis is important to avoid complications particularly tendon necrosis and extension of infection to the adjacent joints [63].

7.11.3
Plantar Fasciitis

This condition, also known as calcaneal periosteitis, can occur as an isolated entity such as occupational injury, degenerative changes or it may accompany spondyloarthropathies. It causes heel pain and can easily diagnosed by planar or pinhole multiphase bone scan by identifying focal usually subtle increases blood pool and delayed uptake at the site of insertion of the long plantar tendon into the calcaneal base (Fig. 7.12).

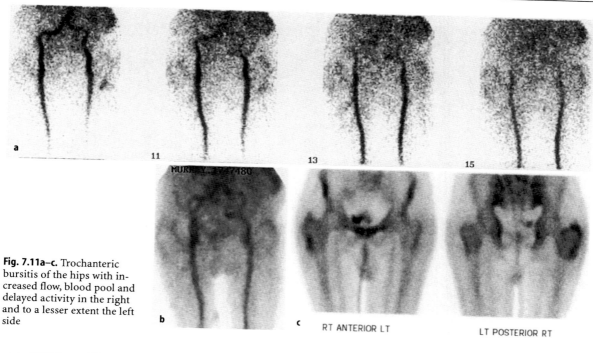

Fig. 7.11a–c. Trochanteric bursitis of the hips with increased flow, blood pool and delayed activity in the right and to a lesser extent the left side

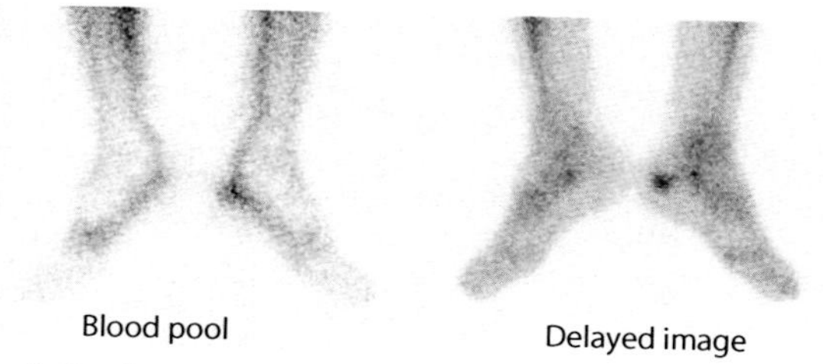

RT ANTERIOR LT   LT POSTERIOR RT

Blood pool   Delayed image

Fig. 7.12. Plantar fasciitis on bone scan. There is linear increased blood pool activity along the plantar aspect of the feet. On delayed images there is a focus of increased uptake in the calcaneus in the left foot but no abnormal uptake in the right foot. This illustrates the two classic scintigraphic patterns of plantar fasciitis

References

1. Duncan I, Dorai-Raj A, Khoo K, Tymms K, Brook A (1999) The utility of bone scans in rheumatology. Clin Nucl Med 24:9–14
2. Bahk Y (2000) Combined scintigraphic and radiographic diagnosis of bone and joint diseases, 2nd edn. Springer, Berlin Heidelberg New York
3. Bahk YW, Kim SH, Chung SK, Kim JH (1998) Dual-head pinhole bone scintigraphy. J Nucl Med 39:1444–1448
4. McCarthy D (ed) (1984) Arthritis and allied conditions. Lea and Fabiger, Philadelphia
5. Vos K, van der Linden E, Pauwels EK (1999) The clinical role of nuclear medicine in rheumatoid arthritis patients. A comparison with other diagnostic imaging modalities. Quart J Nucl Med 43:38–45
6. Cindas A, Gokce-Kustal Y, Kirth PO, Caner B (2001) Scintigraphic evaluation of synovial inflammation in rheumatoid arthritis with (99m)technetium-labelled human polyclonal immunoglobulin G. Rheumatol Int 20:71–77
7. Sahin M, Bernay I, Basoglu T, Canturk F (1999) Comparison of Tc-99m MDP, Tc-99m HSA and Tc-99m HIG uptake in rheumatoid arthritis and its variants. Ann Nucl Med 13:389–395
8. Jamar F, Houssiau FA, Devogelaer JP, Chapman PT, Haskard DO, Beaujean V, Beckers C, Manicourt DH, Peters AM (2002) Scintigraphy using a technetium 99m-labelled anti-E-selectin Fab fragment in rheumatoid arthritis. Rheumatology 41:53–61
9. Gaal J, Mezes A, Siro B, Varga J, Galuska L, Janoky G, Garai I, Bajnok L, Suranyi P (2002) 99m Tc-HMPAO labelled leukocyte scintigraphy in patients with rheumatoid arthritis: a comparison with disease activity. Nucl Med Commun 23:39–46
10. Hoffman GS, Reginato AJ (1994) Arthritis due to deposition of calcium crystals. In: Isselbacher KJ, Braunwald E, Wilson JD, Martin JB, Fauci AS, Kasper DL (eds) Harrison's principles of internal medicine, vol 2, 13th edn. McGraw-Hill, New York, pp 1698–1701
11. Wortmann RL (2002) Gout and hyperuricemia. Curr Opin Rheumatol 14:281–286
12. Urano W, Yamanaka H, Tsutani H, Nakajima H, Matsuda Y, Taniguchi A, Hara M, Kamatani N (2002) The inflammatory process in the mechanism of decreased serum uric acid concentrations during acute gouty arthritis. J Rheumatol 29:1950–1953
13. Kaye JJ (1990) Arthritis: roles of radiography and other imaging techniques in evaluation. Radiology 177:601–608
14. Mijiyawa M (1995) Gout in patients attending the rheumatology unit of Lome Hospital. Br J Rheumatol 34:843–846
15. Koh WH, Seah A, Chai P (1998) Clinical presentation and disease associations of gout: a hospital-based study of 100 patients in Singapore. Ann Acad Med Singapore 27:7–10
16. Sato J, Watanabe H, Shinozaki T, Fukuda T, Shirakura K, Takagishi K (2001) Gouty tophus of the patella evaluated by PET imaging. J Orthop Sci 6:604–607
17. Fink CW, Nelson JD (1986) Septic arthritis and osteomyelitis in children. Clin Rheum Dis 12:243
18. Goldenberg DL (1998) Septic arthritis. Lancet 351:197

19. Pioro MH, Mandel BF (1997) Septic arthritis. Rheum Dis Clin North Am 23:239

20. Welkon CJ, Long SS, Fisher MC et al (1986) Pyogenic arthritis in infants and children: A review of 95 cases. Pediatr Infect Dis; 5:669

21. Tien Y, Chih H, Lin G, Hsien S, Lin S (1999) Clinical application of ultrasonography for detection of septic arthritis in children. Kaohsiung J Med Sci 15:542–549

22. Mah ET, LeQuesne GW, Gent RJ, Paterson DC (1994) Ultrasonic features of acute osteomyelitis in children. J Bone Joint Surg (Br) 76:969–974

23. George E, Creamer P, Dieppe PA (1994) Clinical subsets of osteoarthritis. J Musculoskel Med 11:14

24. McCrae F, Shouls J, Dieppe P, Watt I (1992) Scintigraphic assessment of osteoarthritis of the knee joint. Ann Rheum Dis 51:939–942

25. Coy JT III, Wofl CR, Brower TD, Winter WG Jr (1976) Pyogenic arthritis of the sacro-iliac joint. J Bone Joint Surg 58A:845–849

26. Delbarre F, Rondier J, Delrieu F et al (1975)Pyogenic infection of the sacroiliac joint. Report of thirteen cases. J Bone Joint Surg 57A:819–825

27. Nixon GW (1978) Hematogenous osteomyelitis of metaphyseal-equivalent locations. AJR 130:123–129

28. Bozkurt MF, Ugur O, Ertenli I, Caner B (2001) Combined use of bone and bone marrow scintigraphies for the diagnosis of active sacroiliitis: a new approach. Ann Nucl Med 15:117–121

29. Branson HM, Barnsley L, Duggan JE, Allman KC (2001) A novel pattern of abnormal spinal uptake on Tc-99m MDP skeletal scintigraphy in ankylosing spondylitis. Clin Nucl Med 26:1037–1038

30. Yildiz A, Gungor F, Tuncer T, Karayalcin B (2001) Evaluation of sacroiliitis using 99mTc-nanocolloid and 99mTc-MDP scintigraphy. Nucl Med Commun 22:785–794

31. Schwartz GS, Berenyi MR, Siegel MW (1969) Atrophic arthropathy and diabetic neuritis. Am J Roentgenol Radium Ther Nucl Med106:523–529

32. Horwitz SH (1993) Diabetic neuropathy. Clin Orthop 296:78–85

33. Gold RH, Tang DTF, Crim JR, Seeger LL (1995) Imaging the diabetic foot. Skeletal Radiol 24:563–571

34. Luong AA. Salonen DC (2000) Imaging of the seronegative spondyloarthropathies. Curr Rheumatol Rep 2:288–296

35. Rupani HD, Holder LE, Espinola DA et al (1985) Three phase radionuclide bone imaging in sports medicine. Radiology 156:187–196

36. Yun M, Kim W, Adam LE, Alnafisi N, Herman C, Alavi A (2001) F-18 FDG uptake in a patient with psoriatic arthritis: imaging correlation with patient symptoms. Clin Nucl Med 26:692–693

37. Willkens RF, Arnett FC, Bitter T et al (1981) Reiter's syndrome: evaluation of preliminary criteria for definite disease. Arthritis Rheum 24:844–849

38. Palazzi C, Olivieri I, Salvarani C, D'Amico E, Alleva G, Vitullo P, Petricca A (2002) Reactive arthritis: advances in diagnosis and treatment. Reumatismo 54:105–112

39. Kim SH, Chung SK, Bahk YW et al (1999) Wholebody and pinhole bone scintigraphic manifestation of Reiter's syndrome: distribution patterns and early and characteristic signs. Eur J Nucl Med 26:163–170

40. Resnick D, Niwayama G (1988) Psoriatic arthritis. In: Resnick D, Niwayama G (eds) Diagnosis of bone and joint disorders, 2nd edn. Saunders, Philadelphia

41. Conn DL, Hunder GG, O'Duffy JD (1993) In: Kelley WS, Harris ED, Ruddy S, Sledge CB (eds) Textbook of rheumatology, chap 64. Saunders, Philadelphia

42. Tietze A (1921) Über eine eigenartige Häufung von Fällen mit Dystrophie der Rippenknorpel. Berl Klin Wochenschr 58:829–831

43. Helms CA(1995) Fundamentals of skeletal radiology, 2nd edn. Saunders, Philadelphia, pp 172–173

44. Sain AK (1978) Bone scan in Tietze's syndrome. Clin Nucl Med 3:470–471

45. Yang WJ, Bahk YW, Chung SK et al (1994) Pinhole scintigraphic manifestations of Tietze's disease. Eur J Nucl Med 21:947–952

46. Bhosale P, Barron B, Lamki L (2001) The „SAPHO" syndrome: a case report of a patient with unusual bone scan findings. Clin Nucl Med 26:619–621

47. Rosenthall L (1987) The bone scan in arthritis. In: Fogelman I (ed) Bone scanning in clinical practice. Springer, Berlin Heidelberg New York

48. BahkY (2000) Combined scintigraphic and radiographic diagnosis of bone and joint diseases, 2nd edn. Springer, Berlin Heidelberg New York, pp 73–74

49. Handmaker H, Giammona ST (1984) Improved early diagnosis of acute inflammatory skeletal and articular disease in children: a two radiopharmaceutical approach. Pediatrics 73:661

50. Sullivan DC, Rosenfield NS, Ogden J et al (1980) Problems in the scintigraphic detection of osteomyelitis in children. Radiology 135:731

51. Bravo JF, Herman JH, Smith CH (1967) Musculoskeletal disorders after renal homotransplantation. Ann Intern Med 66:87–104

52. Spencer JD (1986) Bone and joint infection in a renal unit. J Bone Joint Surg (Br) 68:489–493

53. Dorwart RH, Genant HK, Johnston WH, Morris JM (1984) Pigmented villonodular synovitis of synovial joints: clinical, pathologic and radiologic features. AJR 143:877–885

54. Yudd AP, Velchik MG (1985) Pigmented villonodular synovitis of the hip. Clin Nucl Med 10:441–442

55. Makhija M, Stein I, Grossman R (1992) Bone imaging in pigmented villonodular synovitis of the knee. Clin Nucl Med 17:340–343

56. Shanley DJ, Auber AE, Watabe JT, Buckner AB (1992) Pigmented villonodular synovitis of the knee demonstrated on bone scan. Correlation with US, CT, and MRI. Clin Nucl Med 17:901–902

57. Caluser C, Healey J, Macapinlac H, Kostakoglu L, Abdel-Dayem HM, Larson SM, Yeh SD (1992) Tl-201 uptake in recurrent pigmented villonodular synovitis. Correlation with three-phase bone imaging. Clin Nucl Med 17:751–753

58. Craig JG (1999) Infection: ultrasound-guided procedures. Radiol Clin North Am 37:669

59. Cardinol E, Bureau NJ, Aubin B, Chhem RK (2001) Role of ultrasound in musculoskeletal infections. Radiol Clin North Am 39:191–200

60. BahkY (2000) Combined scintigraphic and radiographic diagnosis of bone and joint diseases, 2nd edn. Springer, Berlin Heidelberg New York, pp 148–153

61. Canaso JJ, Barza M (1993) Soft tissue infections. Rheum Dis Clin North Am 19:293

62. Allwright SJ, Cooper RA, Nash P (1988) Trochanteric bursitis: bone scan appearance. Clin Nucl Med 13:561–564

63. Canaso JJ, Barza M (1993) Soft tissue infections. Rheum Dis Clin North Am 19:293

64. Weissman BN (1987) Spondyloarthropathies. Radiol Clin North Am 25:1235–1262

65. Govan A Macfarlane P, Callander R (1988) Pathology illustrated, 2nd edn. Churchill Livingstone, Edinburgh

Diagnosis of Soft Tissue Calcification

8

There are three major types of extraosseous calcification: dystrophic, metastatic and heterotopic. Dystrophic calcification involves the deposition of calcium in damaged tissue and is not usually associated with hypercalcemia. In metastatic calcification, calcium deposition occurs in normal tissue due to hypercalcemia and/or hyperphosphatemia due to a variety of disease conditions, particularly metabolic disorders following renal failure. Heterotopic ossification describes a unique condition that may, or may not, follow trauma and is due to a complex pathogenetic mechanism believed to be due to transformation of certain primitive cells of mesenchymal origin in the connective tissue septa within muscles, into bone-forming cells. Bone scanning can detect all types of soft tissue calcification, usually serendipitously, in cases of dystrophic and metastatic calcification. In the case of heterotopic ossification, bone scanning has a more defined role in early diagnosis of the condition, in follow-up and in determining the proper timing of surgical intervention. Cardiac calcinosis, which is one of the rare findings of metastatic calcification, can be fatal and bone scanning can be a sensitive noninvasive method for its detection; this is in addition to the occasional discovery as an incidental finding on a bone scan performed for other reasons. Calcification of the skin, or calcinosis cutis, can occasionally be seen on bone scans and familiarity with the findings as well as the patterns of other types of calcification help enrich the diagnostic value of the bone scintigraphy. Scintigraphy is useful in evaluating the degree of muscle necrosis of rhabdomyolysis.

8.1
Introduction

Scintigraphy is able to detect certain soft tissue pathologies. Soft-tissue calcification is an important example of a condition that can be suspected during diagnosis or it can be found serendipitously when scintigraphy is performed during the investigation for another suspected pathology. Calcification of soft tissue can be seen using several scintigraphic studies; however, bone scan is the main scintigraphic modality that is able to visualize the condition. Pathological calcification can be classified into three major types: dystrophic calcification, metastatic calcification, and heterotopic bone formation. Certain forms, however, can be difficult to classify into these categories since they may involve more than one variety. One example is calcinosis cutis, which will be considered separately. Familiarity with the appearance of extraskeletal soft-tissue calcification is important since it can help identify certain disease processes and aid in the differential diagnosis of a skeletal abnormality.

8.2
Dystrophic Calcification

This type of calcification occurs in the setting of normal serum calcium and phosphate levels. The primary abnormality is damaged, inflamed, neoplastic, or necrotic tissue. Tissue damage may be from mechanical, chemical, infectious, or other factors. Calcification usually is localized to a specific area of tissue which is

Table 8.1. Causes of dystrophic calcification

Localized
Trauma
Tumors
Necrosis
Inflammation
Degenerative conditions
Chemotherapy-induced tissue damage
Amyloidosis
Repeated heel sticks in the newborn

Generalized
Connective tissue diseases
Dermatomyositis
Lupus erythematosus
Systemic sclerosis
CREST disease (calcinosis cutis, Raynaud phenomenon,
    esophageal dysfunction, sclerodactyly, telangiectasias)
Subcutaneous fat necrosis of the newborn
Pancreatic calcification
Ehlers-Danlos syndrome
Pseudoxanthoma elasticum
Werner syndrome*
Rothmund-Thompson syndrome**

* A rare autosomal recessive disease, characterized by premature ageing of connective tissues caused by a mutation in the
   gene RecQ helicase which is involved in DNA replication
   and cell reproduction.
** A hereditary and familial disease characterized by short
   stature, cataracts, pigmentation of skin, baldness, abnormalities of bones, nails and teeth caused by a mutation in
   the gene RecQ helicase

injured, although it may be generalized in some disorders (Table 8.1). The mechanism appears to be loss of
intracellular calcium in the injured cells with an increased calcium-binding capacity. Examples include
calcification in infarcted myocardial muscle, athero-
mas, amyloid tissue, fibrocystic disease of the breast
and in the centers of tumors such as lymphomas, breast
tumors, ovarian fibroma, hepatoblastoma and other
primary and metastatic tumors (Figs. 8.1, 8.2). In lymphomas it is reported to occur after therapy, and only
rarely before therapy, and it is more commonly seen in
non-Hodgkin's lymphomas [1–6]. Benign and malignant breast disease, in particular fibrocystic disease,
commonly show dystrophic calcification, which can be
seen in many patients on mammography as patterns of
micro-calcification that can differentiate benign from
malignant tumors [7]; it can also be seen incidentally
on bone scans (Fig. 8.3). Certain skin tumors, such as
pilomatrixoma (or calcifying epithelioma of Malherbe)
have a particular tendency to calcify; the syringomas
and basal cell carcinomas less frequently calcify. Arterial calcium deposits detected usually by radiography
and sometimes noted on bone scans (Fig. 8 4), are considered to be a marker of sub-clinical atherosclerotic
disease and an independent predictor of subsequent
vascular morbidity and mortality [8].

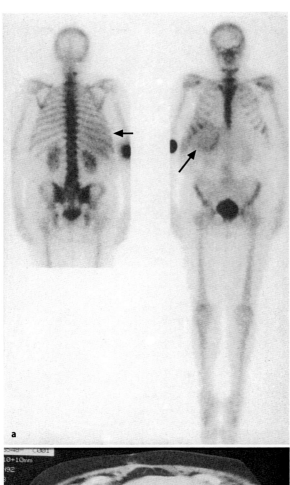

a

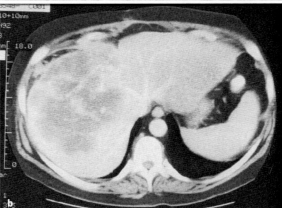

b

Fig. 8.1a, b. Bone scan (**a**) showing calcification in a liver metastases in a patient with breast cancer. CT scan (**b**) illustrates the
hepatic metastases

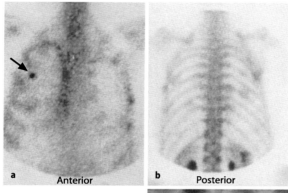

Fig. 8.2a, b. Two examples of breast calcification due to fibrocystic disease seen incidentally on bone scans

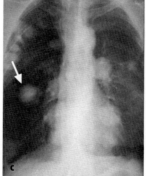

a Anterior   b Posterior

Fig. 8.3a–c. Anterior and posterior chest images of a bone scan (**a–b**) show dystrophic calcification (*arrow*) in lung cancer. Chest x-ray (**c**) shows the tumor (*arrow*)

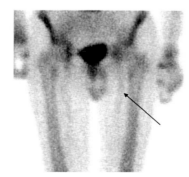

Fig. 8.4. Arterial calcium deposits (*arrow*) seen on bone scan of a diabetic patient

8.3
Metastatic Calcification

Metastatic calcification, first described by Virchow in 1855, describes the calcification of viable undamaged normal tissue as a result of hypercalcemia and/or hyperphosphatemia. This may be associated with an increased calcium phosphate product locally or systemically. This can be due to metabolic alterations such as with renal failure, hemodialysis, hypervitaminosis D and hyperparathyroidism, or it may be due to increased bone demineralization resulting from bone tumors or disseminated metastases (Table 8.2). Therapy with phosphate, steroids, and calcium infusion has also resulted in metastatic calcification. Calcium deposition is frequently widespread. The calcifying process affects principally the blood vessels, periarticular soft tissue, lungs, stomach, kidneys, and the myocardium, and to a lesser extent the skin and skeletal muscles of the extremities (Fig. 8.5). There are diffuse and nodular forms, with the diffuse form being more common [9–11]. Metastatic calcification, affecting the myocardium and lungs is a frequent and potential lethal complication of chronic renal failure (Figs. 8.6, 8.7), which is rarely detected before death because of the absence of specific radiographic abnormalities [11]. When metastatic calcification is peri-articular, large deposits are frequently found around the large joints, such as the knees, elbows, and shoulders, with a symmetrical distribution. A specific form of metastatic calcification that currently has no treatment is calciphylaxis. This condition has a high mortality rate, is often found in patients with renal failure and is characterized by soft tissue calcification and painful skin ulceration. A serum calcium-phosphorus product of more than 60 mg/dl indicates a high risk for calciphylaxis. The diagnosis is made by an incisional biopsy showing calcification of the small, subcutaneous arteries [12].

Table 8.2. Causes of metastatic calcification

Chronic renal failure
Hemodialysis
Hypervitaminosis D
Primary or secondary hyperparathyroidism
Paraneoplastic hypercalcemia
Destructive bone disease
Milk-alkali syndrome
Sarcoidosis
Calciphylaxis*

Tissue calcification in response to administration of an agent after induction of a hypersensitive state.

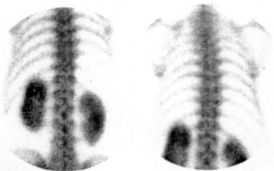

Fig. 8.5. Metastatic calcification affecting kidneys of a patient with hypercalcemia

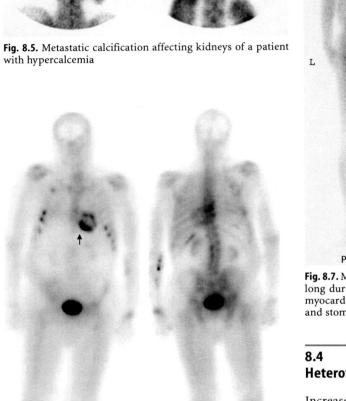

a   Anterior   Posterior

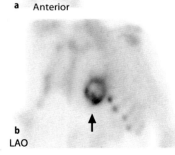

b
LAO

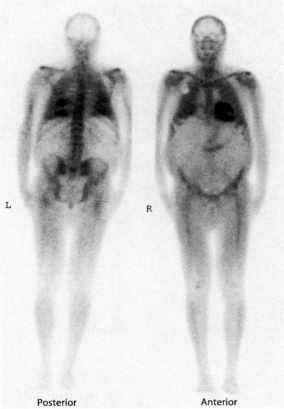

L   R

Posterior   Anterior

Fig. 8.7. Metastatic calcification in a patient with renal failure of long duration with diffuse Tc99m MDP uptake in the lungs, myocardium and stomach uptake in the lungs, myocardium and stomach on whole body bone scan

8.4
Heterotopic Bone Formation

Increased ectopic osteoblastic activity, or heterotopic bone formation (HBF), is defined as the presence of bone in soft tissue where it does not normally exist. HBF was first described in 1883 by Reidel, and in 1918 Dejerne and Ceillier reported that HBF frequently occurred among soldiers who had experienced spinal cord trauma as combatants in World War I [13].

8.4.1
Pathophysiology

There are two major forms of HBF: acquired and hereditary. By far the more common is the acquired form, in which HBF is usually either precipitated by trauma (such as fracture, total hip arthroplasty, or direct mus-

◁

Fig. 8.6a, b. Cardiocalcinosis of an 84-year-old man with a history of longstanding chronic renal failure, history of liver failure and renal transplants. Note the intense uptake (*arrow*) in the heart noted on whole body (**a**) and chest LAO view (**b**) of Tc99m MDP bone scans

cular trauma) or has a neurogenic cause (such as spinal cord injury or central nervous system injury). The rare hereditary form is known as myositis ossificans progressiva. The acquired form of HBF may occur after virtually any type of musculoskeletal trauma. Other conditions associated with HBF include burns, sickle-cell disease, hemophilia, tetanus, poliomyelitis, multiple sclerosis, toxic epidermal necrolysis and cancer. HBF occurs infrequently in the absence of a precipitating event or condition. HBF includes specific entities such as myositis ossificans and neurogenic heterotopic ossification. Myositis ossificans describes a post-traumatic soft-tissue ossification that occurs next to long bones. In many clinical practices, myositis ossificans is usually seen among patients who have sustained trauma such as operative procedures, e.g., total hip arthroplasty (THA), fractures, dislocations, and direct trauma to muscle groups (mainly the quadriceps femoris and brachialis muscles). Other reported sites include abdominal incisions, wounds, and sites in the gastrointestinal tract [14]. The neurogenic form follows trauma to the 'nervous system' and is most commonly seen after spinal cord injury. Patients are typically adolescents, or adults, with 75% of patients below 30 years of age with no sex predominance. This subtype often occurs after closed head injuries, strokes, central nervous system infarctions, and tumors [15, 16]. Tumoral calcinosis, another specific form of HBF, features large amounts of bone formation resembling tumor masses.

The incidence of acquired HBF varies greatly among patient populations. Among patients with spinal cord injury, the incidence ranges from 20% to 30%, and once HBF develops there is up to a 35% chance that the patient will eventually have significantly limited joint motion [17]. Among patients with closed head injury, HBF develops in 10–20%, and in 10% of these patients with HBF, limitations in joint motion will develop [15]. The incidence of HBF after total hip arthroplasty has been reported to range from 0.6% to 90%, although most studies agree that the incidence of HBF is approximately 50–55% [17–19]. The HBF that forms after THA is commonly minor and not clinically significant.

The onset of HBF usually occurs 3–12 weeks after injury, most commonly at 2 months post-injury, although it can occur as late as 1 year, or even later. The most commonly involved areas, in decreasing order of frequency, are hip, knee, shoulder and elbow. Only rarely is the foot involved [20, 21]. In spinal cord injury, HBF always occurs below the level of injury. At the knee, the medial aspect is most commonly affected. In patients with head injury or stroke, HBF almost always occurs on the affected side.

The pathogenesis of HBF is distinct from metastatic and dystrophic soft-tissue calcification and is still debated. However, it is believed to be secondary to transformation of pluripotent mesenchymal cells present in the connective tissue septa within muscle into osteogenic cell line [22]. Chalmers et al. [23] proposed three conditions needed for heterotopic ossification (HO): osteogenic precursor cells, induction agents, and a permissive environment. Urist et al. [22] postulated a small (<0.025 µm), hydrophobic bone morphogenetic protein, which would be capable of changing the development of mesenchymal cells in muscle from fibrous tissue into bone (when respiratory and nutritional requirements are also present) [22]. It has been postulated that the bone morphogenetic protein is liberated from normal bone in response to venous stasis, inflammation, or diseases of the connective tissue attachments to bone, conditions that often accompany immobilization or trauma [22]. Some investigators proposed the presence of a centrally mediated factor [24, 25] and prostaglandin E_2 (PGE_2) has recently been suggested as a mediator in the differentiation of the primitive mesenchymal cells [26]. The heterotopic bone may begin some distance from normal bone, moving towards it later [22]. Interestingly, experiments have also shown that muscle injury alone will not cause the ectopic ossification, concomitant bone damage also being required [22]. Kurer et al. [27] took sera from four paraplegic patients with HBF and four paraplegic patients without HBF; the sera were incubated with human osteoblasts in tissue culture, and their metabolic activity was measured quantitatively. These investigators found that the sera of the patients with HBF had significantly greater levels of osteoblast-stimulating factors, which may contribute to the pathogenesis of HBF. Other contributing factors include hypercalcemia, tissue hypoxia, changes in sympathetic nerve activity, prolonged immobilization, remobilization, and disequilibrium of parathyroid hormone and calcitonin [28, 29].

Early in the course of HBF, edema with exudative cellular infiltrate is present, followed by fibroblastic proliferation and osteoid formation [30]. The distinctive morphological features of myositis ossificans, which are illustrative of HBF as a whole, help the pathologist distinguish myositis ossificans from malignant neoplasms such as parosteal osteosarcoma or osteochondroma. Bone formation occurs in the connective tissue between the muscle planes and not within the muscle itself [30]. Myositis ossificans shows ossification principally in the periphery, so that an ossified and radiopaque peripheral rim surrounds a nonossified and radiolucent center; the opposite is true of osteosarcoma, a malignant tumor that often features dense central ossification [5, 31]. On histological examination, myositis ossificans shows cellular fibrous proliferation, osteoid, and primitive bone, which, if biopsied too early, may be mistaken for that of osteosarcoma [5]. Rossier noted that, after approximately 30 months, the pattern in HBF approached that of normal young adult bone [32]. Anatomically, paraarticular HBF is always

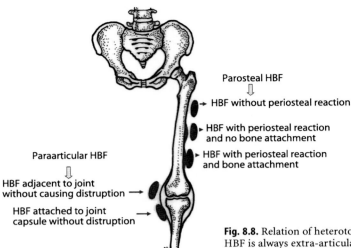

Parosteal HBF
⇩
HBF without periosteal reaction

HBF with periosteal reaction
and no bone attachment

HBF with periosteal reaction
and bone attachment

Paraarticular HBF
⇩
HBF adjacent to joint
without causing distruption →

HBF attached to joint
capsule without distruption →

Fig. 8.8. Relation of heterotopic bone formation to the joints and bone cortex. HBF is always extra-articular, but it may be attached to the joint capsule without disrupting it. Occasionally, HBF may be attached to the cortex of adjacent bone with, or without, cortical disruption

extra-articular [27, 30, 32], but it may be attached to the joint capsule without disrupting it. Occasionally, HBF may be attached to the cortex of adjacent bone with, or without, cortical disruption (Fig. 8.8).

The course of acquired heterotopic bone formation is relatively benign in 80% or more of cases. In the remaining cases, patients often develop significant loss of motion, and ankylosis occurs in up to 10%. Loss of joint mobility and the resulting loss of function are the principal complications of HBF [20, 33, 34]. Other complications include peripheral nerve entrapment and pressure ulcers [35, 36]. HBF following spinal cord injury can lead to various complications, including venous thrombosis, autonomic dysreflexia, and pressure ulcers, and can be refractory to oral indomethacin and local irradiation [37] Mesan and Bassano reported an acute fracture occurring through pre-existing, quiescent, post-traumatic HBF of the gastrocnemius muscle as a rare sequela of HBF [38]. Clinical, laboratory, radiographic and scintigraphic criteria have been used to follow the course of HBF and to assist in its treatment

During formation of HBF, initially immature connective tissue, fibroblasts, ground substance, and collagen fibers are seen. Eventually, usually within 7–14 days, osteoblasts are noted, located irregularly in osteoid. New bone formation may start with multiple foci within the mass of immature connective tissue. Hypervascularity is noted where these centers of ossification appear. As mineralization progresses, amorphous calcium phosphate gradually is replaced by enlarging hydroxyapatite crystals. These multiple foci of osteogenesis may be of simultaneous onset within the lesion, but do not necessarily evolve at identical rates.

Commonly, after approximately 6 months, the appearance of true bone is noted, with cancellous bone, mature lamellar bone and bone marrow which contains predominantly adipose tissue and only a minor amount of hematopoiesis (if any). The mature bone appear intermixed with immature bone until full maturation into lamellar corticospongiosal bone occurs.

Serial serum alkaline phosphatase estimations can be useful. Elevation suggests bone growth, but the amount of increase is not proportional to the extent of HBF. The alkaline phosphatase level also may return to normal before maturity, or it may remain elevated for a prolonged period.

8.4.2
Scintigraphic Evaluation

Multiphase bone scanning is the most useful investigation, as it can detect HBF at the onset of clinical symptoms. These early phases are the most important for early diagnosis and monitoring of the ossification process. Freed [39] evaluated the three-phase bone scan in the detection of HBF and found that a marked vascular blush and increased blood pool about the hips preceded the development of clinical HBF by 2–4 weeks. Assessment of the maturity of the HBF is important because of the fact that resection prior to maturity almost always leads to a recurrence of HBF. Bone scans are currently considered to be the most reliable means of determining the maturity of HO. Serial bone scans, performed weekly for 4–6 weeks, with decreasing uptake over time suggests maturation, although uptake can vary with serial examinations that make assessment of maturation less than 100% accurate.

Blood flow and pool images have detected incipient heterotopic bone formation 2 1/2 weeks after injury, with delayed scintigraphs becoming positive about 1 week later. These scintigraphic findings precede positive radiographs by 1–4 weeks [40]. Scintigraphically,

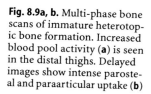

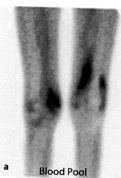

Fig. 8.9a, b. Multi-phase bone scans of immature heterotopic bone formation. Increased blood pool activity (**a**) is seen in the distal thighs. Delayed images show intense parosteal and paraarticular uptake (**b**)

a   Blood Pool

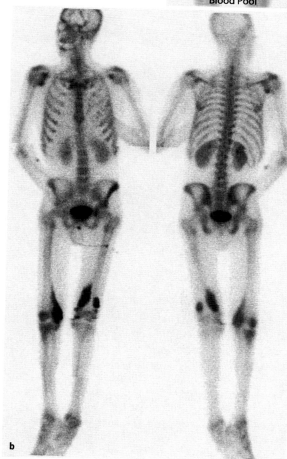

b

during the immature phase often leads to recurrence, serial bone scans are useful in monitoring the activity of the disease in order to determine the appropriate time for the surgical removal of heterotopic bone with minimal risk of recurrence. In several reported series, pre-operative serial bone scans, with quantitation of the uptake ratios between heterotopic and normal bone, have successfully identified those patients who remained free of heterotopic ossification following surgery (i.e. those patients with decreasing, or stable, scintigraphic activity as measured by this quantitative technique). Serial bone scans have been used successfully to monitor the metabolic activity of HBF and determine the appropriate time for surgical resection, if needed, and to predict post-operative recurrence [32, 39, 41, 42]. A technique can be used for the serial quantitative bone scanning to assess the maturity of heterotopic ossification – based on the original 1977 report of Tanaka et al. [42]. The quantitation method of serial bone scans can also be a useful objective means to stage the maturity and can be obtained simply using serial determinations of abnormal uptake relative to a normal skeletal structure. Serial quantitative bone scans that show a sharply decreasing trend followed by a steady state over a 2- to 3-month period are the most reliable scintigraphic parameter for determining whether HBF has reached maturity [43].

Several pathologic conditions can clinically mimic the scintigraphic appearance of early HBF (Table 8.3). Osteomyelitis may represent a difficult diagnostic challenge on scintigraphy, particularly since gallium-67- and, rarely, indium-111-labeled white blood cells accumulate in areas of immature heterotopic bone formation. The uptake of gallium-67 by foci of heterotopic bone formation undergoing osteogenesis, with considerable osteoblastic activity, may be explained by the fact that this radionuclide shares some of the properties of bone imaging agents. Fortunately, gallium-67 uptake in HBF has been found to be proportional to the uptake of Tc-diphosphonates, in contrast to its relatively greater uptake in sites of osteomyelitis. Since gallium-67 uptake otherwise might be mistaken for infection or a tumor, this proportionality can help differentiate HBF from osteomyelitis. Therefore, in the appropriate clinical setting, HBF is a diagnostic consideration for patients with a positive gallium-67 scan [16].

Table 8.3. Conditions clinically mimicking early heterotopic bone formation

Infection
Osteomyelitis
Cellulitis
Thrombophlebitis
Deep vein thrombosis
Neoplasms including recurrent tumors
Osteosarcoma
Osteochondroma

the condition is classified as immature when the blood flow and blood pool activity are increased (Figs. 8.9–8.10). When the blood flow and blood pool patterns normalize, or stabilize, after showing decreasing activity, the condition is considered to be mature. As heterotopic bone progresses from immature to mature, the three-phase bone scan typically shows progressive reduction in the activity of all three phases (Fig. 8.11). The majority of bone scans return to baseline within 12 months, although some patients reach the mature phase much earlier, or later. Since surgical intervention

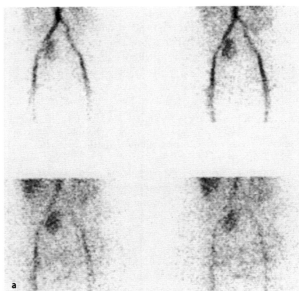

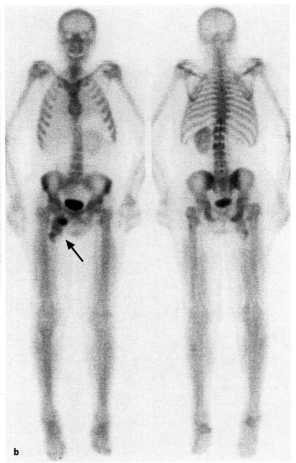

Fig. 8.10a, b. A case of immature heterotopic bone formation of the right groin seen on a flow (**a**) and delayed (**b**) images.

8.4.3
Correlative Imaging

On standard radiographs, soft tissue calcification must occur for radiographic evidence of HBF to be present, radiographs are not helpful in the early stages.

Radiological examinations do not show evidence of HBF until a flocculent patchy appearance develops, as calcium is deposited about 7–10 days after the onset of clinical symptoms. This patchy appearance coalesces and enlarges on subsequent examinations, and, by 2–3 months, the boundaries of the HBF demarcate with the appearance of mature bone. Radiographs, however, are not reliable at assessing maturity of HBF as the more mature areas may hide immature areas. Computed tomography (CT) and magnetic resonance imaging (MRI) may be useful in delineating the local anatomy prior to resection. However, the role of CT and MRI in the evaluation of other aspects of HBF, such as maturity, has not been well established.

8.4.4
Special Forms of Heterotopic Bone Formation
8.4.4.1
Myositis Ossificans Progressiva

One congenital and rare form of HBF is called myositis ossificans progressiva or fibrodysplasia ossificans progressiva [44]. This autosomal dominant congenital disease is often associated with other skeletal abnormalities, including malformation of the great toes and shortening of digits, as well as other clinical features

such as deafness and baldness. Although the symptoms have been reported to develop in patients with this disease prior to 4 years of age, the diagnosis is frequently missed [45]. The soft tissue ossification present may be mistakenly attributed to bruising or even a sarcoma. Initial failure to appreciate the significance of the toe and other digit malformations is also common. Progression to a severely impaired joint mobility with ankylosis by early adulthood is the hallmark of this disease. Radiologically, there are several features including soft tissue calcification of the subcutaneous and fascial connective tissue, tendons, ligaments and skeletal muscles, exostoses, joint malformations, abnormal vertebral bodies and changes to the hands and feet. Scintigraphically some features could be identified (Fig. 8.12), particularly the soft tissue calcification around the joints, mandible, maxilla, shoulders, ribs, parasternal and paraspinal regions, which are seen as areas of increased uptake [44].

Flow   Blood pool   Delayed

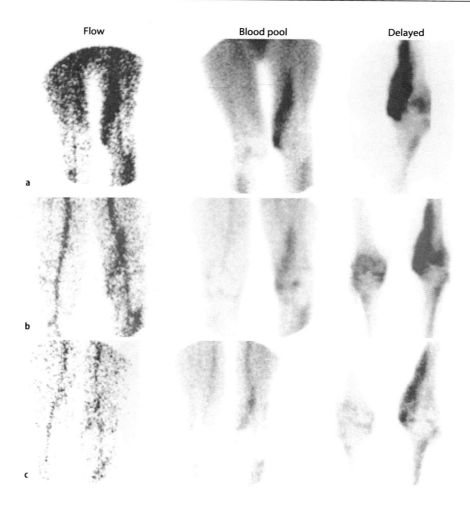

Fig. 8.11. As heterotopic bone develops from immature to mature, the three-phase bone scans typically show a progressive reduction in the activity of all three phases from initial study (**a**) to 12 mo (**b**) and 18 mo (**c**) follow-up studies at teh site of HBF in the medial aspect of the distal left thigh (From [16] with permission)

8.4.4.2
Tumoral Calcinosis

Tumoral calcinosis is an unusual and benign condition characterized by large, calcified, peri-articular soft-tissue masses of calcium phosphate near the large joints such as the hip, the shoulder, and the elbow, in addition to the wrist, feet, and hands. The condition is uncommon in the spine and rarely reported around the temporomandibular joint [46]. This peri-articular calcium deposition can be observed in the absence of vascular, or visceral, calcification and is associated with normocalcemia and normal kidney function which can be sub-classified as a primary form (idiopathic or hereditary). However, the condition may also be found in a wide variety of conditions, such as primary or secondary hyperparathyroidism, scleroderma, renal osteodystrophy associated with chronic renal disease, hypervitaminosis D, milk-alkali syndrome, trauma and sarcoidosis [47–51]. The condition is observed with increasing frequency in patients with chronic renal failure on dialysis. Although tumoral calcinosis has been reported in patients ranging from age 5 months to 83 years, it usually becomes manifest in the second decade of life. Men and nonwhites are affected more commonly than women and Caucasians. A family history is apparent in 30–40% of cases, and an autosomal recessive pattern of inheritance has been suggested [52–54]. Familial cerebral and peripheral vascular aneurysms have also been reported in association with tumoral calcinosis. Patients may be admitted to surgical clinics because of tumor-like painless swellings, which may be solitary or multiple. They may interfere with joint motion, although calcification does not involve the joints and the bones, and before they are diagnosed sufficiently the patients experience repeated surgical excisions associated with loss of function [49]. In a literature review of 121 cases of tumoral calcinosis, Smack et al proposed three pathogenetically distinct subtypes of tumoral calcinosis: (1) primary normophosphatemic tumoral calcinosis, in which patients have normal serum phosphate, normal serum calcium, and no evidence of disorders previously associated with soft tissue calcifica-

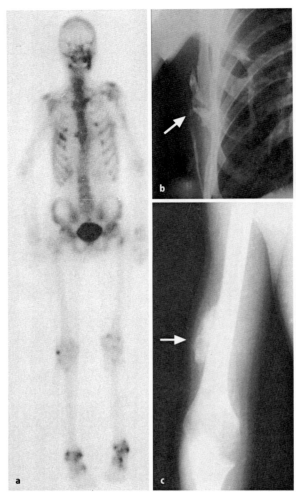

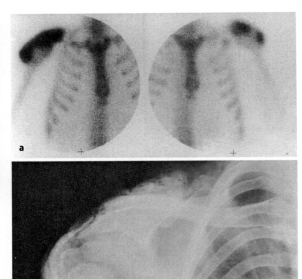

Fig. 8.13a, b. Tumoral calcinosis: selective spot views of Tc99m MDP bone scan of the chest (**a**) showing increase uptake in the right shoulder and to a lesser extent the left shoulder region. Corresponding calcified masses around the right shoulder seen on radiograph (**b**)

Fig. 8.12a–c. A case of myositis ossificans progressiva with a whole body scan (**a**) showing multiple foci of increased uptake in the regions of the mandible bilaterally, chest, mid left arm, left trochanter area, right knee, and feet. Radiographs of the chest (**b**) and left arm (**c**) illustrating the soft tissue calcification (*arrows*) corresponding to the findings of bone scan at these areas. (From [44] with permission)

tion; (2) primary hyperphosphatemic tumoral calcinosis, in which patents have elevated serum phosphate but normal serum calcium, and no evidence of disorders previously associated with soft tissue calcification; and (3) secondary tumoral calcinosis, in which patients have a concurrent disease capable of causing soft tissue calcification [55].

Radionuclide imaging is the most reliable and simplest method of detecting and quantifying the lesions. The calcified masses show increased uptake of Tc-99m diphosphonates (Fig. 8.13). Characteristically, the calcified masses in the appendicular skeleton are visible on plain radiographs. The radiographs usually reveal lobulated, homogeneous, densely calcified peri-articular masses, usually around the large joints, with normal joint spaces. Sometimes the condition may not be apparent on standard radiographs and may not be diagnosed as tumoral calcinosis before surgery. CT can disclose the presence of fluid-calcium levels (sedimentation sign), and MRI displays a low signal density on T1- and T2-weighted images [56, 57].

These radiological characteristics allow tumoral calcinosis to be distinguished in many cases from other diseases which produce soft-tissue calcification, although a biopsy may be needed to exclude musculoskeletal tumor [58, 59].

8.4.4.3
Progressive Osseous Heteroplasia

Progressive osseous heteroplasia is a recently identified disorder characterized by HBF with the development of highly structured, mineralized tissue histologically identifiable as true bone. It is uncommon and can cause a variety of clinical features such as short metacarpals and metatarsals. The condition appears to affect females more than males and is sporadic, although familial associations and atypical phenotypes have been reported [60].

8.4.4.4
Tumoral Calcium Pyrophosphate Dihydrate Crystal Deposition Disease

This rare condition is another variant of HBF that can also produce large masses of calcium deposits simulating tumoral calcinosis. It is seen in adults and is more common in males. Histologically, there is calcification with crystal deposits and chondroid metaplasia. The majority of crystals are rhomboid in shape (characteristic of calcium pyrophosphate dihydrate crystal deposition disease [CPPD]), but some needle-shaped crystals may also be identified, which resembled urate crystals. Yamakawa [61] reviewed 54 reported cases of tumoral CPPD and proposed two categories based on the anatomic location: the central (head and neck) type (33 patients) and the distal (extremity) type (21 patients). The patients in these two groups were not different with respect to age and gender, but those with the central type often presented with a painful mass (15 patients, 46%), or neurological disturbances (11 patients, 33%). Patients with the distal type presented with a painless mass or swelling (12 patients, 57%), but none had neurological signs, although 8 (38.1%) presented with an acute attack similar to tophaceous gout. Tumoral CPPD should be differentiated from tophaceous gout, tumoral calcinosis, and malignant or benign tumors [61].

8.5
Calcinosis Cutis

Calcinosis cutis is a term used to describe a group of disorders in which calcium deposits form in the skin, subcutaneous tissue and connective tissue sheaths around the muscles. Virchow initially described calcinosis cutis in 1855. Calcinosis cutis is presented here separately since is difficult to categorize with the dystrophic, metastatic or heterotopic types of calcification. Etiologically, dystrophic, metastatic, iatrogenic, and idiopathic varieties may be identified. Some rare types may even be variably classified as dystrophic or idiopathic. These include calcinosis cutis circumscripta and calcinosis cutis universalis. Most lesions of calcinosis cutis develop gradually and are asymptomatic. However, the history and evolution of the lesions depends on the etiology of the calcification. Patients with dystrophic calcification may provide a history of an underlying disease, a pre-existing dermal nodule (which represents a tumor), or an inciting traumatic event. Patients with metastatic calcification most frequently have a history of chronic renal failure. Cases of idiopathic calcinosis cutis usually are not associated with prior trauma or disease. Those who develop iatrogenic calcinosis cutis generally have a history of recent hospitalization.

When the calcium deposits are localized to a small area it is called calcinosis cutis circumscripta and if it is diffuse it is called calcinosis cutis universalis. In all cases of calcinosis cutis, insoluble compounds of calcium primarily of hydroxyapatite crystals, or amorphous calcium phosphate, are deposited due to local and/or systemic factors. The pathogenesis of calcinosis cutis is not completely understood and a variety of factors can be recognized. Metabolic and physical factors are most important. Ectopic calcification can occur in the setting of hypercalcemia and/or hyperphosphatemia when the calcium-phosphate product exceeds 70 mg/dl, without preceding tissue damage. These elevated extracellular levels may result in increased intracellular levels, calcium-phosphate nucleation, and crystalline precipitation. Alternatively, damaged tissue may allow an influx of calcium ions, leading to an elevated intracellular calcium level and subsequent crystalline precipitation. Tissue damage also may result in denatured proteins that preferentially bind phosphate. Calcium then reacts with bound phosphate ions, leading to the precipitation of calcium phosphate [55, 62–68].

8.5.1
Calcinosis Cutis Universalis

This entity describes diffuse calcium deposits in the skin, subcutaneous tissue and connective tissue sheaths around the muscles but not within the muscles as is the case with myositis ossificans. It is seen mostly in association with scleroderma and polymyositis [69–72]. On bone scintigraphy it shows uptake of variable degrees in a diffuse fashion in large areas of the skin and subcutaneous regions.

8.5.2
Calcinosis Cutis Circumscripta

This condition is a form of localized calcium deposition in the skin. If dystrophic it is secondary to localized causes of dystrophic calcification such as trauma, insect bites, acne and certain skin tumors. If it is metastatic, or associated with systemic causes of dystrophic calcifications, it generally occurs earlier and tends to involve the extremities, whereas calcinosis universalis occurs later and usually is more widespread [73].

8.6
Rhabdomyolysis

Rhabdomyolysis, also called myoglobulinuria, is a condition that follows muscle damage secondary to infectious and noninfectious injuries including viral infections, electrical injury, certain drugs, trauma and excessive physical activity, as in runners and military re-

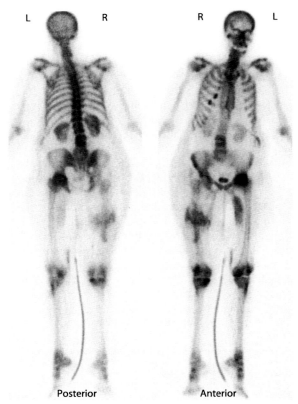

L   R   R   L

Posterior   Anterior

Fig. 8.14. Rhabdomyolysis of both thighs in a patient with a recent history of motor vehicle accident

cruits. The condition can be severe and life threatening. The most severe form is sometimes called crush syndrome. Milder forms are included in compartment syndromes. The condition is characterized by excess myoglobulin in the urine since intracellular muscle protein is released with muscle damage and appears in urine. Certain injuries will cause variable degrees of muscle death. The dead muscle will have an increased calcium content and is sensitively identified using Tc-99m MDP bone scanning which can be used to evaluate the degree of muscle necrosis. The influx of calcium ions into muscle cells occurs secondary to damaged cell membrane integrity which also allows bone seeking radiotracers to form stable complexes inside muscle cells [14]. A variable degree of abnormally increased uptake (Fig. 8.14) is seen in the affected muscle(s) [74–76].

References

1. Elgazzar AH, Jahan S, Motawei S et al (1989) Tc-99m MDP uptake in hepatoblastoma. Clin Nucl Med 14:143
2. Elgazzar AH, Abdel-Dayem HM, Higazi E (1989) Pattern of Tc-99m MDP in inflammatory breast carcinoma. Nucl Compact 20:58
3. Apter S, Avigdor A, Gayer G, Portnoy O, Zissin R, Hertz M (2002) Calcification in lymphoma occurring before therapy: CT features and clinical correlation. Am J Roentgenol 178:935–938
4. Mukhtar AU, Wasswa GM (2001) Non-functioning ovarian fibroma with extensive calcification: case report. East Afr Med J 78:557–558
5. Resnick D, Niwayama G (1988) Soft tissues. In: Resnick D, Niwayama G (eds) Diagnosis of bone and joint disorders, 2nd edn. Saunders, Philadelphia, pp 4171–4294
6. Ohmoto Y, Nishizaki T, Kajiwara K, Nomura S, Kameda H, Suzuki M (2002) Calcified metastatic brain tumor – two case reports. Neurol Med Chir 42:264–267
7. Fondrinier E, Lorimier G, Guerin-Boblet V, Bertrand AF, Mayras C, Dauver N (2002) Breast microcalcifications: multivariate analysis of radiologic and clinical factors for carcinoma. World J Surg 26:290–296
8. Wilson PW, Kauppila LI, O'Donnell CJ, Kiel DP, Hannan M, Polak JM, Cupples LA (2001) Abdominal aortic calcific deposits are an important predictor of vascular morbidity and mortality. Circulation 103:1529–1534
9. Silberstein EB, Elgazzar AH, Fernandez-Uloa M, Nishiyama H (1996) Skeletal scintigraphy in non-neoplatic osseous disorders. In: Henkin RE, Bles MA, Dillehay GL, Halama JR, Karesh SM, Wagner PH, Zimmer AM (eds) Textbook of nuclear medicine. Mosby, New York, pp 1141–1197
10. Nizami MA, Gerntholtz T, Swanepoel CR (2000) The role of bone scanning in the detection of metastatic calcification: a case report. Clin Nucl Med 25:407–409
11. Cesani F, Villanueva-Meyer J (1996) Myocardial and lung uptake of 99m-Tc-pyrophosphate using single photon emission computed tomography in a patient with end-stage renal disease and secondary hyperparathyroidism. Int Urol Nephrol 28:569–574
12. Parker RW, Mouton CP, Young DW, Espino DV (2003) Early recognition and treatment of calciphylaxis. South Med J 96:53–55
13. Dejerne A, Ceillier A (1918) Para-osteo-arthropathies des paraplegiques par lesion medullaire; etude clinique et radiographique. Ann Med 5:497
14. Hakim M. McCarthy EF (2001) Heterotopic mesenteric ossification. Am J Roentgenol 176:260–261
15. Garland D (1991) A clinical perspective on common forms of acquired heterotopic ossification. Clin Orthop Relat Res 263:13-29
16. Nagaraj N, Elgazzar AH, Fernandez-ULLOA M (1995) Heterotopic Ossification Mimicking Infection: Scintigraphic Evaluation. Clin Nucl Med 20:763–766
17. Stover SL, Niemann KM, Tulloss JR (1991) Experience with surgical resection of heterotopic bone in spinal cord injury patients. Clin Orthop 263:71–77
18. Thomas BJ (1992) Heterotopic bone formation after total hip arthroplasty. Orthop Clin North Am 23:347–358
19. Gibson CJ, Poduri KR (1997) Heterotopic ossification as a complication of toxic epidermal necrolysis. Arch Phys Med Rehabil 78:774–776
20. Wharton GW, Morgan TH (1970) Ankylosis in the paralyzed patient. J Bone Joint Surg (Am) 52:105–112
21. Allard MM, Thomas RL, Nicholas RW Jr (1997) Myositis ossification: an unusual presentation in the foot. Foot Ankle Int 18:39–42
22. Urist MR, Nakagawa M, Nakata N, Nogami H (1978) Experimental myositis ossificans: cartilage and bone formation in muscle in response to diffusible bone matrix-derived morphogen. Arch Pathol Lab Med 102:312–316
23. Chalmers J, Gray DH, Rush J (1975) Observations on the induction of bone in soft tissues. J Bone Joint Surg (Br) 57:36–45
24. Craven PL, Urist MR (1971) Osteogenesis by radioisotope labelled cell population in implants of bone matrix under

the influence of ionizing radiation. Clin Orthop 76:231–233

25. Puzas JE, Brand JS, Howard GA, Lio CC, Evarts CM (1984) Heterotopic bone formation after operation: a quantitative, histologic and biochemical study. Surg Forum 35:521–523]

26. Ho SSW, Stern PJ, Bruno LP et al (1988) Pharmacological inhibition of prostaglandin E-2 in bone and its effect on pathological new bone formation in a rat brain model. Trans Orthop Res Soc 13:536

27. Kurer MH, Khoker MA, Dandona P (1992) Human osteoblast stimulation by sera from paraplegic patients with heterotopic ossification. Paraplegia 30:165–168

28. Stover SL, Hataway CJ, Zeiger HE (1975) Heterotopic ossification in spinal cord-injured patients. Arch Phys Med Rehabil 56:199–204

29. Chantraine A, Minaire P (1981) Para-osteo-arthropathies: a new theory and mode of treatment. Scand J Rehabil Med 13:31–37

30. Jensen LL, Halar E, Little J, Brooke MM (1987) Neurogenic heterotopic ossification. Am J Phys Med Rehabil 66:351–363

31. Norman A, Dorfman HD (1970) Juxtacortical circumscribed myositis ossifications: evolution and radiographic features. Radiology 96:301–306

32. Rossier AB, Bussat P, Infante F et al (1973) Current facts on para-osteoarthropathy (POA). Paraplegia 11:36–78

33. Brooker AF, Bowerman JW, Robinson RA, Riley LH Jr (1973) Ectopic ossification following total hip replacement: incidence and method of classification. J Bone Joint Surg (Am) 55:1629–1632

34. Sawyer JR, Myers MA, Rosier RN, Puzas JE (1991) Heterotopic ossification: clinical and cellular aspects. Calcif Tissue Int 49:208–215

35. Brooke MM, Heard DL, de Lateur BJ et al (1991) Heterotopic ossification and peripheral nerve entrapment: early diagnosis and excision. Arch Phys Med Rehabil 72:425–429

36. Hassard GH (1975) Heterotopic bone formation about the hip and unilateral decubitus ulcers in spinal cord injury. Arch Phys Med Rehabil 56:355–358

37. Yin KS, James J, Lew K, Little JW (2001) Refractory heterotopic ossification with complications. J Spin Cord Med 24:119–122

38. Mestan MA. Bassano JM (2001) Fractured heterotopic bone in myositis ossificans traumatica. J Manipul Physiol Ther 24:296–299

39. Freed JH, Hahn H, Menter R, Dillon T (1982) The use of three-phase bone scan in the early diagnosis of heterotopic ossification (HO) and in the evaluation of Didronel therapy. Paraplegia 20:208–221

40. Orzel JA, Redd TG (1985) Heterotopic bone formation: clinical, laboratory and imaging correlation. J Nucl Med 26:125–132

41. Muheim G, Donath A, Rossier AB (1973) Serial scintigrams in the course of ectopic bone formation in paraplegic patients. AJR 118:865–869

42. Tanaka T, Rossier AB, Hussey RW, Ahnberg DS, Treves S (1977) Quantitative assessment of para-osteo-arthropathy and its maturation on serial radionuclide bone images. Radiology 123:217–221

43. Shehab D, Elgazzar A H, Collier B D (2002) Heterotopic ossification. J Nucl Med 43:346–353

44. Elgazzar AH, Martich V, Gelfand MJ (1995) Advanced fibrodysplasia ossificans progressiva. Clin Nucl Med 20:519–521

45. Smith R, Russell RG, Woods CG (1976) Myositis ossificans progressiva: clinical features of eight patients and their response to treatment. J Bone Joint Surg (Br) 58:48–57

46. Noffke C. Raubenheimer E. Fischer E.(2000) Tumoral calcinosis of the temporomandibular joint region. Dento Maxillo Facial Radiol 29:128–130

47. Noyez JF, Murphree SM, Chen K (1990) Tumoral calcinosis. A clinical report of eleven cases. Acta Orthop Belg 59:249–254

48. Steinbach LS, Johnston JO, Tepper EF, Honda GD, Martel W (1995) Tumoral calcinosis: radiologic-pathologic correlation. Skeletal Radiol 24:573–578

49. Savaci N, Avunduk MC, Tosun Z, Hosnuter M (2000) Hyperphosphatemic tumoral calcinosis. Plast Reconstr Surg 105:162–165

50. Arikawa J, Higaki Y, Mizushima J, Nogita T, Kawashima M (2000) Tumoral calcinosis: a case report with an electron microscopic study. Eur J Dermatol 10:52–54

51. García S, Cofán F, Combalia A, Campistol J-M, Oppenheimer F, Ramón R (2000)Compression of the ulnar nerve in Guyon's canal by uremic tumoral calcinosis. Arch Orthop Trauma Surg 120:228–230

52. Thakur A, Hines OJ, Thakur V, Gordon HE (1999) Tumoral calcinosis regression after subtotal parathyroidectomy: a case presentation and review of the literature. Review of reported cases. Surgery 126:95–98

53. Adams WM, Laitt RD, Davies M, O'Donovan DG (1999) Familial tumoral calcinosis: association with cerebral and peripheral aneurysm formation. Neuroradiology 41:351–355

54. Baldursson H, Evans EB, Dodge WF et al (1969) Tumoral calcinosis with hyperphosphatemia: a report of a family with incidence in four siblings. J Bone Joint Surg (Am) 51:913

55. Smack D, Norton SA, Fitzpatrick JE (1996) Proposal for a pathogenesis-based classification of tumoral calcinosis. Int J Dermatol 35:265–271

56. Durant DM, Riley LH III, Burger PC, McCarthy EF (2001) Tumoral calcinosis of the spine: a study of 21 cases. Spine 26:1673–1679

57. Matsukado K, Amano T, Itou O, Yuhi F, Nagata S (2001) Tumoral calcinosis in the upper cervical spine causing progressive radiculomyelopathy – case report. Neurol Med Chir 41:411–444

58. Noyez JF, Murphree SM, Chen K (1990) Tumoral calcinosis. A clinical report of eleven cases. Acta Orthop Belg 59:249–254

59. Steinbach LS, Johnston JO, Tepper EF, Honda GD, Martel W (1995) Tumoral calcinosis: radiologic-pathologic correlation. Skeletal Radiol 24:573–578

60. Stoll C, Javier MR, Bellocq JP (2000) Progressive osseous heteroplasia: an uncommon cause of ossification of soft tissues. Ann Genet 43:75–80

61. Yamakawa K, Iwasaki H, Ohjimi Y, Kikuchi M, Iwashita A, Isayama T, Naito M (2001) Tumoral calcium pyrophosphate dihydrate crystal deposition disease. A clinicopathologic analysis of five cases. Pathol Res Pract 197:499–506

62. Palmieri GM, Sebes JI, Aelion JA (1995) Treatment of calcinosis with diltiazem. Arthritis Rheum 38:1646–1654

63. Plott T, Wiss K, Raimer SS (1988) Recurrent subepidermal calcified nodule of the nose. Pediatr Dermatol 5:107–111

64. Rothe MJ, Grant-Kels JM, Rothfield NF(1995) Extensive calcinosis cutis with systemic lupus erythematosus. Arch Dermatol 126:1060–1063

65. Touart DM, Sau P (1998) Cutaneous deposition diseases, part II. J Am Acad Dermatol 39:527–544

66. Viegas SF, Evans EB, Calhoun J (1985) Tumoral calcinosis: a case report and review of the literature. J Hand Surg (Am) 10:744–748

67. Walsh JS, Fairley JA (1995) Calcifying disorders of the skin. J Am Acad Dermatol 33:693–706

68. Larsen MJ, Adcock KA, Satterlee WG (1985) Dermal up-

take of technetium-99m MDP in calcinosis cutis. Clin Nucl Med 10:780–782]

69. Matsuoka Y, Miyajima S, Okada N (1998) A case of calcinosis universalis successfully treated with low-dose warfarin. J Dermatol 25:716–720

70. Murthy VP. Rao GR. Rao PS (1998) Calcinosis universalis in a case of progressive systemic sclerosis. J Assoc Physic India 46:482–484

71. Eddy MC, Leelawattana R, McAlister WH, Whyte MP (1997) Calcinosis universalis complicating juvenile dermatomyositis: resolution during probenecid therapy. J Clin Endocrinol Metab 82:3536–3542

72. Olhoffer IH, Carroll C, Watsky K (1999) Dermatomyositis sine myositis presenting with calcinosis universalis. Br J Dermatol 141:365–366

73. Mendoza LE, Lavery LA, Adam RC(1990) Calcinosis cutis circumscripta. A literature review and case report. J Am Podiatr Med Assoc 80:97–99

74. Hargens AR, Mubarak SJ (1998) Current concepts in the pathophysiology, evaluation and diagnosis of compartment syndrome. Hand Clin 14:371

75. Hod N, Fishman S, Horne T (2002) Detection of rhabdomyolysis associated with compartment syndrome by bone scintigraphy. Clin Nucl Med 27:885–886

76. Oza UD, Oates E (2003) Rhabdomyolysis of bilateral teres major muscles. Clin Nucl Med 28:126–127

CHAPTER 9

Therapeutic Use of Radionuclides in Bone and Joint Disease

Clinically, bone metastases are manifested by pain and the loss of mechanical stability. Standard treatment options for bone metastases include external beam radiotherapy and analgesics. The use of radionuclides provides an alternative modality for controlling pain. The currently employed agents such as Sr-89, Sm-153, Re-186 and Sn-117 DTPA have only mild side effects and response rates of 70–89% can be achieved. Radionuclide therapy provides an attractive alternative to surgical synovectomy in the management of patients suffering from chronic inflammatory joint disease. It is noninvasive, easily accepted by the patient, and the side effects are related to the leakage of radioactivity from the joint requiring special care and follow-up. New applications of radionuclide therapy for bone tumors such as osteogenic sarcoma and multiple myeloma are being investigated and appear to be promising.

9.1
Introduction

Nuclear medicine therapy uses open radioactive sources for the selective delivery of radiation to tumors or target organs. The basis for successful radionuclide therapy is that sufficient uptake and prolonged retention of the radiopharmaceutical occurs in the target tissues. Until recently, the use of radioisotopes in therapy has been limited to treatment of hyperthyroidism, thyroid cancer and polycythemia rubra vera. In the treatment of bone pain secondary to metastases, the use of strontium 89 (Sr-89), rhenium 186 (Re-186), samarium 153 (Sm-153) and tin 117m (Sn-117m) has been increasingly used. Additionally, I-131 MIBG and pentreotide have been used in the treatment of some neuroendocrine tumors, the use of radiolabeled monoclonal antibodies in treating lymphomas, and radionuclide synovectomy is available for certain arthritides (Table 9.1).

Radionuclide therapy for cancer is viewed as combining the advantage of target selectivity (seen also with techniques such as brachytherapy or external beam radiotherapy) with that of systemic therapy (as with chemotherapy). Short-term side effects are few and are limited to the myelosuppression. When a complete cure is feasible, the long-term consequences of radionuclide therapy, such as fertility disorders and leu-

Table 9.1. Therapeutic applications of nuclear medicine

Oncologic
1. Lymphomas and leukemias
2. Polycythemia rubra vera
3. Solid tumors (thyroid carcinoma, neuroblastoma, ovarian, prostate, breast, osteogenic sarcoma, others)
4. Treatment of metastasis-induced bone pain

Non-oncologic
1. Benign thyroid disease particularly hyperthyroidism
2. Radionuclide synovectomy
3. Bone marrow ablation
4. Intravascular radionuclide therapy for prevention of restenosis

kemia, or other secondary cancers, compare favorably with the risks accepted for chemotherapy and radiotherapy. For benign disorders such as thyrotoxicosis and arthritis radionuclide therapy provides an excellent alternative to surgery or medical treatment.

9.2
Treatment of Cancer-related Bone Pain

9.2.1
Rationale

Approximately 75% of patients with advanced cancer have pain due to skeletal metastases. The pain may be intractable and affect the quality of life of the patients especially if it is associated with immobility, anorexia and anxiety. The mechanism of bone pain induction is not clear in many of these patients (Table 9.2). Cell-secreted pain modulators such as interleukin-1β, interleukin-8 and interferon have been implicated in this respect [1]. Cancer-related bone pain can be controlled by medical treatment; usually narcotics, external beam radiation therapy or radionuclide therapy. Pain relief can be induced in 60–90% of cases by external radiotherapy delivering 2000–3000 rads [2, 3]. Controlling the pain from multiple metastases using external beam radiotherapy is, however, difficult. Hemibody irradiation using 800 rads to the lower half of the body and 600 rads to the upper half have resulted in complete response in 30%, partial response in 50% and no response in 20% of patients. Significant side effects such as nausea, vomiting, diarrhea as well as bone marrow toxicity are observed in one third of patients. In 9% of cases the side effects can be life threatening [4].

Table 9.2. Possible mechanisms of metastases-induced bone pain

1. Stretching periosteum
2. Pressure on nerves
3. Direct bone invasion and local destruction
4. Cell-secreted pain modulators such as interleukin-1 beta, interleukin-8 and interferon

Radionuclide therapy has been gaining popularity in the management of painful osseous metastases. This form of palliative therapy has the advantages of targeting all the involved sites but limiting the dose to normal tissue[5]. The palliative option using radionuclide methods appears underutilized in clinical practice. In a recent study [6], oncologists perceived the systemic radionuclide therapy as being less appropriate for palliation of metastatic bony pain than opioid analgesics. Radionuclide therapy was used in patients with widespread metastatic disease, who would not benefit much from such therapy. On the other hand, oncologists rated the appropriateness of the radionuclide therapy as low in the patient with limited early disease, in whom the greatest benefit would in fact be derived from such intervention [6].

9.2.2
Radiopharmaceuticals

The most frequently used agents for bone palliation today are strontium-89 chloride, rhenium-186 Ethylene Hydroxy Diphosphonate [7] and samarium-153 ethylenediaminetetramethylene phosphonate [8]. The list of radiopharmaceuticals for bone palliation has been increasing including Re-188 and several others such as lutetium-177, which has been investigated recently by Das [9] as a potential agent for bone cancer pain based on an experimental rat study [9].

The uptake of these bone-seeking radiopharmaceuticals by metastases is many (up to 20) times higher than that of normal bone [10]. These agents (Table 9.3) are absorbed into hydroxyapatite crystal at the site of reactive bone formation in a manner similar to Tc-99m diphosphonates. The radiopharmaceuticals, which, are currently used for bone pain control cause only mild transient bone marrow suppression.

9.2.2.1
Strontium-89 Chloride

Systemic radionuclide therapy using Sr-89 chloride was first used to relieve pain from bony metastases in 1937 and regained popularity in the 1980s. It is a pure β-emitter with a relatively long half-life of 50.5 days. It is a chemical analogue of calcium, and accordingly it concentrates avidly in areas of high osteoblastic activity. After intravenous injection, strontium quickly accumulates in the mineral bone matrix where active bone formation takes place. Therefore, there is preferential uptake in and around metastatic tumor deposits. This has been confirmed by external measurements using the gamma emitting radionuclide Sr-85 (with autoradiography) and Sr-89, whose concentration is 2–20 times greater in bone metastases than normal bone [10]. The biological half-life of Sr-89 in bone lesions is about 90

Table 9.3. Radiopharmaceuticals for bone pain palliation

Radiopharma-ceuticals	Physical half-life	Maximum energy of beta-emission (MeV)	Average beta energy	Maxi-mum range in tissue (mm)	Usual dose and route of administration	Appro-ximate efficacy	Toxicity	Dura-tion of effect
Phosphorus-32 Orthophos-phate	10.3 days	1.71	0.695 MeV	8.0	370–777 MBq (10–21 mCi), IV in divided doses	80%	Significant marrow suppression in one third of patients (occasionally up to 36 months)	1.5–11 months
Strontium-89 Chloride	50.5 days	1.46	0.583 MeV	6.8	1.5 MBq/kg (0.04 mCi/kg) or 150 MBq (4 mCi)/ patient, IV	79%	Mild transient marrow suppression, longer than that with Re-186 or Sm-153 and less than with P-32	4–15 months
Rhenium-186-HEDP	3.7 days	1.08	0.346 MeV	4.7	1295 MBq (35 mCi), IV	80%	Mild transient marrow suppression	5 weeks –12 months
Samarium-153 EDTMP	46.3 hours	0.81	0.234 MeV	3.4	37 MBq/kg (1 mCi) i.V.	69%	Mild transient marrow suppression	1–11 months
Tin-117m DTPA	13.6 days	0.13–0.15	Conversion electrons	0.3	5.29–10.58 MBq/kg (0.143–0.286 mCi/kg) i.V.	70%	Mild transient marrow suppression	Not well defined

Modified from Elgazzar and Maxon [28]

days compared to about 2 weeks in normal bone, which can be explained by the immature nature of reactive bone compared to normal lamellar bone. This selective uptake and prolonged retention at sites of increased bone mineral turnover provide precise targeting of bone lesions. The radionuclide is typically administered as a single 150 MBq (4 mCi) intravenous dose. Overall, pain relief occurs in up to 80% of patients, of whom 10–40% became effectively pain free. The mean duration of palliation is 3–4 months [11, 12]. In addition, Sr-89 chloride may cause slowing of the metastatic progression due to inhibition of expression of the cell adhesion molecules (E-selectins) that participate in the metastatic process. A significant transient decrease in serum E-selectin concentration, was observed after systemic radionuclide therapy in a study on 25 men with metastatic prostate carcinoma [13] and may open a window for clinical trials.

9.2.2.2
Phosphorus-32 Orthophosphate

This radionuclide is rarely used for the treatment of bone metastases. Dosimetric studies have demonstrated a relatively high dose to the bone marrow from the highly energetic β-particles of this radionuclide causing myelosuppression with pancytopenia (Table 9.3). An increased incidence of acute leukemia has been reported, although this was following P-32 therapy in patients with polycythemia vera.

9.2.2.3
Samarium-153 Ethylenediaminetetramethylene Phosphonate

Samarium-153 is produced in the nuclear reactor by neutron activation of both natural Sm-203 and 98% enriched Sm-152 targets. It has a relatively short half-life of about 48 h. Coupling of the radionuclide to ethylene diaminetetramethylenephosphonate (EDTMP) leads to the high uptake of the radionuclide by bone. Gamma camera imaging is possible due to the 103-keV gamma ray emitted during decay of Sm-153. The resulting images are similar to those obtained with Tc-99m-MDP, or other diphosphonates, showing increased uptake at the site of metastases. The calculated lesion-to-normal-bone ratio was reported to be 4.0 and the lesion-to-soft-tissue ratio, 6.0 [14].

Administration of Sm-153-EDTMP according to the supplier's recommendations at 37 MBq (1 mCi)/kg would deliver a bone marrow dose of 3.27–5.90 Gy, which would induce myelotoxicity as a side effect. Dosimetric calculation by urine collection and whole body scintigraphy has been used to limit the bone marrow dose to 2 Gy by Cameron and associates [15]. This was achieved by anterior and posterior whole-body images obtained 10 min and 5 h after the intravenous injection of 740 MBq (20 mCi) of Sm-153-EDTMP with determination of the bone activity by imaging and by counting the activity in urine collected for 5 h. The total administered activity of Sm-153-EDTMP predicted on a 2 Gy bone marrow dose was found to be 35–63% of the standard recommended dose of 37 MBq/kg. The authors reported pain relief in eight of the ten patients treated using this dosimetric method [15].

9.2.2.4
Rhenium-186 Ethylene Hydroxy Diphosphonate

In a manner similar to Sm-153, Re-186 has been coupled to a bone-seeking phosphonate, ethylene hydroxy diphosphonate (EHDP). This radionuclide emits β-particles with a maximum energy of 1.07 MeV and γ-photons with an energy of 137 keV which allows bone scanning. Re-186-EHDP undergoes renal excretion within 6 h after intravenous injection, as is the case with the common bone scanning agents. At four days, 14% of the radioactivity remains in bone [16].

Several studies have shown encouraging clinical results of palliative therapy using Re-186-HEDP with an overall response rate of 70% for painful osseous metastases from prostate and breast cancer. Myelosuppression has been limited and reversible, which makes repetitive treatment safe [17]. In a study by Kucuk et al. [18], 31 patients with various cancers (10 prostate, 10 breast, 4 rectum, 5 lung, 2 nasopharynx) and bone metastases were studied. Therapy was delivered using a fixed dose of 1,295 MBq (35 mCi) of Re-186-HEDP. When necessary, the same dose was repeated two to three times after an interval of 10–12 weeks. The mean response rate was 87.5% in patients with breast and prostate cancer, 75% in patients with rectal cancer and 20% in patients with lung cancer. The overall response rate was 67.5% and the palliation period varied between 6 and 10 weeks. The maximal palliation effect was observed between the 3rd and 7th weeks [18].

9.2.2.5
Tin-117m Diethylenetriaminepentaacetic Acid

Tin-117m (Sn-117m) is a reactor-produced radionuclide, with a half-life of 13.6 days. Contrary to the other radionuclides mentioned above, this radionuclide emits internal conversion electrons. Sn-117m is linked to diethylenetriaminepentaacetic acid (DTPA). More than 50% of the administered activity is absorbed by bone in patients with metastatic carcinoma, with a bone-to-red-marrow ratio of up to 9:1. Its 159 keV photon energy allows correlative imaging with a similar uptake pattern as Tc-99m-MDP [19].

In a preliminary study in 10 patients by Atkins et al. [20] none of the patients who received Sn-117m-DTPA for palliation developed marrow toxicity. Another recent study on 47 patients treated with Sn-117m-DTPA, the experimental mean absorbed dose to the femoral marrow was 0.043 cGy/KBq. Compared to 32P-orthophosphate, Sn-117m-DTPA yielded an up to 8-fold therapeutic advantage over the energetic β-emitter P-32. Accordingly, the authors suggested that an internal conversion electron emitter such as Sn-117m offers a large dosimetric advantage over the energetic β-particle emitters permitting higher administered activity for alleviating bone pain, while minimizing marrow toxicity [21].

9.2.2.6
Rhenium-188 Dimercaptosuccinic Acid Complex

Re-188-(V)DMSA, a potential therapeutic analogue of the tumor imaging agent Tc-99m-(V)DMSA, is selectively taken up in bone metastases. In a study by Blower et al. [22] of ten patients with prostate carcinoma and bone metastases studied by Tc-99m-(V)DMSA and Re-188-(V)DMSA to compare their bio-distribution, the authors found only minor differences between both radiopharmaceuticals. Accordingly Tc-99m-(V)DMSA scans are predictive of Re-188-(V)DMSA bio-distribution and can be used to estimate tumor and renal dosimetry and assess suitability of patients for Re-188-(V)DMSA treatment [22]. This advantage makes this tracer a candidate for more trials as a potentially successful agent for bone metastases palliation.

9.2.3
Mechanism of Action

Metastatic bone pain is believed to be due to both mechanical factors (local bony destruction) and due to humoral factors (secretion of certain mediators by tumor and peritumoral cells). Although the mechanism of action is not completely known, radionuclide therapy is thought to deliver sufficient energy from the sites of reactive bone directly to the malignant cells and/or to peritumoral cytokine-secreting cells that may be responsible for the patient's pain.

Pain relief by radiation was found to be independent of the radiosensitivity of the tumor and therefore the mechanism of action does not involve actual killing of the tumor cell. It is more likely that radiation interrupts processes that are maintained by humoral pain mediators in the micro-environment of the tumor [23]. This view is also supported by an absence of a dose-response relationship [24].

9.2.4
Choice of Radiopharmaceutical

It has been demonstrated that myelosuppression is less severe using radionuclides with relatively shorter half lives (Table 9.4). Other physical properties including radiolabeled conjugate biological uptake and clearance, product-specific activity, range and type of emissions, and resultant effects on tumor and normal tissue cellular survival should be all considered along with the clinical outcome to choose a radiopharmaceutical. The response rate of different radiopharmaceuticals currently in use appears not to differ significantly [25]. The side effects, which are mainly hematological, vary

Table 9.4. Dosimetric features of bone pain radiopharmaceuticals

Radiopharma-ceutical	Radiation dose (rad/mCi)		
	Bone	Red marrow	Bone/red marrow ratio
Strontium-89	63	40.7	1.6
Rhenium-186	7.0	3.0	2.3
Samarium-153	15.4	2.8	5.5
Sn-117m	65.1	9.8	6.6

Adapted from [81], with permission

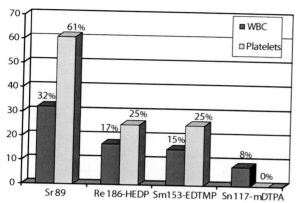

Fig. 9.1. Histogram showing the hematologic effects of common radionuclides used for treating painful metastases

among the agents used (Fig. 9.1), being more pronounced with P-32 than with the newer agents. Sn-117m DTPA differs from the other radiopharmaceuticals in that it emits internal conversion electrons rather than β-particles. Since internal conversion electrons have a low energy and shorter path in tissue, they seem to result in less marrow toxicity.

A multi-center observational study including 29 nuclear medicine departments was conducted by the Italian Association of Nuclear Medicine between 1996 and 1998 to evaluate the efficacy and toxicity of radionuclide therapy of painful bone metastases in a large number of patients. Out of 818 treatments performed using single i.v. doses of 4 mCi (148 MBq) of Sr-89 chloride or 35 mCi (1,295 MBq) of Re-186-HEDP, 610 were suitable for evaluation (527 with Sr-89 and 83 with Re-186-HEDP). Eighty-one patients received up to five treatments with a total number of 100 re-treatments. Patients were followed up for a period of 3–24 months. The results of the clinical outcome were: no response in 19%, mild response in 21.3%, good response in 33.3% and excellent response in 26.4% of cases. Re-treatments showed significantly worse responses (48% with good or excellent response), in comparison to first treatment. The duration of palliation was 5.0+/-3.5 months, and was longer in the cases of patients who had excellent response in the first treatment; in patients with limited metastases; in patients with a good clinical condition; when life expectancy exceeded 3 months; in radiologically osteoblastic or mixed bone lesions and when Sr-89 was used. Overall, mild-to-moderate myelosuppression was observed in 25.5% of cases of first treatment and in 38.9% of re-treatments. Therapy did not seem to prolong life, although scintigraphic regression of bone metastases was observed in some cases. There was no statistically significant difference in the palliative efficacy and toxicity between the two radiopharmaceuticals either in first treatment or in re-treatments [26].

9.2.5
Clinical Use
9.2.5.1
Current Indications

Radiopharmaceutical therapy is indicated for the treatment of patients with painful, multifocal, bone metastases. However, patients with pain that is secondary to either the spinal cord or peripheral nerve invasion by adjacent metastases will not benefit from such treatment.

9.2.5.2
Contraindications

Absolute contraindications are pregnancy and continuing breast feeding. Relative contraindications include pre-existing severe myelosuppression, urinary incontinence, insufficiency or pathological fractures and spinal cord compression. A very short life-expectancy is a relative contraindication since it takes 1–3 weeks for the pain to be relieved by this type of therapy.

9.2.5.3
Clinical Response

The response to these radiopharmaceuticals is more, or less, similar with an average success rate of 70–80% [16, 27–29]. A prospective study of 75 patients with prostatic carcinoma and bone metastases, who were treated with Sr-89 over a 10-year period, was conducted by Windsor [30]. The therapy was successful in 42 (56.0%) patients, unsuccessful in 13 (17.3%) and unchanged in 20 (26.7%). More patients with scintigraphic superscans had an unsuccessful outcome, while the majority of those with fewer metastatic sites had successful outcomes. Patients with a successful outcome had a significantly better survival rate after Sr-89 injection. The study indicated that early treatment with Sr-89 in patients with fewer bone metastases is more likely to be successful, with a longer time before further therapy is required [30]. A retrospective study of 57 patients who received Sr-89 (38 patients), or Sm-153 (19 patients), for prostate cancer with bone metastases was reported by Dickie in 1999 [31]. A total of 40 patients had radionuclide therapy alone, and 28/40 (70%) responded with a beneficial effect on pain. There was no difference in the response rates between the Sm-153 and Sr-89 patients regarding the effect on pain or the time to progression (median of 2–3 months for all patients) [31].

Another study conducted by Sciuto et al. [32] evaluated the therapeutic efficacy of Sr-89 and Re-186 in the palliation of painful bone metastases from breast cancer. A total of 50 patients with painful multi-focal bone metastases from breast cancer were randomized into two groups of 25 patients each according to the radiopharmaceutical used. The overall response rate was 84% (21/25) for Sr-89 and 92% (23/25) for Re-186 respectively. The onset of pain palliation appeared significantly earlier in the group treated with Re-186 (p < 0.0001). The duration of pain relief ranged from 2–14 months in the group treated with Sr-89 and from 1–12 months in the group treated with Re-186 (p = 0.39). A moderate hematological toxicity was apparent in both groups. Platelet and white blood cell counts returned to baseline levels within 12 weeks after Sr-89 administration and 6 weeks after Re-186 administration (p < 0.01). The authors concluded that Re-186 has a significantly faster onset of pain relief [32]. In a recent study, Alshyeri et al reported their experience with the use of Sr-89 in 41 patients with multiple osseous metastases of breast and prostate carcinomas. More than two thirds of patients responded favorably and opioid doses were lowered [33]. Experimentally, the effect of Sr-89, Re-186, Sn-117m or Sm-153 on hematopoietic stem cell survival was found to be mild and comparable [34].

It is clear that the difference in half-life and the extent of bone metastases have an effect both on the onset and the duration of pain relief. Relief rates using the newer agents are not significantly different and is comparable with those of external beam radiotherapy but side-effects are minimal and compare favorably with those of a previously used agent (P-32).

The use of a radionuclide along with chemotherapy for palliation is being investigated and may prove useful. Palmedo et al reported a case of a patient with disseminated bone metastases due to breast cancer and multi-focal pain. Because of persisting pain after a first cycle of chemotherapy, 1295 MBq of Re-186 HEDP was administered and excellent pain relief was observed. Subsequently, the patient received combined chemotherapy and Re-186 HEDP therapy and remained pain free. A follow-up Tc-99m MDP bone scan showed significant regression of osseous metastases. The authors speculated that the combination of Re-186 HEDP and chemotherapy resulted in significantly increased palliation of the metastatic bone disease [35].

9.2.5.4
Precautions and Radiation Safety

All patients must have a bone scan within 8 weeks of the treatment. A complete blood count (CBC) should be obtained before ordering the radiopharmaceutical to ensure suitability of the patient for treatment. An intravenous line should be established and an injection should be given over no less than one minute. Patients with renal failure may need reduction of the administered dose since the radiopharmaceuticals are eliminated by urine. If the patient is on hemodialysis, she/he could receive the therapy, but the radiation safety officer should be notified to oversee the process. If the patient is incontinent, special home instructions should be provided regarding use of a condom catheter, or an indwelling bladder catheter.

In most countries radionuclide treatment for bone pain palliation can be given on an outpatient basis. Moro et al. [36] conducted a series of measurements of the superficial contamination inside the confinement room and also the dose to those individuals close to patients who underwent palliative radionuclide therapy for bone metastases (with Sm-153-EDTMP using radioactivities less than 3 GBq). The results showed that the contamination of the location and objects close to the treated patients was low. Measurements of the external radiation showed that in the proximity of the confinement room the permitted dose to members of the public was not exceeded. The dose to those who took care of the patients including family members was less than 20 µSv. The study confirmed a very low exposure to nearby public, nursing staff, and family members taking care of the patient [36].

The United States Nuclear Regulatory Commission has recently amended its regulations concerning patients who receive therapeutic doses of radioactivity allowing patient release based on a total effective dose equivalent (TEDE) limit of 5 mSv (500 mrem) instead of the activity administered or retained [1,110 MBq (30 mCi)] or the dose rate [0.05 mSv/h (5 mrem/h) at 1 m]. The current TEDE-based release criteria are less restrictive than the previous activity-based or dose rate-based release criteria [37] and allows outpatient treatment using high activity, such as 150 mCi of I-131.

9.3
Radionuclide Synovectomy

There is currently a need for a definitive treatment for joint pain associated with many arthropathies especially rheumatoid arthritis after failure of conventional medications. Therapeutic nuclear medicine offers an alternative to surgical synovectomy. Several radiopharmaceuticals (Table 9.5) can destroy the synovial mem-

Table 9.5. Radiopharmaceuticals used for intra-articular therapy

Colloidal radio-pharmaceutical	Physical half-life in days	Maximum energy Type	Maximum energy β (MeV)	Range in soft tissue (mm) Max.	Range in soft tissue (mm) Mean	Particle size (μm)
Au-198	197	β, γ	0.96	3.6	1.2	20 – 70
P-32	14.0	β	1.7	7.9	2.6	500 – 2000
Re-186 sulfide	3.7	β, γ	0.98	3.6	1.2	5 – 10
Y-90 citrate	2.7	β	2.2	11.0	3.6	100
Dy-165 FHMA	0.1	β, γ	1.29	5.7	1.8	3000 – 8000
Er-169	9.4	β, γ	1.0	1.0	0.3	10
Ho-166	1.12	β, γ	1.85	8.7	4.0*	1200 – 12000

* 2.2 mm in inflamed synovial tissue (modified from [44], with permission)

brane when injected intra-articularly (radionuclide synovectomy or radiosynoviorthesis) and the patients become pain free.

9.3.1
Rationale

The intra-articular administration of radiopharmaceuticals in a colloid form is effective in more than 60% of patients with rheumatoid arthritis and other arthritic diseases. The choice of radionuclide, dose, and injected volume is determined by the size of the joint; and the range of the β-particle spectrum suitable for the thickness of the synovium. Table 9.6 summarizes the major benefits of this technique

Table 9.6. Major benefits of radiosynovectomy

1. Effective	Excellent to good results in approximately 60 – 75% of treated patients
2. Cost-effective	An alternative to surgical synovectomy with significant savings
3. Quality of life	Improvement in approximately 75% of patients with ability to perform new tasks associated with job, school or recreation
4. Additional advantages	No postoperative physical therapy needed to prevent/relieve joint stiffness associated with surgical synovectomy

Adapted from [44], with permission

9.3.2
Radiopharmaceuticals

Several radiopharmaceuticals have been used since radiosynovectomy was first introduced in 1952 by Fellinger and Schmid as a therapy for synovitis. Yttrium-90 colloid, erbium-169 citrate colloid, rhenium-186 colloid and others are used to treat chronic synovial disease [33, 34]. Since these colloid preparations vary in their physical characteristics and accordingly the range of penetration, they are used differently to achieve the therapeutic effects and avoiding injuring the surrounding tissue. Yttrium-90 citrate, or silicate, is generally used for large joints such as the knee; rhenium-186 colloid is used for the shoulder; elbow, hip, and ankle; and erbium-169 citrate for the small joints in the hands and feet (Fig. 9.2).

9.3.2.1
Yttrium-90 Colloid

This radionuclide is used predominantly for radionuclide synovectomy of the knee joint, although it is also used for malignant pleural and peritoneal effusions. The pharmacological characteristics of the silicate and citrate forms are the same. The average range in tissue is 3.6 mm and the maximum is 11 mm. After direct intra-articular administration the colloid penetrates into the superficial cells of the synovia. Small numbers of particles may be transported through the lymphatic system, mainly after active or passive movement of the joint, from the knee to the regional lymph nodes. The safety of this modality of management has been reported, and hence the patient's age should not be regarded as a limiting factor [38]. It is recommended that Y-90 radiosynovectomy can be performed in young patients because the amount of synovium is still moderate. This is because once the degree of synovitis has become severe, the expected results of radioactive synoviorthesis are worse [39].

In a recent study, radioactive Y-90 was injected into 163 joints. Of these patients 115 were hemophiliacs suffering from recurrent hemarthroses. The median age at the time of the initial administration of Y-90 was between 11 and 15 years and the median follow-up period 11 years. Over 80% of the patients with hemophilia reported a decrease in the number of hemarthroses and 15% stopped bleeding altogether in the treated joint [38]. Rodriguez [39] reported the results of 66 Y-90 synoviortheses on 44 persons with hemophilia (45 knees, 12 elbows, 9 ankles). The average age was 21.1 years (range: 9 – 39 years). A quantity of 5 mCi of Y-90 was injected into the knee, and 3 mCi into the elbow and ankle. The average follow-up was 3.5 years (range 1 – 6 years). Of the 45 knees, there were 8 excellent, 10 good, 15 fair and 12 poor results. Of the 12 elbows there were 3 excellent results, 5 good, 3 fair and 2 poor. Of the nine ankles there were no excellent results, four good, three fair and two poor. The elbows had better results

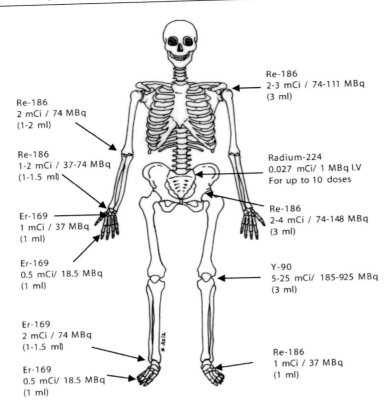

Re-186
2-3 mCi / 74-111 MBq
(3 ml)

Re-186
2 mCi / 74 MBq
(1-2 ml)

Re-186
1-2 mCi / 37-74 MBq
(1-1.5 ml)

Er-169
1 mCi / 37 MBq
(1 ml)

Er-169
0.5 mCi/ 18.5 MBq
(1 ml)

Er-169
2 mCi / 74 MBq
(1-1.5 ml)

Er-169
0.5 mCi/ 18.5 MBq
(1 ml)

Radium-224
0.027 mCi/ 1 MBq I.V
For up to 10 doses

Re-186
2-4 mCi / 74-148 MBq
(3 ml)

Y-90
5-25 mCi/ 185-925 MBq
(3 ml)

Re-186
1 mCi / 37 MBq
(1 ml)

Fig. 9.2. The choice of radiopharmaceutical for different joints

than the knees and ankles. The best results were obtained in the youngest patients, and in those with a moderate degree of synovitis [39].

A study of the efficacy of Y-90 silicate therapy in rheumatoid-knee synovitis was reported by Gencoglu using Tc-99m human polyclonal immunoglobulin G (HIG) scintigraphy for evaluating 15 patients (13 women, 2 men; mean age, 53.5 +/- 8.4 years) with rheumatoid arthritis who had radionuclide synovectomy using 185 MBq (5 mCi) Y-90 silicate in 24 knee joints with chronic persistent synovitis. Radiological and clinical evaluations and Tc-99m HIG scans were performed in each patient before radionuclide synovectomy. Each patient was reassessed 3, 6, 9, and 12 months after therapy using clinical examination and Tc-99m HIG scintigraphy. In 14 of the 24 knee joints that had an excellent, or good, clinical response to Y-90 silicate therapy, the Tc-99m HIG index values at 3 months after treatment were significantly lower than the pretreatment index values. In 13 of these 14 joints, these low index values and clinical results remained constant throughout 1 year of follow-up. The remaining patient experienced severe pain and swelling as a result of recurrent arthritis at 9 months, and the Tc-99m HIG index value increased at 9 months after therapy. In 10 of 24 knee joints that had a fair or poor clinical response, Tc-99m HIG index values were statistically similar before and after radionuclide therapy [40].

9.3.2.2
Rhenium-186 Sulfide (Re-186 Colloid)

This radiopharmaceutical is particularly used for radionuclide synoviorthesis of the hip, shoulder, elbow, wrist or ankle joint. After intra-articular injection, the radiopharmaceutical is absorbed by the superficial cells of the synovia. Beta radiation leads to coagulation necrosis and sloughing of these cells similar to other radionuclides used for synoviorthesis.

9.3.2.3
Erbium-169 Citrate (Er-169 Colloid)

Because of its shorter penetration range in soft tissue this is more suitable for radionuclide synoviorthesis of the metacarpophalangeal, metatarsophalangeal and proximal interphalangeal joints. β-Radiation of the absorbed radiopharmaceutical in the synovia causes coagulation necrosis and sloughing of cells as with other colloid used for other joints. Er-169 colloid has an affinity to chelates, therefore the simultaneous administration of iodine contrast media containing EDTA should be avoided.

9.3.2.4
Phosphorus-32 Chromic Sulfate

P-32 chromic phosphate has a 14-day half-life, has several times larger particles than Y-90 silicate, Re-186,

Er-169, or Au-198 colloids, and emits only β-radiation. The β-radiation from P-32 chromic phosphate has a soft tissue penetration midway between them, at 2 to 3 mm. It has been used by some investigators to treat patients with rheumatoid arthritis and hemophilic arthritis because of these physical advantages [41, 42].

9.3.2.5
Radioactive Gold

Radioactive gold (Au-198), with a mean soft-tissue penetration of only 1–2 mm, has been used also for radiosynovectomy. It has a physical half-life of 197 days and a colloid particle size ranging from 20 to 70 μm.

9.3.2.6
Rhenium-188 Colloid

Since it is a generator-produced β-emitting radionuclide, the importance of Re-188 for radionuclide therapy is increasing rapidly. Jeong [43] prepared Re-188-tin colloid and compared its properties with Re-188-sulfur colloid. The authors found that Re-188 tin colloid was advantageous over Re-188-sulfur colloid since it showed higher labeling efficiency, better control of the particle size, and lower residual activity in the injection syringes [43].

9.3.2.7
Dysprosium-165

This radionuclide has a short half-life of 2.3 h, energetic β-emission with a tissue penetration of 5.7 mm and very large particle size of 3–8 nm. This radionuclide has a 3.6 abundance of γ-emission that can be used by the γ-camera to detect a possible leak. It has been showed to have a response rate of 65–70% with the best results being obtained in patients in early-stage joint disease [44].

9.3.2.8
Holmium-166 Ferric Hydroxide

The first experience with Ho-166 was recently reported by Ofluoglu and colleagues [45]. The knee joints of 22 patients were treated with a mean activity of 1.11 GBq (30 mCi). Ho-166 has a maximum β-energy of 1.85 MeV with a mean penetration in inflamed synovial layer of 2.2 mm and a maximum of 8.7 mm. Its particle size is 1.2–12 nm.

9.3.2.9
Mechanism of Action

Although the mechanism of action cannot be totally explained, the current belief is that after intra-articular administration of the radioactive particles they are ab-

sorbed by the superficial cells of the synovium. β-Radiation leads to coagulation necrosis and sloughing of these cells.

9.3.3
Choice of Radiopharmaceutical

The choice of radiopharmaceutical depends on the physical characteristics and the size of the joint to be treated and the disease status. The therapeutic agents are particulate in nature and labeled with β-emitting radionuclides. The tissue penetration of the radiation is proportional to the energy of the β-particles. For example, yttrium-90, with its highly energetic β-emission has a mean soft tissue penetration of 3–4 mm, while rhenium-186 has a mean penetration of 1–2 mm, the β-emission of phosphorus-32 has a soft-tissue penetration midway between them at 2–3 mm and both radioactive gold and Re-186, have a mean soft-tissue penetration of only 1–2 mm. Such radiopharmaceuticals with a shallow depth of penetration are not optimal for large joints such as the knee, or for patients with an extensively thickened synovium such as the case with rheumatoid arthritis and pigmented villonodular synovitis. Because radiation exposure rate is proportional to the severity of the post-therapy inflammatory reaction, a radionuclide with a moderately long half-life of days may be preferred to that with a half-life of a few hours. Also, it appears that there is an inverse relationship between the size of radioactive particle used and the tendency for the radiocolloid, to leak from the joint space, which in general makes the choice of a relatively large radiocolloid more appropriate. A radionuclide that emits only β-radiation would have more advantages than one that emits both β- and γ-radiation to minimize whole-body radiation.

9.3.4
Clinical Uses
9.3.4.1
Indications

Radionuclide synovectomy is mainly indicated in treating diseased joints in hemophiliac patients and patients with Willebrand's disease with chronic synovitis and hemarthropathy, rheumatoid arthritis, pigmented villonodular synovitis, psoriatic arthritis, ankylosing spondylitis, and collagenosis.

Relative indications include persistent effusion after joint prosthesis [46].

9.3.4.2
Contraindications

The absolute contraindications for the use of the therapeutic radiopharmaceutical colloids for synovectomy are pregnancy and continued breast feeding. Other contraindications include fresh fracture, serious liver disease, myelosuppression and acute infections. The therapy is not contraindicated in children or young adults, but therapy should only be administered if the estimated benefit outweighs the potential risks [46]. The presence of a Baker cyst in the knee joint is considered, by some, as a contraindication. Ultrasonography is particularly important for the knee joint to exclude the presence of a Baker cyst, which is an evagination of the medial dorsal part of the joint capsule in communication with the main joint. If there is inflammation in the knee joint, the effusion can be pumped into the Baker cyst by the enhanced motion. If a valve-mechanism exists in the connection duct, this could have a deleterious effect after radiosynovectomy. The increased pressure in the cyst might lead to its rupture and the radioactive fluid getting into the surrounding tissue of the joint. The consequence could be possible necrosis of the muscles, nerves and blood vessels. Accordingly some authors consider Baker cyst, which is not an uncommon occurrence, a contraindication for a radiosynovectomy of the knee joint. Recent arthroscopy is also a contraindication and radiosynovectomy should be delayed for 4–6 weeks after arthroscopy [46].

9.3.4.3
Patient Preparation

Two- or three-phase bone scan should be obtained before planning therapy in order to assess the degree of inflammation of the joint and soft tissue. It should also be obtained in order to be able to decide if radiosynovectomy is possible and if the patient really could benefit from this kind of therapy. Scintigraphy is particularly important in order to evaluate the extent of abnormalities in the joint to be treated. Quantitation methods could be used before and after therapy. A history of arthroscopy must be checked. Ultrasound or MRI is also helpful to assess the amount of effusion, joint space and the status of the synovium. This ensures the homogeneous distribution of the radiopharmaceutical. A complete blood cell count should be obtained before therapy and a pregnancy test must be obtained for women of child-bearing age. Injections should be performed using aseptic technique. Radiosynovectomy can generally be repeated in 6 months.

9.3.4.4
Treatment Protocol and Clinical Outcome

The protocol of radiosynovectomy varies with the size of the joint treated. Generally radiosynovectomy of the knees, elbows, ankles and joints of the hands and feet are performed on an outpatient basis under local anesthesia. Sedation, or general anesthesia, is used for chil-

dren. Shoulder and hip treatment can also be performed as an outpatient but is recommended to be performed under radiographic guidance [39]. The injection technique also depends on the joint (Figs. 9.3–9.7).

The largest number of treated patients are those with rheumatoid arthritis and hemophilia. Generally good results are obtained among these patients as well as those with psoriatic arthropathy. On the other hand, in osteoarthritis with recurrent joint effusion radiosynovectomy has not been as successful in relieving the symptoms and a good response is reported in 40–70% of patients [47]. In patients with advanced cartilage destruction or bone-on-bone interaction, the synovial membrane is likely to be practically non-existent. Accordingly, patients with less radiological damage generally show better results than those with more severe damage. If there is initially a poor response or a relapse, more than half the patients may benefit from a re-injection [48, 49]. In a recent review of literature [50] of 2,190 joints treated with radiosynovectomy, with a minimum of one year follow up but without specifying the radiopharmaceutical used, the overall success rate was 73%. For rheumatoid arthritis it was 67%, whereas it was 56% for osteoarthritis, 91% for hemophilia and Willebrand's disease and 77% for pigmented villonodular synovitis [50].

Hemophilia

Good results in patients with hemophilia have been reported using Y-90 [44]. Heim et al. [38] used Y-90 in the knees of 58 patients with hemophilia and a favorable response was noted in 84% of patients after 34 months of follow-up. In 1996 a small study consisting of 10 joints in 10 patients with hemophilia was performed by Fernandez-Palazzi et al. with Re-186 [51]. Excellent results were reported in 9/10 patients (90%) following treatment. The authors chose to use Re-186 because its physical properties are similar to those of Au-198, but without the γ-radiation, thereby minimizing whole body radiation.

Some authors prefer P-32 for hemophilia because of its physical characteristics (the half life of 14 days) which provide a theoretical advantage of a more gradual deposition of energy and a minimization of the severity of potentially acute inflammatory reactions. Additionally, the relatively large size of the P-32 colloid minimizes the potential for joint leakage. Furthermore P-32 is a pure β-emitter with only 2.6 mm of radiation penetration in soft tissue, which minimizes radiation dose. Table 9.7 summarizes the efficiency of radiosynovectomy in treating hemophilic joints.

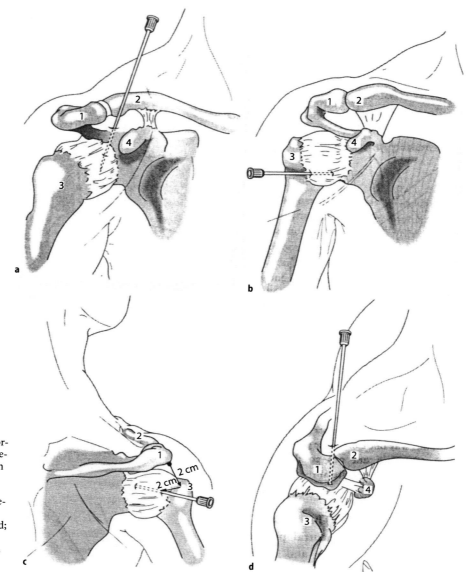

Fig. 9.3a–d. Shoulder synoviorthesis: **a** Injection by the antero-superior route; **b** injection by the antero-inferior route; **c** injection by the posterior route; **d** injection by the superior route (*1* = acromion; *2* = clavicle; *3* = humeral head; *4* = coracoid process). From Fernandez-Palazzi et al. [51], with permission

Table 9.7. Results of radiosynovectomy in hemophiliac patients

Author	Year	Radio-nuclide	Favorable response
Erkon [84]	1991	Y-90	81%
Fernandez-Palazzi [51]	1996	Re-186	90%
Siegel [85]	1994	P-32	80%
Rivard [42]	1994	P-32	78%
Heim [83]	2001	Y-90	80%
Siegel [44]	1997	P-32	75%
Chew [86]	2004	P-32/Re-186	80%

Arthritis

Rheumatoid Arthritis

Rheumatoid arthritis affects 1–2% of the population worldwide. The inflammatory process of the arthritic joint is characterized by cellular proliferation with the synovial lining becoming hyperplastic and may thicken to 10–12 cells in thickness with a large increase in the percentage of macrophage-like cells associated with an increased secretion of synovial fluid and secretion of cytokines and enzymes that are capable of degrading cartilage matrix and bone, leading to joint destruction. There is also formation of synovial granulation tissue (pannus) (see Fig. 7.1, Chapter 7) [52, 53].

Surgical synovectomy for treating intractable rheumatoid joint disease has the disadvantages of the risks of complications from anesthesia, the need for an approximately 2 week post-operative hospitalization, the need for rehabilitation that may take as long as 6 months, and frequent loss of motion as the final result.

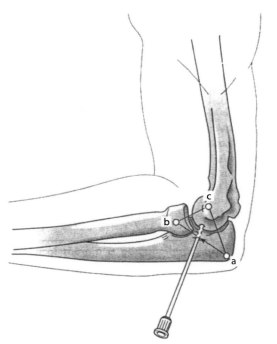

Fig. 9.4a, b. Elbow synoviorthesis: with the elbow in lateral view the needle should be inserted in the center of the triangle formed by the olecranon (*a*), the radial head (*b*) and the lateral epicondyle (*c*). From [51], with permission

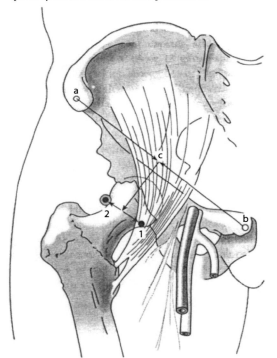

Fig. 9.5a–c. Hip synoviorthesis should be carried out with the help of two important cutaneous landmarks: the antero-superior iliac spine (*a*) and the pubic tubercle (*b*). In this way one can get the position of the center of the femoral neck (*c*). Then one can proceed via the inferomedial route (*1*) or through the supero-lateral route (*2*). From [51], with permission

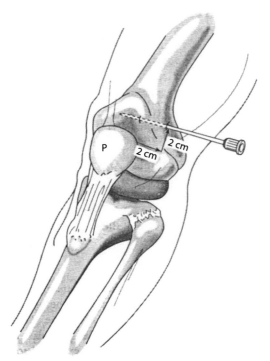

Fig. 9.6. Knee synoviorthesis (right knee) through the suprapatellar-lateral route. The injection is made above the lateral corner of the patella (*P*) and directly into the supra patellar pouch. From [51], with permission

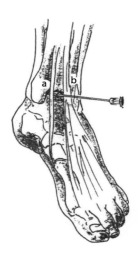

Fig. 9.7a, b. Ankle synoviorthesis through the anterior route. Note the site of injection between the tibialis anterior tendon (*a*) and the extensor digitorum longus (*b*). From [51], with permission

The success rate for therapy of rheumatoid arthritis using Re-186 is 86% and using Er-169 is 82% [54, 55]. Using Au-198, approximately 70% of rheumatoid patients benefited, with the most benefit from the procedure being obtained in the early stages of the disease [56–58]. However, the γ-radiation and leakage of the small Au-198 colloid from the joint lead to some concerns regarding whole body radiation. Moreover, the maximum tissue range is 4 mm and the average tissue penetration depth is approximately 1 mm; this may be inadequate to treat an extremely inflamed synovial lining, which may be greater than 5 mm in thickness. Y-90 may be preferred for these reasons [56–61]. Yttrium-90 has the advantage of being a pure β-emitter, with a higher energy and a greater maximum tissue penetration than Au-198 (11 mm versus 4 mm), making it an attractive agent for radiosynovectomy. Using Y-90 for the knee joint, decrease in pain, joint effusion, and motility are reported in 60% of patients 6 months after radiosynovectomy.

The results of the treatment of approximately 1500 rheumatoid joints by Grove, using Y-90, were good in approximately 67% of joints and no side effects were noted over a follow-up of several years [62].

Other Arthopathies
Arthopathies in which radiosynovectomy may prove to be successful include pigmented villonodular synovitis, psoriatic arthritis, ankylosing spondylitis, osteoarthritis and collagenosis. Franssen et al. [63], using Y-90 in the treatment of pigmented villonodular synovitis of the knee, showed improvement in 50% of patients with a 32-month follow-up. Additionally, Alexieva and Kunnev [64] showed favorable results in 80% of patients treated with Y-90 for ankylosing spondylitis, psoriatic arthritis, and collagenosis involving the knee joint. Radium-224 has also been used successfully to treat ankylosing spondylitis. It is a decay product of thorium-232, emits both α- and β-particles with a mean range in soft tissue of 50 μm and 8 mm respectively. It has a physical half-life of 3.64 days and is administered as 10 intravenous injections at intervals of 1 week. The cumulative total activity administered should not exceed 10 MBq. Approximately 90% of treated patients become pain free for many years [65]. Patients with psoriatic arthropathies also show satisfying and encouraging results [66] after radiosynonectomy.

9.3.4.5
Side Effects of Radiosynovectomy

The side effects of radiosynovectomy depend on the radiopharmaceutical used, the activity administered and more importantly the technique of administering the dose. The side effects include necrosis of the extra-articular soft tissue, febrile reaction, local pain and leakage of radiopharmaceutical from the joint via lymph nodes.

The most important side effect is the leakage of the radioactivity from the joint since it has the potential of causing infertility [67], although there is no evidence of patients treated for arthritis [68].

Radiopharmaceutical Leakage

Leakage of the radionuclide from the treated joint has limited the use of radiation synovectomy as an alterna-

tive to surgical treatment. Unconjugated radionuclides will diffuse through the joint and they must therefore be conjugated with a non-diffusible particle to prevent leaking. Accordingly, the currently used therapeutic radionuclides are in colloidal form, where the particles are small enough to be phagocytized by the synovial tissue, but not small enough to escape from the joint before being phagocytized. Thus, the particle size is critical in limiting the leakage from a synovial joint. Immobilization of the treated joint for 48–72 h is necessary to minimize the leakage by means of blood and lymphatic transport [69]. To avoid radionecrosis, needle placement is confirmed by fluoroscopy and flushing the needle with saline prior to removal to avoid needle tract necrosis. Rivard reported leakage in only 3 of 71 radiosynovectomies using P-32 colloid with a mean percentage leakage of 0.6% (range 0.1–2%) [42]. In a review of 100 radiosynovectomies [70], the maximum leakage was 2.5% of the target dose and it occurred in one patient. Winston et al. [71], using P-32 in rheumatoids, reported a maximum leakage of 3.2% in only one patient.

Post-therapeutic Regional Inflammatory Reaction

Further side-effects can be painful reactions in the treated joint (treated with a cold pad and analgesia), edema of the forearm after treatment of the wrist joint and exceptional joint infection.

Somatic and Genetic Effects

Available data point to a negligible somatic and genetic risk [72]. Therefore younger patients may be treated with radiosynovectomy if the benefit outweighs the risk. Because the whole body dose from the β-emitting radionuclides used for radiation synovectomy is low, the effects, if any, on chromosomes are considered to be a result of the leakage to the inguinal lymph nodes. The hypothetical disadvantage of radiosynovectomy is that the radioactivity may theoretically diffuse from the joint and adversely affect chromosomal material, or induce late radiation-induced neoplasms. Rivard et al. [42] reported that perhaps the strongest argument for the safety of intra-articular radiocolloids is the long-term follow-up of the more than 5000 radiosynovectomies performed since 1971, mainly in patients with rheumatoid arthritis, none of whom have been reported to have developed radiation-induced malignancies. Early studies with Au-198 reported that greater than 10% and as much as 60% of the activity was found in the draining lymph nodes, and yet there have been no reports linking the use of this agent to hematogenous malignancies or sarcomas. De la Chapelle et al. also noted no correlation between any detectable lymph node activity and the detection of chromosomal aberrations [67]. Rivard et al. [42] found no chromosomal aberrations at 1 week or at 6 months after P32 chromic phosphate injection in the knees of seven hemophiliac patients [42].

Radiation Sickness

This is a rare side effect seen in about 3% of patients after radiosynovectomy. Patients transiently have a slightly increased temperature and feel sick, but no special therapy is necessary.

9.4
Other Radionuclide Therapies

Certain promising radionuclide therapies are being tried both on animals and humans. These are focused on treating certain primary and metastatic malignancies such as neuroblastoma, multiple myeloma, osteosarcoma and metastatic prostatic cancer.

9.4.1
Treatment of Osteogenic Sarcoma

Targeted radionuclide therapy using Sm-153-EDTMP was reported to provide a substantial palliative effect in a case of primary osteogenic sarcoma in the first lumbar vertebra which had relapsed with progressive back pain after conventional treatment modalities had failed. The patient was bed-ridden, and developed paraparesis and impaired bladder function. On a diagnostic bone scan intense radioactivity was localized in the tumor. The patient was twice treated with Sm-153-EDTMP , 8 weeks apart using 35 and 32 MBq/kg body weight respectively. After a few days the pain was significantly relieved and by the second radionuclide treatment the paresis subsided. For 6 months he was 'up and about' without any neurological signs or detectable metastases. Eventually, however, the patient redeveloped local pain and paraparesis, was re-operated and died 4 months later. The authors concluded that this dramatic transient improvement observed in this case warrants further exploration using 3Sm-153-EDTMP as a boost technique, supplementary to conventional external radiotherapy [73].

Another case was also reported which illustrated high-activity Sm-153-EDTMP therapy within a multi-modal therapy concept to improve local control of an unresectable osteogenic sarcoma with poor response to initial polychemotherapy. A 21-year-old woman with an extended, unresectable pelvic osteogenic sarcoma and multiple pulmonary metastases was treated with high activity of Sm-153-EDTMP. Afterwards, external radiotherapy of the primary tumor site was performed and polychemotherapy continued, followed by autologous peripheral blood stem cell reinfusion. Within 48 h after Sm-153-EDTMP treatment the patient had complete pain relief. After 3 weeks the response was documented by three-phase Tc-99m-MDP bone scintigraphy with a decrease in the tracer uptake in the primary tumor and metastases and whole-body F-18-FDG-PET with an interval decrease of uptake. Accordingly, further evaluation of the feasibility and efficacy of this multimodal therapy combination of high-activity Sm-153-EDTMP therapy, external radiation, polychemotherapy and stem cell support for unresectable osteogenic sarcoma is warranted [74].

An animal study was conducted on 15 dogs with spontaneous osteogenic sarcoma, and local pain, who were treated with Sm-153-EDTMP. The tumors were located in the extremities, scapula, maxilla, and the frontal bone. The dogs were injected intravenously one to four times with Sm-153-EDTMP; 36–57 MBq/kg body weight. Three dogs had surgery in addition to the radionuclide treatment. Platelet and white blood cell counts showed a moderate and transient decrease with no other toxicity observed. The average tumor dose after a single injection was approximately 20 Gy. Seven dogs had metastases on autopsies. Although none of the dogs was cured, nine dogs had obvious pain relief, and five of them seemed pain-free: one for 20 months and one for 48 months. The authors suggested that high tumor radiation doses may be deposited in dog osteosarcomas by Sm-153-EDTMP, and the ratio between the tumor dose and the dose to surrounding tissues is favorable. The treatment gives pain relief and may cause tumor growth delay, and the combination of surgery and Sm-153-EDTMP may prolong life significantly and possibly cure the disease, because the development of metastases appears to be postponed [75].

9.4.2
Metastatic Prostate Carcinoma

A study was conducted to explore the effects of Re-186-HEDP treatment on the progression of lumbar-skeletal metastasis in an animal model (Copenhagen rat) and to correlate the eventual treatment efficacy with the radionuclide tissue distribution. The Re-186-HEDP administration, given either 1 day or 8 days after surgical induction of lumbar metastasis, was found to significantly increase the symptom-free survival of the animals. These results were confirmed by a significant decrease in the presence of histologically detectable tumor tissue. Bio-distribution studies demonstrated the uptake of the major part of the radionuclide within bone tissue, concentrated in areas of bone formation and turnover. These results show that radionuclide treatment with Re-186-HEDP is a potentially efficacious treatment option in prostate cancer disseminated to the skeleton [76].

9.4.3
Multiple Myeloma

Recent use of high dose Ho-166-DOTMP (Ho-166-1,4,7,10-tetraazocyclododecane-1,4,7,10-tetramethylene-phosphonic acid) in treating patients with multiple myeloma has been reported [77]. Thirty-two patients were treated with 581 – 3,987 mCi with an average of 2,007 mCi (74.3 GBq). Ho-166 has a half-life of 26.8 h and a β-emission of 1.85 MeV (51%) and 177 MeV (48%) as well as a 80.6 keV (6.6%) β-emission suitable for a γ-camera imaging. The β-particles have a mean range of 4 mm in soft tissue and can deliver high levels of radiation to the marrow and trabecular bone [77]. The radiopharmaceutical has selective bone uptake and rapid urinary excretion of the remaining activity. However, due to the high doses used, catheterization and continuous irrigation of the urinary bladder after therapy has to be used to reduce radiation dose to the bladder mucosa. This agent has a potential to treat patients with resistant multiple myeloma. However, clinical studies with an emphasis on the outcome in comparison with the currently used high dose of chemo-radiotherapy with or without stem cell rescue are warranted to evaluate the impact on the poor survival of patients affected by the tumor. Also more studies are needed to compare the adverse effects of this agent to the incidence of systemic toxicities of the currently available radiopharmaceuticals [78, 79].

9.4.5
Treatment of Neuroblastoma with MIBG

Iodine-131-MIBG has been used to treat patients with stage 4 neuroblastoma including those with bone metastases after failure of all other modalities of therapy. The response rate is approximately 35% [80]. I-125-MIBG has also been used for bone marrow infiltrates.

References

1. Ferreira SH, Lorenzethi BB, Bristow AF et al (1988) Interleukin-1 beta as a potent hyperalgesic agent antagonized by a tripeptide analogue. Nature 334:698–700
2. Poulson HS, Nielsen OS, Klee M et al (1989) Palliative irradiation of bone metastases. Cancer Treatment Rev 16:41–48
3. Tong D, Gillick L, Hendrickson FR (1982) Palliation of symptomatic osseous metastases. Cancer 50:893–899
4. Salazar OM, Rubin P, Hendrickson FR et al (1986) Single dose half-body irradiation for palliations of multiple bone metastases from solid tumors. Final radiation therapy oncology group report. Cancer 58:29–36
5. Robinson RG, Preston DF, Schiefelbein M et al (1995) Strontium-89 therapy for the palliation of pain due to osseous metastases. JAMA 274:420–424
6. Papatheofanis FJ (1999) Variation in oncologic opinion regarding management of metastatic bone pain with systemic radionuclide therapy. J Nucl Med 40:1420–1423
7. Quirijnen JP, Han SH, Zonnenberg M et al (1996) Efficacy of rhenium-186-etidronate in prostate cancer patients with metastatic bone pain. J Nucl Med 37:1511–1515
8. Serafini AN, Houston SJ, Resche I et al (1998) Palliation of pain associated with metastatic bone cancer using samarium-153 Lexidronam: a double-blind placebo-controlled clinical trial. J Clin Oncol 16:1574–1581
9. Das T, Chakraborty S, Unni PR, et al (2002) 177Lu-labeled cyclic polyaminophosphonates as potenzial agents for bone pain palliation. Appl radiat Isot 51:177–184
10. Pauwels EKJ, Stokkel MPM (2001) Radiopharmaceuticals for bone lesions Imaging and therapy in clinical practice. Q J Nucl Med 45:18–26
11. Giammarile F, Mognetti T, Resche I (2001) Bone pain palliation with strontium-89 in cancer patients with bone metastases. Quart J Nucl Med 45:78–83
12. Patel BR, Flowers WM Jr (1997) Systemic radionuclide therapy with strontium chloride Sr 89 for painful skeletal metastases in prostate and breast cancer. South Med J 90:506–508
13. Papatheofanis FJ (2000) Decreased serum E-selectin concentration after 89Sr-chloride therapy for metastatic prostate cancer bone pain. J Nucl Med 41:1021–1024
14. Ramamoorthy N, Saraswathy P, Das MK, Mehra KS, Ananthakrishnan M (2002) Production logistics and radionuclidie purity aspects of 153Sm for radionuclide therapy. Nucl Med Commun 23:83–89
15. Cameron PJ, Klemp PF, Martindale AA, Turner JH (1999) Prospective 153Sm-EDTMP therapy dosimetry by wholebody scintigraphy. Nucl Med Commun 20:609–615
16. Maxon HR, Thomas S, Hertzberg VS, Schroder LE, Englaro EE, Samaratunga R et al. (1992) Rhenium-186 hydroxyethylidene diphosphonate for the treatment of painful osseous metastases. Semin Nucl Med 22:33–40
17. Han SH, De Klerk JM, Zonnenberg BA, Tan S, van Rijk PP (2001) 186Re-etidronate. Efficacy of palliative radionuclide therapy for painful bone metastases. Quart J Nucl Med 45:84–90
18. Kucuk NO, Ibis E, Aras G, Baltaci S, Ozalp G, Beduk Y, Canakci N, Soylu A (2000) Palliative analgesic effect of Re-186 HEDP in various cancer patients with bone metastases. Ann Nucl Med 14:239–245
19. Atkins HL, Mausner LF, Srivastava SC, Meinken GE, Cabahug CJ, D'Alessandro T (1995) Tin-117m (4+)-DTPA for palliation of pain from osseous metastases: a pilot study. J Nucl Med 36:725–729
20. Atkins HL, Mausner LF, Srivastava SC, Meinken GE, Straub RF, Cabahug CJ et al (1993) Biodistribution of Sn-117m DTPA for palliative therapy of painful osseous metastases. Radiology 186:279–283
21. Bishayee A, Rao DV, Srivastava SC, Bouchet LG, Bolch WE, Howell RW (2000) Marrow-sparing effects of 117mSn-diethylenetriaminepentaacetic acid for radionuclide therapy of bone cancer. J Nucl Med 41:2043–2050
22. Blower PJ, Kettle AG, O'Doherty MJ, Coakley AJ, Knapp FF Jr (2000) 99mTc(V)DMSA quantitatively predicts 188Re(V)DMSA distribution in patients with prostate cancer metastatic to bone. Eur J Nucl Med 27:1405–1409
23. Krishnamurthy GT, Krishnamurthy S (2000) Radionuclides for metastatic bone pain palliation: a need for rational re-evaluation in the new millennium (comment). J Nucl Med 41:688–691
24. Hoskin PJ, Ford HT, Harmer CL (1989) Hemibody irradiation (HBI) for metastatic bone pain in two histologically distinct groups of patients. Clin Oncol R Coll Radiol 1:67–69
25. Wessels BW, Meares CF (2000) Physical and chemical properties of radionuclide therapy. Semin Radiat Oncol 10:115–122

26. Dafermou A, Colamussi P, Giganti M, Cittanti C, Bestagno M, Piffanelli A (2001) A multicenter observational study of radionuclide therapy in patients with painful bone metastases of prostate cancer. Eur J Nucl Med 28:788–798

27. Silberstein EB, Elgazzar AH, Kapilivsky A (1992) Phosphorus-32 radiopharmaceuticals for the treatment of painful osseous metastases. Semin Nucl Med 17:17–27

28. Elgazzar AH, Maxon HR (1993) Radioisotope therapy for cancer related bone pain. Imaging Insights 2:1–6

29. Quilty PM, Kirk D, Bolger JJ, Dearnaley DP, Lewington VJ, Mason MD, Reed NS, Russell JM, Yardley J (1994) A comparison of the palliative effects of strontium-89 and external beam radiotherapy in metastatic prostate cancer. Radiother Oncol 31:33–40

30. Windsor PM (2001)Predictors of response to strontium-89 (Metastron) in skeletal metastases from prostate cancer: report of a single centre's 10-year experience. Clin Oncol (R Coll Radiol) 13:219–227

31. Dickie GJ, Macfarlane D (1999) Strontium and samarium therapy for bone metastases from prostate carcinoma. Austr Radiol 43:476–479

32. Sciuto R, Festa A, Pasqualoni R, Semprebene A, Rea S, Bergomi S, Maini CL (2001) Metastatic bone pain palliation with 89-Sr and 186-Re-HEDP in breast cancer patients. Breast Cancer Res Treat 66:101–109

33. Ashayeri E, Omogbehin A, Sridhar R, Shakar RA (2002) Stronium-89 in the treatment of pain due to diffuse osseous metastses: a university hospital experience. J Natl Med Assoc 94:706–711

34. Kvinnsland Y, Skretting A, Bruland OS (2001) Radionuclide therapy with bone- seeking compounds: Monte Carlo calculations of dose-volume histograms for bone marrow in trabecular bone. Phys Med Biol 46:1149–1161

35. Palmedo H, Grunwald F, Wagner U, Kohler S, Krebs D, Biersack HJ (1998) Remission of bone metastases after combined chemotherapy and radionuclide therapy with Re-186 HEDP. Clin Nucl Med 23:501–504

36. Moro L, Fantinato D, Aprile C, Preti P, Robustelli della Cuna G (2001) 153Sm-EDTMP radionuclide treatment of bony metastatic disease: a radiation protection evaluation. G Ital Med Lav Ed Ergon 23:435–437

37. Zanzonico PB, Siegel JA, St Germain J (2000) A generalized algorithm for determining the time of release and the duration of post-release radiation precautions following radionuclide therapy. Health Phys 78:648–659

38. Heim M, Goshen E, Amit Y, Martinowitz U (2001) Synoviorthesis with radioactive yttrium in haemophilia: Israel experience. Haemophilia 7 [Suppl 2]:36–39

39. Rodriguez-Merchan EC, Jimenez-Yuste V, Villar A, Quintana M, Lopez-Cabarcos C, Hernandez-Navarro F (2001) Yttrium-90 synoviorthesis for chronic haemophilic synovitis: Madrid experience. Haemophilia 7 [Suppl 2]:34–35

40. Gencoglu EA, Aras G, Kucuk O, Atay G, Tutak I, Ataman S, Soylu A, Ibis E (2002) Utility of Tc-99m human polyclonal immunoglobulin G scintigraphy for assessing the efficacy of yttrium-90 silicate therapy in rheumatoid knee synovitis. Clin Nucl Med 27:395–400

41. Onetti CM, Guyierrez F, Hiba E et al (1982) Synoviorthesis with P-32 colloid chromic phosphate in rheumatoid arthritis and hemophilia, clinical, histopathological and arthographic changes. J Rheumatol 9:229–238

42. Rivard GE, Givard M, Belanger R et al (1994) Synoviortheses with colloidal P-32 chromic phosphate for the treatment of hemophilc arthropathy. J Bone Joint Surg (Am) 76:482–487

43. Jeong JM, Lee YJ, Kim YJ, Chang YS, Lee DS, Chung JK, Song YW, Lee MC (2000) Preparation of rhenium-188-tin colloid as a radiation synovectomy agent and comparison with rhenium-188-sulfur colloid. Appl Radiat Isot 52:851–855

44. Siegel ME, Siegel HJ, Luck JV Jr (1997) Radiosynovectomy's clinical applications and cost effectiveness: a review. Semin Nucl Med 28:364–371

45. Ofluoglu S, Schwameis E, Zehetagruber I, Havlic E, Wanivenhaus A, Schweeger I, Weiss K et al (2002) Radiation synovectomy with Ho-166-Ferric hydroxide: a first experience. J Nucl Med 43:1489–1494

46. Fischer M, Modder G (2002) Radionuclide therapy of inflammatory joint disease. Nucl Med Commun 23:829–831

47. Hauss F (1992) Radiosynoviorthese in der Orthopadie. Aktuel Rheumatol 17:64–66

48. Asavatanabodee P, Sholter D, Davis P (1997) Yttrium-90 radiochemical synovectomy in chronic knee synovitis: a one year retrospective review of 133 treatment interventions. J Rheumatol 24:639–642

49. Deutsch E, Brodack JW, Deutsch KF (1993) Radiation synovectomy revisited. Eur J Nucl Med 20:1113–1127

50. Kresnik E, Mikososch P, Gallowitsch HJ, Jesenko R, Just H, Kogler D, Gasser J, Heinisch M, Unterweger O, Kumnig G, Gomez I, Lind P (2002) Clinical outcome of radiosynoviorthesis: a meta-analysis including 2190 treated joints. Nucl Med Commun 23:683–688

51. Fernandez-Palazzi F, Rivas S, Ciberia JL et al (1996) Radioactive synoviorthesis in hemophiliac hemarthrosis: materials, techniques and dangers. Clin Orthop 328:14–18

52. Athanasou NA, Quinn J, Heryet A et al (1988) The immunohistology of synovial lining cells in normal and inflamed synovium. J Pathol 155:133–142

53. Henderson B, Edwards JCW (1987) The synovial lining, in health and disease. Chapman and Hall, London

54. Gobel D, Gratz S, von Rothkirch T, Becker W (1997) Chronische Polyarthritis und Radiosynoviorthese: eine prospektive, kontrollierte Studie der Injektionstherapie mit Erbium-169 und Rhenium-186. Z Rheumatol 56:207–213

55. Gobel D, Gratz S, von Rothkirch T, Becker W, Willert HG (1997) Radiosynoviorthesis with rhenium-186 in rheumatoid arthritis: a prospective study of three treatment regiment. Rheumatol Int 17:105–108

56. Ahlberg A, Mikulowski P, Odelberg-Johnson O (1969) Intra-articular injection of radioactive gold in treatment of chronic synovial effusion in the knee. Acta Rheum Scand 15:81–89

57. Ansell BM, Crook A, Mallard JR et al (1966) Treatment of persistent knee effusions with intra-articular radioactive gold. In: Studies of rheumatic disease. Proceedings of 3rd Canadian Conference on Research in Rheumatic Disease. University of Toronto Press, Toronto

58. Ansell BM, Crook A, Mallard JR et al (1963) Evaluation of intra-articular colloidal gold Au-198 in the treatment of persistent knee effusion. Ann Rheum Dis 22:435–439

59. Jalava S (1973) Irradiation synovectomy: clinical study of 67 knee effusions in intra-articularly irradiated with Y-90 resin. Curr Ther Res 15:395–401

60. Menkes CJ, Tubiana R, Galmiche B et al (1973) Intra-articular injection of radio-isotopic beta emitters. Orthop Clin North Am 4:1113–1125

61. Gumpel JM, Williams ED, Glass HI (1973) Use of yttrium-90 in persistent synovitis of the knee. I. Retention in the knee and spread in the body after injection. Ann Rheum 32:223–227

62. Grove F (1995) Radio synovectomy: clinical review. Presented at the world congress of nuclear medicine and biology, Sydney, Australia

63. Franssen MJAM, Boerboom ANT, Kerthaus RP et al (1989) Treatment of pig mounted vilonodular synovitis of the knee with Y-90 silicate. Ann Rheum Dis 48:1007–1013

64. Alexieva T, Kunnev K (1990) The treatment of gonathritis with y-90. Vutr Voles 29:59–61
65. Fischer M (1999) Society of Nuclear Medicine, Proceedings, pp 353–355
66. Panholzer PJ et al (2000) Effiziente Lokalbehandlung der Psoriasis-Arthritis mit der Radiosynoviorthese (RSO). DGN 29:13–14
67. De la Chapelle A, Oka M, Rekonen A, Ruotsi A (1972) Chromosome damage after intra articular injection of radioactive yttrium. Ann Rheum Dis 31:508–512
68. Gumpel JM (1978) Radiosynoviorthesis. Clin Rheum Dis 41:311–326
69. Noble J, Jones AG, Davies MA et al (1983) Leakage of radioactive particle systems from a synovial joint studied with a gamma camera. J Bone Joint Surg 65-A:381–389
70. Siegel ME, Luck JV Jr, Siegel HJ et al (1997) Radiosynoviorthesis for chronic hemophilic hemarthrosis and synovitis: efficacy and cost analysis. J Nucl Med 38:120–121
71. Winston MA, Bluestone R, Cracchiolo A III et al (1973) Radioisotope synovectomy with P-32 chromic phosphate-kinetic studies. J Nucl Med 14:886–889
72. Klett R, Puille M, Matter HP, Steiner D, Sturz H, Bauer R et al. (1999) Aktivitatsa tansport und Strahlenexposition durch die Radiosynoviorthese des Kniegelenks: Einfluss unterschiedlicher Therapiemodalitaten. Z Rheumatol 58:207–212
73. Bruland OS, Skretting A, Solheim OP, Aas M (1996) Targeted radiotherapy of osteosarcoma using 153 Sm-EDTMP. A new promising approach. Acta Oncol 35:381–384
74. Franzius C, Bielack S, Sciuk J, Vollet B, Jurgens H, Schober O (1999) High-activity samarium-153-EDTMP therapy in unresectable osteosarcoma. Nuclear-Medizin 38:337–340
75. Aas M, Moe L, Gamlem H, Skretting A, Ottesen N, Bruland OS (1999) Internal radionuclide therapy of primary osteosarcoma in dogs, using 153Sm-ethylene-diamino-tetramethylene-phosphonate (EDTMP). Clin Cancer Res 5 [Suppl 10]:3148s–3152s
76. Geldof AA, van den Tillaar PL, Newling DW, Teule GJ (1997) Radionuclide therapy for prostate cancer lumbar metastasis prolongs symptom-free survival in a rat model. Urology 49:795–801
77. Rajendran JG, Eary JF, Bensinger W, Durack LD, Vernon C, Fritzberg A (2002) High-dose 166Ho-DOTMP in myeloablative treatment of multiple myeloma: pharmacokinetics, biodistribution, and absorbed dose estimation. J Nucl Med 43:1383–1390
78. Alexanan R, Dimopoulos M (1994) The treatment of multiple myeloma. N Engl J Med 330:484–489
79. Barlogie B, Alexanian R, Dick KA et al (1987) High dose chemotherapy and autologous bone marrow transplantation for resistant myeloma. Blood 70:869–872
80. Hoefnagel CA (1988) radionuclide cancer therapy. Ann Nucl Med 12:61–70
81. Srivastava S, Dadachova E(2001) Recent advances in radionuclide therapy. Semin Nucl Med 31:330–341
82. Owunwanne A, Sadek S, Patel M (1995) The handbook of radiopharmaceuticals. London, Chapman and Hall medical publishers
83. Heim H, Goshen E, Amit Y, Martinowitz U (2001) Synoviorthesis with radioactive Yttrium in haemophilia: Israel experience. Hemophilia 7:36–39
84. Erkon EHW (1991) Radiocolloids in the management of hemophilic arthropathy in children and adolescents. Clin Orthop 264:129–134
85. Siegel HJ, Luck JV Jr, Siegel ME, Quines C, Anderson E (1994) Hemarthrosis and synovitis associated with hemophilia: clinical use of P-32 chromic phosphate synoviorthesis for treatment. Radiology 190:297–261
86. Chew EM, Tien SL, Sundram FX et al (2003) Radionuclide synovectomy and chronic haemophilic synovitis in Asians: a retrospective study. Haemophilia 9:632–637

Glossary

Ankylosing spondylitis: The most common type of spondyloarthropathies with chronic inflammatory changes leading to stiffening and fusion (ankylosis) of the spine and sacroiliac with a strong genetic predisposition associated with HLA B27. Other joints, such as hips, knees and shoulders, are involved in approximately 30% of patients.

Apophysis: An accessory secondary ossification center that develops late and forms a protrusion from the growing bone where tendons and ligaments insert or originate.

Avulsion: Complete separation of tendons or ligaments, with or without a portion of bone and/or cartilage.

Behçet's syndrome: An uncommon disorder characterized by recurrent oral and genital ulceration, uveitis, or retinal vasculitis, cutaneous pustules or erythema nodosum and synovitis. The disease is more common in Mediterranean countries and Japan than in the United States.

Bone contusion (bone bruise): A term describing microfractures of trabecular bone together with edema or hemorrhage within the marrow.

Brodie's abscess: An intraosseous abscess in the cortex that becomes walled off by reactive bone.

Calciphylaxis: Soft tissue calcification in response to administration of an agent after induction of a hypersensitive state.

Calcinosis cutis: A term used to describe a group of disorders in which calcium deposits form in the skin, subcutaneous tissue and connective tissue sheaths around the muscles but not within the muscles.

Costochondritis (Tietze's syndrome): A common painful condition that affects the costochondral junction, usually in young patients, and is self-limiting. The etiology remains unknown, although trauma and infection have been proposed. It can affect any rib, but the first and second ribs are most commonly involved.

Complex regional pain syndrome type I (reflex sympathetic dystrophy): A pain syndrome that usually develops after an initiating noxious event with no identifiable major nerve injury, is not limited to the distribution of a single peripheral nerve, and is disproportional to the inciting event or expected healing response.

CPPD: Calcium pyrophosphate dihydrate deposition disease, also called pseudogout and chondrocalcinosis: a type of crystal deposition arthropathy with such crystals deposited in cartilage, synovium, tendons, and ligaments.

Dystrophic calcification: A type of soft tissue calcification that occurs in the setting of normal serum calcium and phosphate levels and occurs in damaged, inflamed, neoplastic or necrotic tissue.

Endochondral ossification: Most of the skeleton forms by this type of ossification, where a pre-existing cartilage forms first and then undergoes ossification.

Enteropathic arthropathies: Arthropathies associated with inflammatory bowel diseases, including ulcerative colitis, Crohn's disease, Whipple's disease, intestinal bypass surgery and celiac disease.

Entheses: The sites of insertion of tendons, ligaments and articular capsule to bone.

Enthesopathy: A pathologic process affecting entheses particularly trauma and or inflammation resulting in regional periosteal reaction with osteoblastic bone activity.

Fibrous dysplasia: A benign bone disorder characterized by the presence in the fibrous tissue in lesions of trabeculae of non-lamellar bone (woven bone) which remains essentially unchanged.

Flare pattern on bone scan: An initial apparent deterioration of primary or some or all metastatic lesions on the bone scan, followed by improvement usually accompanying successful treatment.

Fracture delayed union: Delay of fracture union beyond the expected time (usually 9 months).

Fracture non-union: Complete cessation of repair process of a fracture.

Fracture: A break in the continuity of a bone.

Gout: A metabolic disorder that results in hyperuricemia and leads to deposition of monosodium urate monohydrate crystals in various sites in the body, especially joint cartilage.

Heterotopic ossification: A specific type of soft tissue calcification that may or may not follow trauma and is due to a complex pathogenetic mechanism believed to be due to transformation of certain primitive cells of mesenchyma origin in the connective tissue septa within muscles into bone-forming cells.

Hypertrophic osteoarthropathy: A form of periostitis that may be painful and may be associated with clubbing of fingers and toes, sweating, and thickening of skin. It may be primary or may follows a variety of pathologic conditions, predominantly intra thoracic, and is characterized by periosteal new bone formation.

Impingement syndromes: A group of painful conditions caused by friction of joint tissue, which include bone impingement, soft tissue impingement and entrapment neuropathy, depending on the type of tissue involved.

Inflammation: A complex non-specific tissue reaction to injury caused by many agents such as living agents such as bacteria and viruses, leading to infection, or non-living agents, including chemical, physical, and immunologic factors or radiation.

Intramembranous ossification: Occurs through the transformation of mesenchymal cells into osteoblasts, seen in flat bones of the skull, part of the mandible and part of the clavicle.

Involucrum: A layer of new bone formation around the site of skeletal infection formed secondary to the body's response to that infection.

Lisfranc injury: Fracture or fracture-dislocation of tarsometatarsal joints.

Malunion: Healing of a bone in a non-anatomic orientation.

Metastatic calcification: The type of soft tissue calcification that involves viable undamaged normal tissue as a result of hypercalcemia and/or hyperphosphatemia associated with increased calcium phosphate product locally or systematically.

Myositis ossificans progressiva: The congenital and rare form of heterotopic ossification.

Osteochondritis dissecans: Transchondral fracture with fragmentation and separation of portions of cartilage or cartilage and bone; most prevalent in adolescents.

Osteomalacia: Abnormal mineralization of bone with a decrease in bone density secondary to lack of both calcium and phosphorus with no decrease in the amount of osteoid (bone formation).

Osteomyelitis: A term applied to skeletal infection when it involves the bone marrow.

Osteopetrosis: A rare inherited metabolic bone disease characterized by a generalized increase in skeletal mass due to a congenital defect in the development or function of the osteoclasts, leading to defective bone resorption.

Osteoporosis: Reduction of bone tissue amount increasing the likelihood of fractures.

Oxalosis: Deposition of calcium oxalate crystals that leads to arthropathy.

Pathologic fracture: A fracture at a site of preexisting abnormalities that weaken bone.

Plantar fasciitis (calcaneal periosteitis): An inflammatory condition that can occur as an isolated entity, e.g., secondary to occupation or degenerative, or may accompany spondylarthropathies.

Podagra: A term describing affection of the metatarsophalangeal joint of the great toe in gout, the most typical finding of gouty arthritis.

Pseudoarthrosis: A gap between the fracture bone ends containing a space filled with fluid. Also termed „false joint".

Reactive arthritis (Reiter's disease): A syndrome characterized by a combination of nongonococcal urethritis, arthritis and conjunctivitis.

Renal osteodystrophy: A metabolic condition of bone associated with chronic renal failure.

Rheumatoid arthritis: An autoimmune disease causing inflammation of connective tissue, mainly in the joints, with synovial inflammatory response triggered by immune complexes in the blood and synovial tissue through activation of plasma protein complement. This inflammation spreads from the synovial membrane to the articular cartilage, joint capsule and the surrounding tendons and ligaments, leading to pain, loss of function and joint deformity.

SAPHO syndrome: A syndrome characterized by synovitis, acne, palmoplantar pustulosis, hyperostosis, and osteitis. The small and large joints of the feet, the ankles, knees, hips, right sacroiliac joints and shoulders are affected by the synovitis.

Scheuermann disease: A destructive form of osteochondrosis with erosions of the endplates of two adjacent vertebrae and anterior wedging of thoracic vertebrae.

Septic tenosynovitis: An inflammatory condition affecting generally the flexor tendons of the hands and feet of diabetic patients and resulting from penetrating injuries or spread of infection from a contiguous focus of infection.

Sequestrum: Segmental bone necrosis that develops when normal blood supply to the bone is interrupted by the edema and ischemia produced by the inflammation.

Shin splints: Periosteal elevation with reactive bone formation secondary to extreme tension on muscles or muscle groups inserting on bones.

Slipped capital femoral epiphysis: Displacement of the femoral head from the femoral neck at the site of the growth plate during growth.

Spondyloarthropathies: A group of seronegative arthropathies formerly called rheumatoid variants that share common clinical and radiographic features with characteristic involvement of the sacroiliac joints, spine, and to various degrees, the peripheral joints, are linked to HLA B27 histocompatibility antigen and include ankylosing spondylitis, psoriatic arthritis, reactive arthritis (Reiter's disease), enteropathic spondylitis.

Spondylolysis: A loss of continuity of bone of the neuroarch of the vertebra due to stress or trauma.

Spondylolysthesis: Forward movement of one vertebra on another, usually as a result of fracture of the neuroarch.

Sprains: Tears of tendons.

Strains: Tears of ligaments.

Stress fracture: A pathologic condition of bone due to repeated episodes of stress, each less forceful than that needed to cause acute fracture of the bony cortex.

Synovial joints: Specialized joints that are found mainly in the appendicular skeleton and allow free motion.

Tarsal coalition: Fusion of the talus and calcaneus or of the navicular and calcaneus due to failure of normal segmentation of their ossification centers during embryogenesis.

Toddler's fracture: Fracture in preschool children which is typically a non-displaced spiral fracture of the mid-tibia but also includes fractures of other bones, such as the fibula, calcaneus, talus, metatarsal and cuboid bones.

Transient synovitis: A joint inflammation of unknown origin and self-limiting course affecting most frequently boys between 5 and 10 years of age. It was previously known as toxic synovitis and affects preferentially the hip or knee and subsides without antibiotics.

T-score: A parameter used to express bone mineral density by relating an individual's bone density to the mean BMD of healthy young adults, matched for gender and ethnic group.

Tumoral calcinosis: A type of soft tissue calcification characterized by large, calcified, periarticular soft-tissue masses of calcium phosphate near the large joints such as the hip, the shoulder, and the elbow, in addition to the wrist, hands and feet.

Woven bone: Immature non-lamellar bone that is later normally converted to lamellar bone.

Z-score: A parameter used to express bone mineral density by comparing the bone density value of an individual to the mean value expected for his/her age group.

Subject Index